Ped Clinics

CME on Line

Wafa

215 - 239 - 6084

P'word = Paulasteel
Claim.online.access
Act # 1941632-2

Adolescents and Sports

Guest Editors

DILIP R. PATEL, MD, FAAP, FACSM, FAACPDM, FSAM
DONALD E. GREYDANUS, MD, FAAP, FSAM, FIAP (H)

PEDIATRIC CLINICS OF NORTH AMERICA

www.pediatric.theclinics.com

June 2010 • Volume 57 • Number 3

SAUNDERS an imprint of ELSEVIER, Inc.

W.B. SAUNDERS COMPANY
A Division of Elsevier Inc.

1600 John F. Kennedy Boulevard ● Suite 1800 ● Philadelphia, Pennsylvania 19103-2899

http://www.theclinics.com

THE PEDIATRIC CLINICS OF NORTH AMERICA Volume 57, Number 3
June 2010 ISSN 0031-3955, ISBN-13: 978-1-4377-2006-8

Editor: Carla Holloway
Developmental Editor: Theresa Collier

Photocopying
Single photocopies of single articles may be made for personal use as allowed by national copyright laws. Permission of the Publisher and payment of a fee is required for all other photocopying, including multiple or systematic copying, copying for advertising or promotional purposes, resale, and all forms of document delivery. Special rates are available for educational institutions that wish to make photocopies for non-profit educational classroom use. For information on how to seek permission visit www.elsevier.com/permissions or call: (+44) 1865 843830 (UK)/(+1) 215 239 3804 (USA).

Derivative Works
Subscribers may reproduce tables of contents or prepare lists of articles including abstracts for internal circulation within their institutions. Permission of the Publisher is required for resale or distribution outside the institution. Permission of the Publisher is required for all other derivative works, including compilations and translations (please consult www.elsevier.com/permissions).

Electronic Storage or Usage
Permission of the Publisher is required to store or use electronically any material contained in this journal, including any article or part of an article (please consult www.elsevier.com/permissions). Except as outlined above, no part of this publication may be reproduced, stored in a retrieval system or transmitted in any form or by any means, electronic, mechanical, photocopying, recording or otherwise, without prior written permission of the Publisher.

Notice
No responsibility is assumed by the Publisher for any injury and/or damage to persons or property as a matter of products liability, negligence or otherwise, or from any use or operation of any methods, products, instructions or ideas contained in the material herein. Because of rapid advances in the medical sciences, in particular, independent verification of diagnoses and drug dosages should be made.

Although all advertising material is expected to conform to ethical (medical) standards, inclusion in this publication does not constitute a guarantee or endorsement of the quality or value of such product or of the claims made of it by its manufacturer.

The Pediatric Clinics of North America (ISSN 0031-3955) is published bimonthly by Elsevier Inc., 360 Park Avenue South, New York, NY 10010-1710. Months of issue are February, April, June, August, October, and December. Periodicals postage paid at New York, NY and additional mailing offices. Subscription prices are $167.00 per year (US individuals), $378.00 per year (US institutions), $227.00 per year (Canadian individuals), $503.00 per year (Canadian institutions), $270.00 per year (international individuals), $503.00 per year (international institutions), $83.00 per year (US students and residents), and $142.00 per year (international and Canadian residents and students). To receive students/resident rare, orders must be accompanied by name of affiliated institution, date of term, and the signature of program/residency coordinator on institution letterhead. Orders will be billed at individual rate until proof of status is received. Foreign air speed delivery is included in all *Clinics* subscription prices. All prices are subject to change without notice. **POSTMASTER:** Send address changes to *The Pediatric Clinics of North America*, Elsevier Health Sciences Division, Subscription Customer Service, 3251 Riverport Lane, Maryland Heights, MO 63043. **Customer Service: 1-800-654-2452 (US and Canada). From outside of the US and Canada: 1-314-447-8871. Fax: 1-314-447-8029. For print support, E-mail: JournalsCustomerService-usa@elsevier.com. For online support, E-mail: JournalsOnlineSupport-usa@elsevier.com.**

Reprints. For copies of 100 or more, of articles in this publication, please contact the Commercial Reprints Department, Elsevier Inc., 360 Park Avenue South, New York, NY 10010-1710. Tel.: 212-633-3812; Fax: 212-462-1935; E-mail: reprints@elsevier.com.

The Pediatric Clinics of North America is also published in Spanish by McGraw-Hill Inter-americana Editores S.A., Mexico City, Mexico; in Portuguese by Riechmann and Affonso Editores, Rua Comandante Coelho 1085, CEP 21250, Rio de Janeiro, Brazil; and in Greek by Althayia SA, Athens, Greece.

The Pediatric Clinics of North America is covered in *MEDLINE/PubMed (Index Medicus)*, *Excerpta Medica*, *Current Contents*, *Current Contents/Clinical Medicine*, *Science Citation Index*, *ASCA*, *ISI/BIOMED*, and *BIOSIS*.

Printed in the United States of America.

GOAL STATEMENT

The goal of *Pediatric Clinics of North America* is to keep practicing physicians up to date with current clinical practice in pediatrics by providing timely articles reviewing the state of the art in patient care.

ACCREDITATION

The *Pediatric Clinics of North America* is planned and implemented in accordance with the Essential Areas and Policies of the Accreditation Council for Continuing Medical Education (ACCME) through the joint sponsorship of the University Of Virginia School Of Medicine and Elsevier. The University Of Virginia School of Medicine is accredited by the ACCME to provide continuing medical education for physicians.

The University of Virginia School of Medicine designates this educational activity for a maximum of 15 *AMA PRA Category 1 Credits*™ for each issue, 90 credits per year. Physicians should only claim credit commensurate with the extent of their participation in the activity.

The American Medical Association has determined that physicians not licensed in the US who participate in this CME activity are eligible for a maximum of 15 *AMA PRA Category 1 Credits*™ for each issue, 90 credits per year.

Credit can be earned by reading the text material, taking the CME examination online at http://www.theclinics.com/home/cme, and completing the evaluation. After taking the test, you will be required to review any and all incorrect answers. Following completion of the test and evaluation, your credit will be awarded and you may print your certificate.

FACULTY DISCLOSURE/CONFLICT OF INTEREST

The University of Virginia School of Medicine, as an ACCME accredited provider, endorses and strives to comply with the Accreditation Council for Continuing Medical Education (ACCME) Standards of Commercial Support, Commonwealth of Virginia statutes, University of Virginia policies and procedures, and associated federal and private regulations and guidelines on the need for disclosure and monitoring of proprietary and financial interests that may affect the scientific integrity and balance of content delivered in continuing medical education activities under our auspices.

The University of Virginia School of Medicine requires that all CME activities accredited through this institution be developed independently and be scientifically rigorous, balanced and objective in the presentation/discussion of its content, theories and practices.

All authors/editors participating in an accredited CME activity are expected to disclose to the readers relevant financial relationships with commercial entities occurring within the past 12 months (such as grants or research support, employee, consultant, stock holder, member of speakers bureau, etc.). The University of Virginia School of Medicine will employ appropriate mechanisms to resolve potential conflicts of interest to maintain the standards of fair and balanced education to the reader. Questions about specific strategies can be directed to the Office of Continuing Medical Education, University of Virginia School of Medicine, Charlottesville, Virginia.

The faculty and staff of the University of Virginia Office of Continuing Medical Education have no financial affiliations to disclose.

The authors/editors listed below have identified no financial or professional relationships for themselves or their spouse/partner:
David Angert, BS; Magdalena Bartoszewska, BA; Delmas J. Bolin, MD, PhD; Christopher C. Cheatham, PhD; Eugene Diokno, MD; Martin B. Draznin, MD; Donald E. Greydanus, MD (Guest Editor); Carla Holloway (Acquisitions Editor); Trudy A. McKanna, MS; Michael G. Miller, EdD, ATC, CSCS; Hatim Omar, MD; Dilip R. Patel, MD, FSAM; Neil D. Patel; Helen D. Pratt, PhD; Vinay Reddy, MD; Karen Rheuban, MD (Test Author); Dale Rowe, MD; Eric A. Schaff, MD; Saad Siddiqui, MD; and Helga V. Toriello, PhD.

The authors/editors listed below identified the following professional or financial affiliations for themselves or their spouse/partner:
Cnythia L. Feucht, PharmD, BCPS's spouse serves on the Speakers Bureau for Wyeth.
Manmohan Kamboj, MD serves on the speakers bureau for Pfizer.

Disclosure of Discussion of Non-FDA Approved Uses for Pharmaceutical Products and/or Medical Devices
The University of Virginia School of Medicine, as an ACCME provider, requires that all faculty presenters identify and disclose any off-label uses for pharmaceutical and medical device products. The University of Virginia School of Medicine recommends that each physician fully review all the available data on new products or procedures prior to clinical use.

TO ENROLL

To enroll in the Pediatric Clinics of North America Continuing Medical Education program, call customer service at 1-800-654-2452 or visit us online at www.theclinics.com/home/cme. The CME program is available to subscribers for an additional fee of $223.00

Contributors

GUEST EDITORS

DILIP R. PATEL, MD, FAAP, FACSM, FAACPDM, FSAM
Professor, Department of Pediatrics and Human Development, Michigan State University College of Human Medicine, East Lansing, Michigan

DONALD E. GREYDANUS, MD, FAAP, FSAM, FIAP (H)
Professor, Department of Pediatrics and Human Development, Michigan State University College of Human Medicine, East Lansing; Pediatrics Program Director, Kalamazoo Center for Medial Studies, Kalamazoo, Michigan

AUTHORS

DAVID ANGERT, BS
Department of Physiology, Cardiovascular Research Center, Temple University School of Medicine, Philadelphia, Pennsylvania

MAGDALENA BARTOSZEWSKA, BA
Michigan State University College of Human Medicine, East Lansing, Michigan; Michigan State University Kalamazoo Center for Medical Studies, Kalamazoo, Michigan

DELMAS J. BOLIN, MD, PhD
Associate Professor, Departments of Sports, Family Medicine, and Osteopathic Manipulative Medicine, The Via College of Osteopathic Medicine, Blacksburg, Virginia; Head Team Physician, Radford University, Radford, Virginia; Director, PCA Center for Sports Medicine, Salem, Virginia

CHRISTOPHER C. CHEATHAM, PhD
HPER Department, Western Michigan University, Kalamazoo, Michigan

EUGENE DIOKNO, MD
Primary Care Sports Medicine Program, Arnold Palmer Sports Health Center, Baltimore, Maryland

MARTIN B. DRAZNIN, MD
Director, Pediatric Endocrine Subspecialty Clinics, Michigan State University Kalamazoo Center for Medical Studies; Professor of Pediatrics and Human Development, Michigan State University College of Human Medicine, Kalamazoo, Michigan

CYNTHIA L. FEUCHT, PharmD, BCPS
Assistant Professor, Department of Pharmacy Practice, Ferris State University, Kalamazoo, Michigan; MSU/KCMS, Kalamazoo, Michigan

DONALD E. GREYDANUS, MD, FAAP, FSAM, FIAP (H)
Professor, Department of Pediatrics and Human Development, Michigan State University College of Human Medicine, East Lansing; Pediatrics Program Director, Kalamazoo Center for Medial Studies, Kalamazoo, Michigan

MANMOHAN KAMBOJ, MD
Associate Professor, Department of Pediatrics and Human Development, Michigan State University College of Human Medicine, East Lansing, Michigan; Pediatrics Residency Program, Division of Pediatric Endocrinology, Michigan State University, Kalamazoo Center for Medical Studies, Kalamazoo, Michigan

TRUDY A. MCKANNA, MS
Certified Genetic Counselor, Spectrum Health Genetic Services, Grand Rapids, Michigan

MICHAEL G. MILLER, EdD
HPER Department, Western Michigan University, Kalamazoo, Michigan

HATIM OMAR, MD
Chief, Division of Adolescent Medicine, Department of Pediatrics; Professor, Department of Obstetrics and Gynecology, University of Kentucky, Lexington, Kentucky

DILIP R. PATEL, MD, FAAP, FACSM, FAACPDM, FSAM
Professor, Department of Pediatrics and Human Development, Michigan State University College of Human Medicine, East Lansing, Michigan

NEIL D. PATEL
Human Resuscitation Learning Laboratory, Department of Emergency Medicine, Michigan State University Kalamazoo Center for Medical Studies, Kalamazoo, Michigan

HELEN D. PRATT, PhD
Professor, Department of Pediatrics and Human Development, Michigan State University College of Human Medicine, East Lansing, Michigan; Director, Behavioral-Developmental Pediatrics, Michigan State University, Kalamazoo Center for Medical Studies, Kalamazoo, Michigan

VINAY REDDY, MD
Associate Professor, Department of Pediatrics and Human Development, Michigan State University College of Human Medicine, Kalamazoo Center for Medical Studies, Kalamazoo, Michigan

DALE ROWE, MD
Professor, Department of Orthopedic Surgery, Michigan State University College of Human Medicine, East Lansing, Michigan; Program Director, Orthopedic Residency Program, Kalamazoo Center for Medical Studies, Kalamazoo, Michigan

ERIC A. SCHAFF, MD
Assistant Professor and Director of Adolescent Medicine, Department of Pediatrics, Temple University School of Medicine, Philadelphia, Pennsylvania

SAAD SIDDIQUI, MD
Fellow, Pediatric Cardiology, Hope Children's Hospital, Oak Lawn, Illinois

HELGA V. TORIELLO, PhD
Director of Clinical Genetics, Spectrum Health Genetic Services, Grand Rapids, Michigan

Contents

A preparticipation cardiovascular screening is recommended for all athletes with the aim of identifying conditions that increase the risk for adverse cardiac event, including sudden death. History and physical examination are the mainstay of cardiovascular screening of young athletes. The ability to identify athletes at risk, however, based on history and physical examination alone is low, and inclusion of an electrocardiogram as a screening tool has been suggested to improve the sensitivity of screening. This article provides an overview of key aspects of cardiovascular screening currently recommended in the United States for young athletes.

Sport-related concussion is a common problem encountered by pediatricians and other primary care physicians. Assessment of concussion is based on clinical evaluation. The Zurich consensus statement provides a basic framework to guide concussion management decisions and recommends an individualized approach and the exercising of clinical judgment in return-to-play decisions. This article reviews practice aspects of concussion for the adolescent athletes who present in the primary care office or clinic setting.

The benefits and possible detriments of resistance training have been noted extensively in the literature. Although the benefits of resistance training are well known, many professionals fail to heed scientific advice or follow appropriate recommendations for resistance training in adolescents. When developing a resistance training program for adolescents, be cognizant of any pre-existing health conditions and experience level of the adolescent. For strength training, the adolescent should begin with exercises that involve all major muscle groups with relatively light weight, one to three sets of 6 to 15 repetitions, 2 to 3 non-consecutive days per week. As the adolescent becomes more experienced, gradually increase loads and add multijoint exercises. Each exercise session should be properly supervised for safety, and to provide feedback on technique and form, regardless of the resistance training experience of the adolescent. This article reviews the guidelines for resistance training for health-related fitness for adolescents.

have been used include anabolic steroids, anabolic-like agents, designer steroids, creatine, protein and amino acid supplements, minerals, antioxidants, stimulants, blood doping, erythropoietin, β-blockers, and others. The use of these agents has considerable potential to cause physical and psychological damage. Use and misuse of drugs in this sports doping process should be discouraged. This discussion reviews some of the agents that are currently being used. Clinicians providing sports medicine care to youth, whether through anticipatory guidance or direct sports medicine management, should educate their young patients about the hype and hyperbole of these products that may keep them out instead of in the game at considerable financial cost to the unwary consumer.

Both acute and overuse musculoskeletal injuries are common in adolescent athletes. Pharmacologic agents including nonsteroidal anti-inflammatory drugs, acetaminophen, and topical over-the-counter agents have been shown to be effective in controlling pain, but data regarding their efficacy in expediting healing and time to recovery continue to be debated. Studies indicate that adolescents consume analgesic agents on their own and may be unaware of their potential toxicities. Data also indicate that adolescent athletes use medications in hopes of alleviating pain and allowing continuation of sports without adequate time for healing. This article reviews the mechanisms, toxicity, drug interactions, efficacy, and abuse potential of commonly used analgesic and anti-inflammatory drugs.

The application of manual techniques to pediatric athletic injuries has been considered alternative medicine. There are many injuries that are associated with loss of normal motion. Altered biomechanics can be readily identified and treated using manual methods. These include articular or thrust techniques, muscle energy, strain-counterstrain, and myofascial treatments, among others. Although there are few high-quality studies available, most available literature reports effectiveness of manual techniques in combination with therapeutic exercise for common pediatric motion restrictions.

Many physically and cognitively challenged athletes participate in organized and recreational sports. Health benefits of sport participation by athletes with disabilities have been well recognized. A careful preparticipation evaluation and proper classification of athletes ensures safe sports participation by athletes with disabilities. Some conditions in these athletes, such as problems with thermoregulation, autonomic control, neurogenic bladder and bowel, latex allergy, and many associated and secondary complications deserve special consideration. This article reviews common medical issues that relate to sport participation by athletes with physical and cognitive disabilities.

RELATED INTEREST

Physical Medicine and Rehabilitation Clinics of North America Volume 19, Issue 2
(May 2008)
The Child and Adolescent Athlete
Brian J. Krabak, MD, MBA, *Guest Editor*
www.pmr.theclinics.com

Pediatric Clinics of North America Volume 54, Issue 4 (August 2007)
Performance Enhancing Drugs
Peter D. Rogers, MD, MPH, and Brian Hardin, MD, *Guest Editors*
www.pediatric.theclinics.com

THE CLINICS ARE NOW AVAILABLE ONLINE!

Access your subscription at:
www.theclinics.com

Preface: Adolescents and Sports

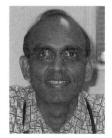
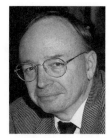

Dilip R. Patel, MD, FSAM   Donald E. Greydanus, MD,
FSAM, FIAP (H)

Guest Editors

Dr Nathan J. Smith was the guest editor for the December 1982 issue of *Pediatric Clinics of North America* devoted to sports medicine. This was followed by publication of an issue of *Pediatric Clinics of North America* devoted to sports medicine in October 1990, coedited by Dr Albert Hergenroeder and Dr James Garrick, and in August and October 2002 issues edited by Dr Eugene F. Luckstead Sr. It has been a humbling experience for us to follow such giants in the field. We consider it a great privilege and honor to be guest editors of this issue of *Pediatric Clinics of North America* devoted to the adolescent athlete. Our goal is to provide reviews of selected topics of relevance to pediatricians and other primary care physicians in their daily practice.

We thank all the authors for sacrificing their time and sharing their expertise to contribute articles to this issue. We thank Carla Holloway, editor, for her guidance and patience during this project from start to finish. Dilip Patel especially appreciates continued professional guidance and support from Dr Hergenroeder.

On a personal level, we would like to especially note that we have enjoyed our years of friendship with Dr Luckstead (Gene)—thank you Gene for years of wisdom, friendship, and collegiality—looking forward to many more years of the same.

Dilip R. Patel, MD, FSAM
Donald E. Greydanus, MD, FSAM, FIAP (H)
Department of Pediatrics and Human Development
Michigan State University College of Human Medicine
MSU/Kalamazoo Center for Medical Studies
1000 Oakland Drive
Kalamazoo, MI 49008-1284, USA

E-mail addresses:
patel@kcms.msu.edu (D.R. Patel)
greydanus@kcms.msu.edu (D.E. Greydanus)

Pediatr Clin N Am 57 (2010) xv
doi:10.1016/j.pcl.2010.03.007   **pediatric.theclinics.com**
0031-3955/10/$ – see front matter © 2010 Elsevier Inc. All rights reserved.

Cardiovascular Screening of Adolescent Athletes

Saad Siddiqui, MD[a],*, Dilip R. Patel, MD, FAAP, FACSM, FAACPDM, FSAM[b]

KEYWORDS

• Young athletes • Electrocardiography • Sudden cardiac death
• Preparticipation screening

Preparticipation screening of competitive athletes refers to the "systematic practice of medically screening large populations of athletes before participation in sports for the purpose of identifying abnormalities that could provoke disease progression or sudden death."[1] The main objective of screening is to identify athletes who have cardiovascular risk factors so that timely evaluation and management can be initiated and appropriate decisions made about the level of physical activity or sport participation.[1–6]

Screening and prevention are the most important strategies for several reasons.[7–13] It is commonly believed that automated external defibrillators (AEDs) placed at strategic locations at athletic venues and public places will help in improving survival after a sudden cardiac arrest (SCA).[7] Results of studies done to evaluate survival after an SCA on the athletic field with timely use of an AED by reasonably trained personnel are at best equivocal.[7–13] Thirty percent to 50% of all sudden cardiac deaths (SCDs) are the first clinical manifestation of an underlying pathology.[12] Various aspects related to cardiovascular screening of young athletes and SCD are subjects of a voluminous published research and excellent reviews, commentaries, and editorials.[1–6,14–21] This article provides an overview of key aspects of cardiovascular screening currently recommended in the United States for young athletes. The main concern and impetus for such an intense focus on cardiovascular screening is the risk of SCD during sport participation.

SCD

SCD refers to "nontraumatic and unexpected sudden death that may occur from a cardiac arrest, within 6 hours of a previously normal state of health."[3] In the modern

[a] Pediatric Cardiology, Hope Children's Hospital, 4440 West 95th Street, Oak Lawn, IL, USA
[b] Department of Pediatrics and Human Development, Michigan State University College of Human Medicine, Kalamazoo Center for Medical Studies, 1000 Oakland Drive, Kalamazoo, MI 49024, USA
* Corresponding author.
E-mail address: siddiq27@msu.edu

Pediatr Clin N Am 57 (2010) 635–647
doi:10.1016/j.pcl.2010.03.001
0031-3955/10/$ – see front matter © 2010 Elsevier Inc. All rights reserved.

era of competitive sports, there have been instances of athlete deaths in almost all sports but more commonly in basketball, soccer, and football.[1–4] Sudden death in athletes is especially disconcerting because exercise has proved to decrease the risk of life-threatening cardiovascular disease.[1]

Epidemiology

Although the exact incidence of SCD during sport participation in young athletes is not known, several studies provide an estimate of the incidence and data on other epidemiologic characteristics of SCD.[1–6,22–24] The incidence of SCD is estimated to be 1 in 200,000 in high school athletes and 1 in 65,000 in collegiate athletes in the United States.[1–6,22] The incidence of cardiovascular collapse as the cause of athletic fatalities is twice that of death caused by trauma.[14,15] SCD is more common in men than in women at a ratio ranging from 5:1 to 9:1; this may be because of the higher participation rate in men in competitive sports.[1,5,16] The incidence is higher in African American athletes; the disparity could be because of a higher number of competitive athletes (almost 40%) who are African American.[1,5,23] In previous studies from Italy, the incidence of SCD in athletes was reported at 3 in 100,000.[2,25] This difference between the United States and Italy is thought to be due to the younger age of the American athletes and the inclusion of a larger number of female athletes.[2,18] In the United States, the most common sports associated with SCA are football, basketball, and ice hockey whereas in Europe it is soccer.[1–6]

Causes

Pathophysiology of SCD is explained by exercise acting as a trigger for precipitation of sometimes lethal arrhythmias in the presence of underlying structural heart diseases or other susceptibilities.[1–6,25,26] In the United States, the most common cause of SCD in young athletes (26%) is hypertrophic cardiomyopathy (HCM).[1–6,27–31] The second most frequent cause of SCD in athletes (14%) is anomalous origin of the coronary artery, most commonly the left coronary artery arising from the right sinus of Valsalva.[32,33] This group of patients may have a completely normal electrocardiogram (ECG) and exercise stress test and first manifests symptoms with exertion while playing sport.[32] Other heart-related conditions that increase the risk for SCA in young athletes are listed in **Box 1**.[1–6,10,11]

In young children, commotio cordis is an important cause of sudden death. Commotios cordis results from a blunt trauma to the chest by a fast moving projectile, such as a baseball or ice hockey puck.[10,11] The mechanism of cardiac arrest is ventricular fibrillation. The blow should be inflicted within a narrow window of time (within 10–30 milliseconds) just before the peak of the T wave during repolarization.[1,10,11] Commotio cordis accounts for 20% of SCD in children on the field.[1,10,11]

CARDIOVASCULAR SCREENING
History and Physical Examination

The current American Heart Association (AHA) recommendations for cardiovascular screening of competitive young athletes consist of a review of 12 items (**Box 2**).[1] A positive response to 1 or more of these items is considered an indication for additional cardiovascular evaluation. Information that should be ascertained in the cardiovascular screening history of young athletes is listed in **Box 3**.[1–6]

In the United States there is no mandate or law regarding preparticipation screening. The responsibility of providing screening services for student athletes rests with the institutions organizing sports. Personal physicians are expected to conduct

---

Box 1
Conditions affecting the heart that increase young athletes' risk for SCD

Anomalous origin of coronary artery (second most common cause in the United States)

Aortic stenosis

Aortic dissection (usually complication in Marfan syndrome)

ARVC (most common cause in Italy)

Brugada syndrome (most prevalent in those of Asian descent)

HCM

Dilated cardiomyopathy

Coarctation of aorta

Congenital heart block (Mobitz type II, complete, or third degree)

Congenital or acquired long QT syndromes

Short QT syndrome

Coronary artery disease (rare in those younger than 35)

Restrictive cardiomyopathy

Endocarditis

Ehlers-Danlos syndrome

Mitral valve prolapse

Myocarditis

Pericarditis

Postoperative congenital heart disease

Status post heart transplant

Kawasaki disease (coronary artery abnormalities)

---

the 12-point screening evaluation in cases of high school athletes. At higher levels of athletic participation, it is the team physician who decides appropriate medical screening procedures.

In the United States, history and physical examination (H&P) has been the standard of cardiovascular screening for competitive athletes, although several studies have questioned the efficacy of the screening H&P alone in identifying athletes at risk for cardiovascular adverse events.[1,4,18,34–38] A study of 134 cases of SCD who had undergone a screening H&P reports that only 3% of patients were suspected of having cardiac disease and eventually only fewer than 1% received an accurate diagnosis.[34] This conferred a low sensitivity to H&P as a screening tool. The investigators also reported that at the high school level, the H&P was not being administered as recommended by the AHA.[34] The low sensitivity of the H&P is partly explained by suboptimal ascertainment of information. Surveys have reported that a significant percentage of H&P forms used by high schools do not include all 12 AHA-recommended screening items (see **Box 2**). Another issue relates to who is responsible for administering the H&P. H&P is administered by professionals with different levels of qualifications. In 64% of states in the United States, nonphysicians can administer the H&P.[38] In cases of college athletics, 25% of colleges were judged to have inadequate screening H&P forms. The National Collegiate Athletic Association H&P form includes 10 of 12 items from the AHA recommendations.[36]

Box 2
The 12-element AHA recommendations for preparticipaton cardiovascular screening of competitive athletes

Personal history

1. Exertional chest pain/discomfort

2. Unexplained syncope/near syncope (judged not to be neurocardiogenic or vasovagal, of particular concern when related to exertion)

3. Excessive exertional and unexplained dyspnea/fatigue associated with exercise

4. Prior recognition of a heart murmur

5. Elevated systemic blood pressure

Family history

6. Premature death (sudden and unexplained or otherwise) before age 50 because of heart disease in 1 or more relative

7. Disability from heart disease in a close relative younger than 50

8. Specific knowledge of certain cardiac conditions in family members: HCM or dilated cardiomyopathy, long QT syndrome, other ion channelopathies, Marfan syndrome, or clinically important arrhythmias

Physical examination

9. Heart murmur (auscultation should be performed in supine and standing positions [or with Valsalva maneuver], specifically to identify murmurs of dynamic left ventricular outflow tract obstruction)

10. Femoral pulses to exclude aortic coarctation

11. Physical stigmata of Marfan syndrome

12. Brachial artery blood pressure (sitting position) preferably taken in both arms

---

The H&P has come under scrutiny for having low sensitivity for identifying athletes with cardiovascular risk factors. The most frequently reported causes of SCD in young athletes, HCM and anomalous origin of coronary artery, are generally asymptomatic and have normal findings on examination. The advantages of H&P include cost effectiveness, need for minimal resources, and efficiency in administration with reasonable sensitivity. Several studies have reported data substantiating the higher efficacy of ECG in identifying athletes with HCM, channelopathies, and other clinically silent cardiovascular diseases that increase the risk for SCD in young athletes.[18,20,21,25,28,39–44]

Electrocardiogram

The 12-lead ECG obtained at rest on a nontraining day has received a lot of attention as a screening tool consequent to the Italian experience showing marked decrease in SCD rates after making ECG part of standard screening.[44] The International Olympic Committee and the European Sports Council require an ECG before sports participation.[2,20,21] Japan has been subjecting all first, seventh, and tenth graders to an ECG since 1973.[40] An ECG is abnormal in 90% of patients with HCM.[1,44] Other ECG detectable diseases causing SCD include arrythmogenic right ventricular cardiomyopathy (ARVC), ion channelopathies, dilated cardiomyopathy, and Wolff-Parkinson-White syndrome (WPW).[44,45]

Corrado and colleagues[28] showed that they were able to identify 22 asymptomatic athletes (of 33,735 athletes screened) with HCM based on screening ECG, later

Box 3
Cardiovascular preparticipation screening history

Symptoms

Unusual (more than or different from others) fatigue associated with physical activities

Pain, discomfort, or feeling of pressure in chest during exercise

Presyncope or syncope (fainting) during or after exercise, emotion, or startle

Exercise-associated dizziness

Exercise-associated shortness of breath

Heart racing or skipping beats

Medical or personal history and review of systems

Unexplained seizures or seizure-like episodes

Unexplained episodes of exercise-induced asthma or asthma-like symptoms

Recent febrile illness

Detailed history of any congenital structural heart disease

Use of a cardiac pacemaker or implanted cardiac defibrillator

History of Kawasaki disease

History of rheumatic fever

Known heart murmur

Known high cholesterol or lipid disorder

Systemic hypertension

Diabetes mellitus

Thyroid disease

Any previous recommendations to restrict physical activity

Use of therapeutic medications

Use of dietary supplements or over-the-counter medications

Substance abuse or tobacco use

Use of excessive caffeine or energy drinks

Family history

Sudden or unexpected death of family members before age 50 (include deaths due to possible sudden infant death syndrome, automobile accident, or drowning)

Coronary artery disease before age 50

Family members using pacemaker or implanted cardiac defibrillator

Family history of congenital deafness

Family history of certain cardiovascular diseases, such as Marfan syndrome, cardiomyopathies, long QT syndrome, short QT syndrome, or Brugada syndrome

Family history of lipid disorders, diabetes mellitus, or systemic hypertension

Family history of primary pulmonary hypertension

confirmed with an echocardiogram (ECHO). Eighty-two percent of the patients had abnormal ECG whereas 23% had some suggestions of underlying disease based on family history, a murmur, or both. In an extension of that, Corrado and colleagues[20,39] showed an 89% decrease in the incidence of SCD in athletes screened with ECG in Italy. A study of more than 5000 Nevada high school athletes showed the sensitivity of ECGs at 78% in detecting athletes at risk; this compares to 3% sensitivity for the H&P alone.[38] The specificity seems to increase when ECG changes considered grossly abnormal are pursued with additional studies.

In the United States, routine ECG is not currently recommended as part of cardiovascular screening of young asymptomatic athletes.[1,3] Reasons cited for not including ECG include cost, need for trained personnel, need for appropriate infrastructure, false-positive findings (in 10%–40%) warranting further unnecessary testing, and potential to cause anxiety in otherwise healthy athletes and their families.[1,3,4,46] Current recommendations include improving and standardizing the existing H&P forms, thus improving their yield, and creating a national data registry for reporting SCDs to better assess the epidemiology of SCD in the US athletic population. Because SCD is a rare event in young athletes, with a large number of athletes (5–10 million), it is estimated that it would cost $3.4 million to save 1 athlete's life from SCD and $330,000 to identify 1 athlete at risk for SCD.[1] The sensitivity of the screening ECG depends on appropriate interpretation by qualified professionals. The knowledge of specific ECG findings in healthy adolescents and ECG changes in athletes is imperative to determine what constitutes an abnormal and clinically significant change.[44,47–49]

There have been several questions raised regarding the Italian experience, which is cited most frequently as the basis for including ECG as a screening tool. One argument against that study is that it is an observational study and not a prospective study with a control population.[1] Also, the incidence rates that the Italians have managed to achieve after almost 25 years of ECG screening are not significantly different from the existing SCD rates in the United States.

Myerburg and Vetter[41] make several points in favor of including ECG for cardiovascular screening of competitive athletes. They contend that the false-positive rate of 10% to 25% cited in the AHA recommendations for abnormal findings on ECG is too high and according to their estimate it is approximately 4.8%.[41,42] Myerburg and Vetter[41] have suggested that all school athletes receive ECGs only twice during their school athletic career. This would mitigate the need for annual ECG for each athlete and significantly bring down the cost of such a program. With regards to personnel, the argument is that ancillary health staff with an interest in SCA should be recruited and trained to provide for the numbers required for a functional screening strategy that includes ECG. Fuller and colleagues,[38] based on their study of more than 5000 high school athletes, estimated that including an ECG in the screening protocol would cost $44,000 for each life saved. Fuller and colleagues[38] report that screening 700,000 high school athletes annually results in 1080 years of life gained when an ECG is used compared with 92 years of life gained when the AHA-recommended H&P alone is used. The average cost of screening in Japan is $8800 per life saved and in Italy a similar type of program cost $15,926 per life saved; both include screening ECG.[43,50] With government subsidy and more realistic cost assessment, it has been surmised that a screening program with ECG can be put in place at 20% to 25% of the cost presented in the AHA report.[1,41]

Currently, there is no consensus regarding whether or not routine ECG screening is prudent to apply to the US athlete population. The AHA report provides the framework for cardiovascular screening.[1,3] Large prospective studies are needed to evaluate the value of screening ECGs in the US population. In more recent publications, Maron and colleagues[1,6] have reviewed the recommendations for and against including an ECG in preparticipation screening. Maron and colleagues[1,6] note the potential usefulness of ECGs in identifying athletes at risk but also cite lack of infrastructure (including trained personnel) and the demographics of the athletic population as the principle barriers to implementing a large-scale screening program that includes ECG. Maron and colleagues[1,6,22] in their study comparing the rate of SCD in similar-sized populations in Minnesota, United States, and Veneto, Italy, reported that the rate of SCD was not significantly different between the 2 groups. The investigators, however, note that the rate of SCD has declined in Veneto, Italy, after implementation of an ECG-based screening program. In Italy, a specialist who has received training for 4 years administers the sports screening. Such a person is well trained in reading ECG of athletes, decreasing the false-positive rates and keeping the costs down. Based on many reports, including that of the AHA, inclusion of an ECG in routine screening of asymptomatic young athletes presents considerable economic and logistical challenges. Therefore, at present, ECG is indicated based on abnormal findings of H&P.

Physiology and cardiac remodeling

Knowledge of cardiovascular changes that result from regular exercise is essential in the interpretation of ECG changes in athletes.[44,51] The term, *athlete's heart*, refers to the changes that result from regular exercise, characterized by a benign increase in cardiac mass and specific circulatory and cardiac morphologic alterations that represent a physiologic adaptation to systematic training.[47,49,51–62] Endurance training (dynamic, isotonic, or aerobic), such as running or swimming, and resistance training (static, isometric, or anaerobic), such as weight training, result in different training effects on the cardiovascular system (**Table 1**).[1] In most sports, however, there is some overlap of endurance and resistance training. This is exemplified in sports, such as skiing, rowing, cycling, and triathlon. It is, therefore, expected that with regular exercise training there is some combination of cardiac chamber dilation and increase in wall thickness.[1]

The cardiac remodeling associated with regular exercise training in athletes is not a uniform phenomenon. Fifty percent of athletes may show some cardiac remodeling that includes 1 or all of the following: increase left ventricle, right ventricle, or left atrium chamber size. Ventricular wall thickness may or may not be increased. These changes are usually associated with normal systolic and diastolic function. Remodeling may occur rapidly or more gradually. Most of these changes are still within normal limits when compared with age- and gender-matched sedentary individuals.[47]

Table 1 Cardiovascular adaptation from training	
Type of Training	**Training Adaptations**
Endurance	Increased oxygen use
	Decreased peripheral vascular resistance
	Increased stroke volume
	Increased cardiac output
	Volume overload–induced ventricular dilatation
Resistance	No change in oxygen use
	No change in cardiac output
	Increased peripheral vascular resistance
	Increased heart rate
	Pressure overload–induced ventricular hypertrophy

The degree of structural change in the heart may correlate with the type of sport that an athlete is involved in, but this is not proved conclusively.[48,49,52–54] The clinical variables that may play a role in influencing the degree of structural change in the heart include body size (50%), type of sport (14%), gender (7%), age (4%), and unknown factors (25%).[48–55] Genetics also plays a role and may be responsible for some of the unknown variables.[48–55]

Often the changes in ventricular chamber size and wall thickness seen in competitive athletes may mimic structural heart disease. A ventricular wall thickness between 13 and 15 mm and left ventricular end-diastolic size greater than or equal to 55 mm but less than or equal to 60 mm constitute the gray zone of overlap between physiologic change and structural heart disease.[1,3,48,55] In these cases, it is often difficult to make a decision whether or not to allow continued competitive sport participation. One option is to discontinue training and serially measure these variables.[27,48,62] Normalization would suggest physiologic change and an athlete might be allowed to resume competitive sport participation.[42,48,62]

Several changes are noted on an ECG due to cardiac remodeling with regular exercise training. Approximately 60% of athletes have a normal ECG whereas 15% may have ECG changes suggestive of an underlying heart disease.[44,47,48] The most commonly observed ECG changes in athletes include early repolarization, increased QRS voltages, diffuse T-wave inversion, and deep Q waves.[44,47] The most common rhythm abnormalities in athletes include bradycardia, first-degree heart block, and Wenckebach phenomenon.[44,47] Recent studies with Holter monitor have identified more complex ventricular arrhythmias, which are usually abolished on discontinuing training and may be of no clinical significance. These may be considered part of the spectrum that constitutes an athlete's heart.[44,47]

In most athletes, the changes in the heart that occur with regular training and conditioning regress with deconditioning; however, in 20% of these athletes, the changes may be permanent.[1,47] There is no evidence to show that the cardiac remodeling in an athlete has a disabling, permanent, or detrimental course.[47]

2-D ECHO

2-D ECHO is most useful for the diagnosis of structural heart disease.[45,63] Diastolic and systolic function, wall motion abnormalities, wall thickness, valve morphology, and internal chamber size can be assessed with confidence with ECHO. ECHO has also been shown to be useful in visualizing the origin of the coronary arteries.[64,65] Including contrast and tissue Doppler greatly increases the likelihood of diagnosing ARVC while using the ECHO.[63,64] Adding an ECHO to a cardiovascular screening program increases the likelihood of identifying structural abnormalities of the heart. The added cost of screening and the scarcity of resources, equipment, and personnel are significant barriers to recommend routine use of ECHO for screening. An ECHO can be considered a good confirmatory test after abnormal findings on H&P or ECG.

Genetic Testing

There have been significant advances in the identification of genetic causes for cardiovascular diseases,[66–69] leading to the question of present or future methods involving identification of genetic risk factors for cardiovascular disease using genetic testing as a screening tool. Even though progress has been made in identification of these genetic mutations, the genotype-phenotype correlation is still poor. It cannot be reliably predicted if an identified mutation will eventually lead to an expression of disease. This may lead to a high false-positive rate. With more mutations identified, the battery of tests is ever-increasing and to apply the entire set to an athlete is not prudent, which leads back to the need for a good H&P as an initial screening tool with emphasis on family history to identify individuals at risk. Once a proband is identified, an entire family can be screened for that specific mutation that has been identified.[64,68]

Other Tests

Exercise stress testing is of limited value as a screening tool but has a role in risk stratification.[45] Exercise stress testing has been recommended in athletes older than 35. This is also part of the extended Italian recommendation for athletes older than 35.[2] Maximal exercise testing is an integral component to unmask arrhythmia in ARVC, familial catecholaminergic polymorphic ventricular tachycardia, and long QT syndrome. Frequent ventricular extrasystoles during exercise indicate underlying cardiac disease.[45]

Several other tests are available for identification of certain specific conditions.[45,70] These include Holter monitoring (quantification of extrasystoles and identification of tachy- and bradyarrythmias), cardiac MRI scan (ARVC, HCM, and myocarditis), tissue Doppler (ARVC), sodium channel blocker challenge (Brugada syndrome), and adenosine challenge for pre-excitation (familial risk of WPW syndrome and supraventricular tachycardia). These tests are not appropriate for mass screening due to low yield and also due to the need for expertise to successfully obtain and interpret the results. They become important after screening has raised concerns for specific problems.

SUMMARY

Identification of young athletes at risk for an adverse cardiovascular event during sport participation is a challenging task. Even in the best of circumstances, outcome of SCA on the field remains poor; therefore, prevention is critical. Cardiovascular screening of young athletes is based on ascertaining specific history and a thorough physical examination. Although inclusion of an ECG in screening asymptomatic athletes has been shown to increase the likelihood of identifying athletes at risk, considerable logistical and economic challenges remain, including using ECG as a screening tool. Even the most ideal screening strategy may not identify all athletes at risk for SCA on the field, and unfortunately SCD may be the first clinical manifestation of some cardiac conditions.

ACKNOWLEDGMENTS

Parts of this article are updated and adapted from authors' previous work, Siddiqui SA, Patel DR. Prevention of sudden cardiac death in young athletes: impact and limitations of preparticipation screening. International Public Health Journal 2009;1(4): 379–88, with permission.

REFERENCES

1. Maron BJ, Thompson PD, Ackerman MJ, et al. Recommendations and considerations related to preparticipation screening for cardiovascular abnormalities in competitive athletes: 2007 update. Circulation 2007;115:1643–55.
2. Corrado D, Pelliccia A, Bjornstad HH, et al. Cardiovascular pre-participation screening of young competitive athletes for prevention of sudden death: proposal for a common European protocol. Consensus Statement of the Study Group of Sport Cardiology of the Working Group of Cardiac Rehabilitation and Exercise Physiology and the Working Group of Myocardial and Pericardial Diseases of the European Society of Cardiology. Eur Heart J 2005;26:516–24.

3. American College of Cardiology 36th Bethesda Conference: eligibility recommendations for competitive athletes with cardiovascular abnormalities. J Am Coll Cardiol 2005;45(8):1317–75.
4. Berger S, Kugler JD, Thomas JA, et al. Sudden cardiac death in children and adolescents: introduction and overview. Pediatr Clin North Am 2004;51(5):1201–9.
5. Maron BJ, Doerer JJ, Haas TS, et al. Sudden deaths in young athletes: analysis of 1866 death in the United States, 1980–2006. Circulation 2009;119:1085–92.
6. Maron BJ, Haas TS, Doerer JJ, et al. Comparison of US and Italian experiences with sudden cardiac deaths in young competitive athletes and implications for preparticipation screening strategies. Am J Cardiol 2009;104:276–80.
7. Drezner JA. Preparing for sudden cardiac arrest—the essential role of automated external defibrillators in athletic medicine: a critical review. Br J Sports Med 2009; 43:702–7.
8. Germann CA. Sudden cardiac death in athletes: a guide for emergency physicians. Am J Emerg Med 2005;23:504–9.
9. Drezner JA, Courson RW, Roberts WO, et al. Inter-association task force recommendations on emergency preparedness and management of sudden cardiac arrest in high school and college athletic programs: a consensus statement. J Athl Train 2007;42(1):143–58.
10. Maron BJ, Gohman TF, Kyle SB, et al. Clinical profile and spectrum of Commtio Cordis. JAMA 2002;287:1142–6.
11. Maron BJ, Wentzel DC, Zenovich AG, et al. Death in a young athlete due to commotio cordis despite prompt external defibrillation. Heart Rhythm 2005;2:991–3.
12. Myerburg RJ. Sudden cardiac death: exploring the limits of our knowledge. J Cardiovasc Electrophysiol 2001;12:369–81.
13. Harmon KG, Drezner JA. Update on sideline and event preparation for management of sudden cardiac arrest in athletes. Curr Sports Med Rep 2007;6(3):170–6.
14. Basilico FC. Cardiovascular disease in athletes. Am J Sports Med 1999;27: 108–21.
15. Cantu RC. Congenital cardiovascular disease: the major cause of athletic death in high school and college. Med Sci Sports Exerc 1992;24:279–80.
16. Maron BJ, Shirani J, Poliac LC, et al. Sudden death in young competitive athletes: clinical, demographic, and pathological profiles. JAMA 1996;276:199–204.
17. Maron BJ. Sudden death in young athletes. N Engl J Med 2003;349:1064–75.
18. Corrado D, Basso C, Schiavon M, et al. Pre-participation screening of young competitive athletes for prevention of sudden cardiac death. J Am Coll Cardiol 2008;52(24):1981–9.
19. Thompson PD, Levine BD. Protecting athletes from sudden cardiac death. JAMA 2006;296(13):1648–50.
20. Corrado D, Basso C, Pavei A, et al. Trends in sudden cardiovascular death in young competitive athletes after implementation of a preparticipation screening program. JAMA 2006;296(13):1593–601.
21. Bille K, Figueiras D, Schamasch P, et al. Position paper: sudden cardiac death in athletes: the Lausanne recommendations. Eur J Cardiovasc Prev Rehabil 2006; 13:859–75.
22. Maron BJ, Gohman TC, Aeppli D. Prevalence of sudden cardiac death during competitive sports activities in Minnesota high school athletes. J Am Coll Cardiol 1998;32:1881–4.
23. Maron BJ, Carney KP, Lever HM. Relationship of race to sudden cardiac death in competitive athletes with hypertrophic cardiomyopathy. J Am Coll Cardiol 2003; 41:974–80.

24. Van Camp SP, Bloor CM, Mueller FO, et al. Non-traumatic sports death in high schools and college athletes. Med Sci Sports Exerc 1995;27:641–7.
25. Corrado D, Basso C, Rizzoli G, et al. Does sports activity enhance the risk of sudden death in adolescents and young adults? J Am Coll Cardiol 2003; 42(11):1959–63.
26. Maron BJ. Triggers for sudden cardiac death in athlete. Cardiol Clin 1996;14: 195–210.
27. Maron BJ, Pelliccia A, Spirito P. Cardiac disease in young trained athletes. Insights into methods for distinguishing athlete's heart from structural heart disease, with particular emphasis on hypertrophic cardiomyopathy. Circulation 1995;91(5):1596–601.
28. Corrado D, Basso C, Schiavon M, et al. Screening for hypertrophic cardiomyopathy in young athletes. N Engl J Med 1998;339(6):364–9.
29. Maron MS, Olivotto I, Zenovich AG, et al. Hypertrophic cardiomyopathy is predominantly a disease of left ventricular outflow tract obstruction. Circulation 2006;114(21):2232–9.
30. Maron BJ. Hypertrophic cardiomyopathy: a systematic review. JAMA 2002; 287(10):1308–20.
31. Maron BJ. Hypertrophic cardiomyopathy. Curr Probl Cardiol 1993;18:639–704.
32. Basso C, Maron BJ, Corrado D, et al. Clinical profile of congenital coronary artery anomalies with origin from the wrong aortic sinus leading to sudden death in young competitive athletes. J Am Coll Cardiol 2000;35:1493–501.
33. Link MS, Wang P, Pandian NG, et al. An experimental model of sudden death due to low-energy chest-wall impact (commotio cordis). N Engl J Med 1998;338: 1805–11.
34. Glover DW, Maron BJ. Profile of preparticipation cardiovascular screening for high school athletes. JAMA 1998;279(22):1817–9.
35. Glover DW, Maron BJ. Evolution over 8 years of the US preparticipation screening process for undetected cardiovascular disease in US high school athletes. Circulation 2006;114(Suppl II):II502.
36. Pfister GC, Puffer JC, Maron BJ. Preparticipation cardiovascular screening for US collegiate student-athletes. JAMA 2000;283(12):1597–9.
37. Preparticipation physical evaluation. 3rd edition. Minneapolis (MN): McGraw-Hill/The Physican and Sports Medicine; 2005.
38. Fuller CM, McNulty CM, Spring DA, et al. Prospective screening of 5,615 high school athletes for risk of sudden cardiac death. Med Sci Sports Exerc 1997; 29:1131–8.
39. Corrado D, McKenna WJ. Appropriate interpretation of the athlete's electrocardiogram saves lives as well as money. Eur Heart J 2007;28(16):1920–2.
40. Tasaki H, Hamasaki Y, Ichimaru T. Mass screening for heart disease of school children in Saga city: 7-year follow up study. Jpn Circ J 1987;51:1415–20.
41. Myerburg RJ, Vetter VL. Electrocardiograms should be included in preparticipation screening of athletes. Circulation 2007;116(22):2616–26.
42. Pelliccia A, Culasso F, Di Paolo FM, et al. Prevalence of abnormal electrocardiograms in a large, unselected population undergoing pre-participation cardiovascular screening. Eur Heart J 2007;28:2006–10.
43. Tanaka Y, Yoshinaga M, Anan R, et al. Usefulness and cost effectiveness of cardiovascular screening of young adolescents. Med Sci Sports Exerc 2006; 38:2–6.
44. Corrado D, Pelliccia A, Heidbuchel H, et al. Recommendations for interpretation of 12-lead electrocardiogram in the athlete. Eur Heart J 2010;31(2):243–59.

45. Attari M, Dhala A. Role of invasive and noninvasive testing in risk stratification of sudden cardiac death in children and young adults: an electrophysiologic perspective. Pediatr Clin North Am 2004;51:1355–78.

46. Sen-choudary S, McKenna WJ. Sudden cardiac death in the young: a strategy for prevention by targeted evaluation. Cardiology 2006;105(4):196–206.

47. Maron BJ, Pelliccia A. The heart of trained athletes: cardiac remodeling and the risk of sports, including sudden death. Circulation 2006;114:1633–44.

48. Abernethy WB, Choo JK, Hutter AM Jr. Echocardiographic characteristics of professional football players. J Am Coll Cardiol 2003;41(2):280–4.

49. Fagard R. Athlete's heart. Heart 2003;89(12):1455–61.

50. Quaglini S, Rognoni C, Spazzolini C, et al. Cost-effectiveness of neonatal ECG screening for the long QT syndrome. Eur Heart J 2006;27:1824–32.

51. Rost R. The athlete's heart: historical perspective. Cardiol Clin 1992;10(2):197–207.

52. Spirito P, Pelliccia A, Proschan MA, et al. Morphology of the "athlete's heart" assessed by echocardiography in 947 elite athletes representing 27 sports. Am J Cardiol 1994;74(8):802–6.

53. Pelliccia A, Culasso F, Di Paolo FM, et al. Physiologic left ventricular cavity dilatation in elite athletes. Ann Intern Med 1999;130(1):23–31.

54. Pelliccia A, Maron BJ, Culasso F, et al. Clinical significance of abnormal electrocardiographic patterns in trained athletes. Circulation 2000;102(3):278–84.

55. Huston TP, Puffer JC, Rodney WM. The athletic heart syndrome. N Engl J Med 1985;313(1):24–32.

56. Choo JK, Abernethy WB 3rd, Hutter AM Jr. Electrocardiographic observations in professional football players. Am J Cardiol 2002;90(2):198–200.

57. Balady GJ, Cadigan JB, Ryan TJ. Electrocardiogram of the athlete: an analysis of 289 professional football players. Am J Cardiol 1984;53(9):1339–43.

58. Biffi A, Pelliccia A, Verdile L, et al. Long-term clinical significance of frequent and complex ventricular tachyarrhythmias in trained athletes. J Am Coll Cardiol 2002;40(3):446–52.

59. Biffi A, Maron BJ, Verdile L, et al. Impact of physical deconditioning on ventricular tachyarrhythmias in trained athletes. J Am Coll Cardiol 2004;44(5):1053–8.

60. Pelliccia A, Maron BJ, Culasso F, et al. Athlete's heart in women. Echocardiographic characterization of highly trained elite female athletes. JAMA 1996;276(3):211–5.

61. Sharma S, Maron BJ, Whyte G, et al. Physiologic limits of left ventricular hypertrophy in elite junior athletes: relevance to differential diagnosis of athlete's heart and hypertrophic cardiomyopathy. J Am Coll Cardiol 2002;40(8):1431–6.

62. Pelliccia A, Maron BJ, De Luca R, et al. Remodeling of left ventricular hypertrophy in elite athletes after long-term deconditioning. Circulation 2002;105(8):944–9.

63. Cava JR, Danduran MJ, Fedderly RT, et al. Exercise recommendations and risk factors for sudden cardiac death. Pediatr Clin North Am 2004;51:1401–20.

64. Zeppilli P, dello Russo A, Santini C, et al. In vivo detection of coronary artery anomalies in asymptomatic athletes by echocardiographic screening. Chest 1998;114:89–93.

65. Crispell KA, Hanson EL, Coates K, et al. Periodic rescreening is indicated for family members at risk of developing familial dilated cardiomyopathy. J Am Coll Cardiol 2002;39:1503–7.

66. Brugada R, Hong K, Dumaine R, et al. Sudden death associated with short-QTsyndrome linked to mutations in HERG. Circulation 2004;109:30–5.

67. Schimpf R, Wolpert C, Gaita F, et al. Short QT syndrome. Cardiovasc Res 2005; 67:357–66.
68. Tan H, Hofman N, van Langen I, et al. Sudden unexplained death: heritability and diagnostic yield of cardiological and genetic examination in surviving relatives. Circulation 2005;112:207–13.
69. Tester D, Kopplin L, Creighton W, et al. Pathogenesis of unexplained drowning: new insights from a molecular autopsy. Mayo Clin Proc 2005;80:596–600.
70. Prakken NH, Velthuis BK, Cramer MJ, et al. Advances in cardiac imaging: the role of magnetic imaging and computed tomography in identifying athletes at risk. Br J Sports Med 2009;43:677–84.

Sport-related Concussion in Adolescents

Dilip R. Patel, MD, FAAP, FACSM, FAACPDM, FSAM*, Vinay Reddy, MD

KEYWORDS

- Concussion • Neuropsychological testing
- Balance Error Scoring System
- Sport Concussion Assessment Tool

Sport-related concussions are common in adolescents and can have significant acute and long-term adverse effects on the developing brain of the young athlete.[1–8] This review discusses the practical aspects of sport-related concussions that are most relevant in the management of young athletes who present in the office. The Zurich consensus statement on concussion in sport provides a basic framework and a reference point for the evaluation and management of sport-related concussion in adolescents and adults.[7] The Sport Concussion Assessment Tool 2 (SCAT2) (Appendix 1), developed as part of the Zurich guidelines, provides a convenient and standard format for clinical evaluation and serial documentation of symptoms and examination findings of concussion.[7] However, each athlete should be individually assessed, and clinical judgment ultimately supersedes in making management and return-to-play decisions.

DEFINITION

In its practice parameter on concussion management in sports, the American Academy of Neurology defined concussion as a trauma-induced alteration in mental status that may or may not be associated with loss of consciousness.[9] Confusion, loss of memory, and reduced speed of information processing, which may occur immediately or several minutes later, are considered to be the key features of concussion seen in most cases.[3–12]

Concussion is defined by the Zurich consensus statement as a complex pathophysiological process affecting the brain, induced by traumatic biomechanical forces.[7] Certain common clinical, pathologic, and biomechanical features of concussion that form the basis of this definition are listed in **Box 1**.[7]

Department of Pediatrics and Human Development, Michigan State University College of Human Medicine, Kalamazoo Center for Medical Studies, 1000 Oakland Drive, Kalamazoo, MI 49008, USA
* Corresponding author.
E-mail address: patel@kcms.msu.edu

Pediatr Clin N Am 57 (2010) 649–670
doi:10.1016/j.pcl.2010.03.006
0031-3955/10/$ – see front matter © 2010 Elsevier Inc. All rights reserved.
pediatric.theclinics.com

> **Box 1**
> **The Zurich consensus statement common features associated with sport-related concussion**
>
> 1. Concussion may be caused by a direct blow to the head, face, neck, or elsewhere on the body with impulsive force transmitted to the head.
>
> 2. Concussion typically results in the rapid onset of short-lived impairment of neurologic function that resolves spontaneously.
>
> 3. Concussion may result in neuropathological changes, but the acute clinical symptoms largely reflect a functional disturbance rather than structural injury.
>
> 4. Concussion may result in a graded set of clinical syndromes that may or may not involve loss of consciousness. Resolution of the clinical and cognitive symptoms typically follows a sequential course; however, in a small percentage of cases, postconcussive symptoms may be prolonged.
>
> 5. No abnormality on standard structural neuroimaging studies is seen in concussion.

EPIDEMIOLOGY

The Centers for Disease Control and Prevention, in the United States, reported 300,000 head injuries in a year in high-school sports, 90% of which are concussions.[1,3] Reported incidence of concussions at high-school level is 0.14 to 3.66 concussions per 100 player seasons accounting from 3% to 5% of all sport-related injuries.[12] Gessel and colleagues,[13] using data from the High School Reporting Information Online and National Collegiate Athletic Association Injury Surveillance, reported that concussions represented 8.9% (n = 396) of all high-school athletic injuries and 5.8% (482) of all collegiate athletic injuries. The highest number of concussions has been reported in American football, followed by (in decreasing order of risk) ice hockey, soccer, wrestling, basketball, field hockey, baseball, and softball.[6]

Symptoms and signs of concussion are often not recognized by the athlete or by medical personnel, and the athlete may fail to grasp the significance of head trauma and subsequent symptoms of concussion and not seek timely medical attention.[14–23] Some athletes may not report symptoms or head injury for fear of being excluded from further sport participation. For these reasons it is generally accepted that the reported incidence of concussion is a gross underestimate.[14–24]

MECHANISM AND PATHOPHYSIOLOGY

In addition to direct impact to the head or other parts of the body in contact or collision sports, concussion can also occur in noncontact sports as a result of sudden acceleration, deceleration, or rotational forces imparted to the brain.[1] Thus, absence of a history of direct impact to the head or elsewhere on the body does not rule out the possibility of a concussion.[2]

The biomechanics and pathophysiology of concussion have been elucidated by many investigators in animal models as well as in humans.[6,8,10–27] Pathophysiology of concussion on a cellular level is characterized by disruption and increased permeability of neuronal cell membranes.[6,8] This results in an efflux of potassium into extracellular spaces, resulting in a calcium-dependent release of excitatory amino acids, specifically glutamate.[6] The increase in extracellular potassium triggers neuronal cell-membrane depolarization resulting in neuronal suppression. Sodium-potassium pump is activated to restore homeostasis. The increased cellular metabolic activity increases the need for energy and glucose, and leads to hyperglycolysis. To meet the increased metabolic demands in the brain, an increase in cerebral blood flow is expected; however, a decrease in cerebral blood flow is observed in concussive injury of the brain.[6,8] A mismatch between metabolic demands and supply results in neuronal dysfunction that can last from 1 to 10 days or more following the concussion, during which time the brain is more vulnerable to further injury.[6,8]

HISTORY

In the primary care setting the athlete with a concussion is seen in the office setting when they present for a follow-up of head injury and need a medical clearance to return to sport.[28–30] On the other hand, some athletes may initially present with symptoms or signs of concussion several days or weeks after the head injury; many may not realize the significance of the initial symptoms and delay seeking medical attention or seek medical attention because of persistence or worsening or onset of new symptoms.[1,2] Parents may first seek a pediatrician's advice when they notice deterioration of academic performance and changes in behavior, mood, or personality in the athlete; in these cases a history of antecedent head trauma should be ascertained.[1,2]

The athlete may give a history of direct blow to the head or other part of the body, a collision with another player, a fall to the ground, or being struck by an object such as a ball, puck, or a bat.[1,2] There may not be any history of direct impact to the head or other part of the body, and concussion can result from indirect shearing or rotational forces imparted to the brain without direct impact.[1] Not uncommonly, a teammate may notice that something is not right with the athlete and communicate that to the trainer on the sideline. The athletic trainer or the coach or, less commonly, a spectator may see a collision and observe that the player is confused, disoriented, and not able to execute tasks or follow commands as expected within the context of the play at the time.[3]

The athlete with concussion may manifest any 1 or more of several symptoms or signs (**Table 1**)[1–5,7,10]; some develop immediately after the injury to the brain, whereas others may be delayed for days or weeks.[9] Because no single symptom or set of symptoms and signs is pathognomonic of concussion, and many symptoms are nonspecific in nature, a contemporaneous relationship between the time of initial head injury and subsequent development of symptoms and signs should be established based on history and examination.[1] Several symptom checklists or scales are used in the evaluation of concussion; however, none is specifically validated for such use.[31–41] SCAT2 includes one such symptom evaluation scheme.[7] Increasing evidence suggests that concussion rating scales based on athlete self-report of multiple symptoms are a more reliable and practical way of detecting concussion and monitoring progress during the recovery phase.[31–41]

Details of any previous head injury should be ascertained. Detailed history should include the date of injury, symptoms or signs, recovery time, and results of any neuropsychological (NP) testing.[1,2,28,30] If multiple concussions have occurred in the past, obtain similar details for each concussion and document the interval between successive concussions.[1,2]

REVIEW OF SYSTEMS

A relevant review of systems should include any known (preinjury) neurologic condition or learning disability, attention deficit/hyperactivity disorder, depression, academic function before and since the injury, use of drugs or performance-enhancing supplements, and use of therapeutic medications.[1–3] Psychosocial history should assess the athlete's interest in sports and any evidence of parental pressure to return to sport.[1,3,42]

Table 1 Symptoms and signs of concussion	
Mental status changes	Amnesia Confusion Disorientation Easily distracted Excessive drowsiness Feeing dinged, stunned, or foggy Impaired level of consciousness Inappropriate play behaviors Poor concentration and attention Seeing stars or flashing lights Slow to answer questions or follow directions
Physical or somatic	Ataxia or loss of balance Blurry vision Decreased performance or playing ability Dizziness Double vision Fatigue Headache Lightheadedness Nausea, vomiting Poor coordination Ringing in the ears Seizures Slurred, incoherent speech Vacant stare/glassy eyed Vertigo
Behavioral or psychosomatic	Emotional lability Irritability Low frustration tolerance Personality changes Nervousness, anxiety Sadness, depressed mood

Data from Refs.[1–5,7,10]

NEUROLOGIC EXAMINATION

A complete neurologic examination is essential in the evaluation of athletes with concussion, with specific attention to speech, visual acuity, visual fields, ocular fundi, pupillary reaction, extraocular movements, muscle strength, deep-tendon reflexes, tandem gait, finger-nose test, pronator drift, and Romberg test.[2,3,10,43,44] Postural stability has been shown to be a sensitive indicator of sensory-motor dysfunction in concussion.[33–36] SCAT2 includes the Balance Error Scoring System to assess balance, and finger-to-nose task to assess coordination.[7] Abnormal or focal findings on neurologic examination should prompt consideration of a focal intracranial pathology and emergent evaluation and management of the athlete. Findings on neurologic examination should be normal in athletes with concussion, other than the mental status or cognitive functions.

COGNITIVE FUNCTION

Assessment of cognitive functions, assessed clinically or by formal NP tests (conventional or computer based), is an essential component of the evaluation of concussion.[7,45–51] Cognitive function can be affected by many factors other than the effects of concussion, such as baseline (preinjury) intellectual ability, learning disability, attention deficit/hyperactivity disorder, substance abuse, level of education, cultural background, lack of sleep, fatigue, anxiety, age, and developmental stage.[1–3,46,47] Cognitive assessment techniques should be appropriate for the athlete's age, level of education, and developmental stage or maturity. SCAT2 provides a method or format for clinically assessing cognitive function.[7] An athlete with concussion may continue to manifest somatic or behavioral symptoms even after resolution of cognitive deficits.

NP TESTING

Conventional (paper-and-pencil) or computer-based NP testing can be used to formally assess the cognitive functions (**Box 2**) of athletes who have concussion.[41,52–57] Conventional NP testing uses a battery of tests administered in 1 or more sessions (several hours) and interpreted by neuropsychologists.[1,2,46,54,55] Conventional NP tests have not been traditionally designed or validated to assess athletes with sport-related concussion, cannot be easily adapted for mass application, and are expensive and labor intensive.

Computerized NP testing specifically designed to assess athletes with sport-related concussion is now being used at high-school, collegiate, and professional levels to obtain baseline as well as postconcussion NP profiles of athletes to monitor recovery.[1–4,47,53–55] Some of the advantages of computerized testing include ease of administration, cost-effectiveness, and ease of interpretation. Examples of currently available computerized NP tests are listed in **Box 3**. For interested physicians, detailed information on each of the tests is available at their Web sites.

It is possible to use NP testing to monitor an athlete's recovery from a concussion, but data obtained from such tests after a concussion are most useful when compared with an injured athlete's performance on those tests before injury (baseline profile model).[4,58] This requires preparticipation baseline testing for all athletes in sports in which the risk of concussion is high. Computer-based tests make preparticipation testing more feasible by reducing the time involved in testing and by reducing observer bias in test results. These tests can also minimize the effect of repeated practice on an

---

Box 2
Major cognitive functions assessed by NP testing

Amnesia after trauma

Attention span (focused, sustained, and visual)

Mental flexibility

Motor coordination

Motor speed

Orientation to person, place, and time

Processing speed

Reaction time

Verbal memory, immediate and delayed

Visual scanning

Box 3
Examples of computerized NP test suites
Automated Neuropsychological Assessment Metrics (ANAM)
CogSport (formerly Concussion Sentinel)
Concussion Resolution Index (CRI)
Immediate Measurement of Performance and Cognitive Testing (ImPACT)
Standardized Assessment of Concussion (SAC) and its electronic version eSAC

athlete's performance on specific tests and detect attempts by an athlete to do poorly on baseline testing so that they will be more easily cleared to return to play after a concussion.

ANAM

The ANAM (www.armymedicine.army.mil/prr/anam.html) suite was developed primarily by the United States Department of Defense.[59,60] The original purpose of ANAM was to assess how normal physical and cognitive performance might be affected by chemical warfare agents, and many of the component tests were taken from batteries of NP and psychomotor tests developed by different branches of the United States Armed Forces. However, ANAM has been used for evaluation of other types of injuries, including concussion in athletes. Retest reliability needed for baseline measurements has been studied, but ANAM scores do not measure or indicate return to baseline after a concussion.[61,62]

CogSport

CogSport (CogState Limited: www.cogstate.com; known in an earlier version as Concussion Sentinel) is a suite of 4 tests that measure psychomotor function, processing speed, visual attention, vigilance, visual learning, verbal learning, and memory.[57,63] The suite is sensitive to cognitive changes seen in sport-related concussions compared with baseline performance, which is necessary for the evaluation of an athlete after concussion.[64,65]

CRI

CRI[8,10] (HeadMinder, Inc: www.headminder.com) is a Web-based NP test that includes measures of cognitive functions related to postconcussion syndrome, including memory, reaction time, and speed of decision making and of information processing.[58,63] As with several similar test suites, CRI was developed specifically to allow for comparison of an athlete's baseline and postconcussion performance.[57,58,66]

Immediate Postconcussion Assessment and Cognitive Testing (ImPACT)

ImPACT (ImPACT Applications, Inc: www.impacttest.com; the acronym also stands for Immediate Measurement of Performance and Cognitive Testing) was the first test suite designed specifically to evaluate NP function in athletes, at baseline and after concussive injury, and is one of the most widely used test suites for evaluation of concussion in athletes, including professional players.[67,68] ImPACT evaluates multiple neurocognitive skills, and assesses changes in processing speed as a test subject becomes fatigued. It can also vary stimuli randomly, which reduces the effect of practice on the athlete's score, and can detect attempts by an athlete to reduce baseline performance deliberately so that postconcussion changes are masked.

SAC, eSAC

SAC (www.csmisolutions.com) is a brief examination intended for use at the sideline, and is based on the American Academy of Neurology's 1997 Practice Parameter for management of sports-related concussion.[9,69,70] The original SAC, which is still available, was a paper-and-pencil test that measures orientation, immediate and delayed memory, and concentration. Unlike other paper-and-pencil and performance tests, evaluation with SAC does not show a practice effect on repeated administration.[71] An electronic version operating on handheld personal digital assistants is also available.

Validity of Computer-based NP Testing

The validity of computer-based NP testing in the evaluation of sport-related concussions remains a subject of intense debate and remains unsettled.[57] Some investigators have questioned the value of baseline testing because of lack of clear evidence that such testing helps to positively affect the outcome of concussion.[57] The performance of currently available NP tests for the evaluation of athletes after concussion seems to be variable, but better than pencil-and-paper tests. In one study, sensitivity of 2 different neurocognitive tests (CRI and ImPACT) to concussion were 78.6% and 79.2% respectively when used as the sole instrument for detection of concussion, compared with 43.5% for pencil-and-paper tests.[71] When combined in a battery with reports of concussion-related symptoms (which had a stand-alone sensitivity of 68.0%), evaluation of postural control (stand-alone sensitivity 61.9%), and the pencil-and-paper tests, overall sensitivity ranged from 89% to 96%, suggesting that a battery of several tests including NP tests is preferable for detection of concussion effects.

Test-retest reliability has also been shown to be low to moderate over a 5- to 50-day interval between initial and later testing with ImPACT, CRI, and Concussion Sentinel.[72,73] None of these tests reached the correlation coefficient of 0.75 considered acceptable for test-retest reliability. A head-to-head comparison of CogSport, ImPACT, and CRI showed significant but modest correlation in assessment of complex reaction time between ImPACT and CogSport and between ImPACT and CRI, but not between CogSport and CRI, and no significant correlation in assessment of memory indices between any pair of programs.[74] This suggests that the same NP test suite needs to be used for baseline and postinjury evaluation. Self-reported previous histories of concussion do not correlate with performance on pencil-and-paper or computer-based NP tests.[73,75]

One problem frequently encountered in concussion evaluation by comparison of baseline and postconcussion assessment is sandbagging, or performance deliberately reduced by an athlete during baseline testing with the intent of being able to return to play after a concussion without adequate recovery. Manual timing of an athlete during a paper-and-pencil test is difficult and may not have sufficient resolution to detect sandbagging. However, computer-based test suites can be designed to time tasks to high resolution, sometimes on the order of milliseconds, and tests can be designed to detect poor performance (ImPACT, in particular, contains tests that are intended to detect sandbagging); variability in time taken for a task, as well as in responses, is also associated with concussion.[64,67]

Another issue is the effect of repeated practice on an athlete's ability to perform tasks included in a test suite. Because paper-and-pencil tests are limited in their item variability, the practice effect is more pronounced with such tests, although one study showed little such effect with the SAC.[71] Computer-based test suites can and should be designed so as to vary aspects of each individual test in the suite, and many of these tests, including ImPACT, CogState, and ANAM, provide for such variation.[59,64,73]

Applications of Computer-based NP Testing

In the last 10 years NP evaluation of sports-related brain injury has become widespread. The management decisions in concussion should not be guided solely by the results of NP testing, and NP testing should be used as 1 tool in the overall assessment along with clinical evaluation.[2,7,54] Such testing provides at least some objective data on cognitive function in concussion. Computer-based testing reduces interobserver variability in the gathering of test data and makes test results less dependent on the competence of test administrators. Accurate interpretation of the results of these tests requires knowledge of the tests used and of their limitations, in general use and with players in different sports, on different teams, and in different situations.

Adolescence is developmentally characterized by continued neurologic maturation associated with increased acquisition of neurocognitive abilities as well as rapid acquisition of new skills and knowledge.[1–3] Therefore, continued improvement in measures of NP tests is expected through adolescence. A return to baseline NP profile may not necessarily indicate full recovery.[3] This confounding factor should be taken into account in interpreting the results of NP tests in adolescents.

Brief mental status evaluations and assessments of cognitive function that can be administered easily on the sideline immediately after a head injury were among the initial applications of computer-based NP testing. Some of these tests, including SAC and ImPACT, were originally developed as pencil-and-paper tests; their adaptation to electronic testing increases precision, repeatability, and objectivity of test results while reducing the practice effect seen with repetitive administration of the same test items. In particular, the high precision of timing, to fractions of a second, possible in computer-based testing allows for better comparison of pre- and postconcussion performance and improved detection of subtle cognitive defects.

Another advantage of computer-based testing for evaluation of concussion is that the ability to test athletes without neuropsychologists having to administer the tests makes NP testing more accessible.[4] Some of the available test suites, in particular ImPACT, can also detect sandbagging or other non–trauma-related changes in test performance, which is especially important during baseline testing.

Computer-based NP testing has been shown to provide valid and repeatable information on the effects of concussion on an athlete, and can be used in conjunction with baseline (before the season) test results to assess changes over time in cognitive functions. Formal NP testing is useful to delineate specific impairments in athletes who fail to recover as expected, or who deteriorate, or those who have had multiple concussions.[3] NP testing can be useful in guiding the management of academic difficulties in children and adolescents. Computerized NP testing can be done on an individual basis in an office or clinic setting; however, in most communities it is done through the school system. Pediatricians are increasingly likely to see athletes who present with such baseline and postinjury test reports (**Fig. 1**).

NEUROIMAGING

Neuroimaging is indicated in athletes with focal neurologic signs, those with progressively worsening symptoms and signs, failure of clinical resolution of symptoms (typically more than 2 weeks), severe acute headache, and loss of consciousness greater than a few seconds.[1–3,52] Static imaging with magnetic resonance imaging (MRI) or computerized tomography does not show any structural abnormalities of the brain in concussion.[1–7] Imaging modalities such as positron emission tomography,

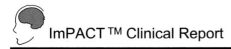
ImPACT ™ Clinical Report

Exam Type	Base line	Post -Injury 1	Post -Injury 2	Post -Injury 3	
Date Tested	12/03/2007	01/17/2008	01/22/2008	01/26/2008	
Last concission			01/12/2008	02/02/2008	
Exam Language	English	English	English	English	
Test Version	2.0	2.0	2.0	2.0	

Composite Score									
Memory composite (verbal)	78	27%	53	<1%	81	37%	96	88%	
Memory composite (visual)	66	22%	39	<1%	72	38%	55	6%	
Vis. motor speed composite	50.97	98%	11.75	<1%	51	96%	51.43	97%	
Reaction time composite	0.57	54%	0.95	1%	0.54	69%	0.58	69%	
Impulse control composite	10		6		8		2		
Total symptom Score	12		12		4		1		

Fig. 1. An ImPACT clinical report showing the composite scores of a 17-year hockey player who sustained 2 concussions in a short period of time. The scores that exceed the Reliable Change Index are highlighted in the report. Percentile scores, if available, are shown as small numbers to the right of the composite score. Percentile scores reflect the percentile rank of the athlete for their gender and age at the time of testing. The full report contains detailed clinical history and detailed analysis of scores for individual modules and subsets.

functional MRI, or single photon emission computed tomography provide information on brain metabolism and regional blood flow; however, their application in clinical evaluation and management of athletes with concussion is limited.[3,7,34,35]

DIFFERENTIAL DIAGNOSIS

In the evaluation of an athlete with symptoms and signs of concussion, the physician should consider other conditions that can present with similar clinical features. In the acute setting, heat-related illness, dehydration, hypoglycemia, and acute exertional migraine can mimic concussion.[1–4] Many of the delayed symptoms of concussion are nonspecific, making it necessary to carefully delineate concomitant conditions such as headache disorders, conduct disorder, depression, attention deficit/hyperactivity disorder, sleep disorder, cerebellar or brain stem lesions, or psychosomatic disorder.[3]

MANAGEMENT
Adolescent Development

Normal psychological and social development has implications for the management of concussion in adolescents.[3] Concrete thinking and concerns about one's physical appearance are characteristics of early adolescence (generally 12–14 years). The adolescent at this stage of development may not fully comprehend the significance of long-term adverse effects of concussion and therefore not report head injury or its symptoms. For the same reason, they may also fail to adhere to the treatment plan. Questions during history taking and instructions for treatment should be framed in simple, direct, and concrete language.

During middle adolescence (generally 15–16 years), the adolescent is highly susceptible to the influence of peers and media. The adolescent at this stage is also becoming more independent from parents and other adults in their life. Because of a sense of invulnerability, risk taking is common. Despite advice against it, the adolescent may continue to participate in sports for peer acceptance. The adolescent may find it difficult to cope with their inability to continue to play and, in some cases, may become depressed. When treating adolescents at this stage of development, the treating physician should take into account the psychosocial significance of sport participation in the adolescent's life.

Abstract thinking, future perspectives, life career, and interpersonal and social relationships are characteristics of late adolescence (generally 17–19 years). Because the adolescent at this stage is able to comprehend the potential for adverse long-term consequences of concussion, they are more likely to seek timely medical attention and adhere to a treatment plan.

Severity Grading

Concussion grading schemes based on the presence or absence and duration of loss of consciousness, confusion, and posttraumatic amnesia have not been shown to be clinically useful in the management of concussion.[1–10,12,52] Although the duration of certain symptoms and signs, such as the loss of consciousness or amnesia, may suggest the severity of concussion, the severity of concussion in an individual athlete can only be ascertained retrospectively after full clinical recovery has occurred.[1,2,7,10,52] Therefore, severity grading of concussion is not a main consideration in the initial management of most cases.

Return to Play

Each athlete follows a variable time course to recovery from acute cerebral concussion, so an individualized, stepwise plan for return to play is now considered the preferred practice, rather than following the conventional return-to-play guidelines.[1–3,7] Although most athletes recover in a period of between 2 to 3 weeks and 1 to 3 months, each athlete follows a variable trajectory to recovery following a concussion, making any fixed period of time out before return to play (used in the past in conventional concussion severity-based guidelines) a less valid approach.[1–4,7–12]

Following a concussion, complete physical and cognitive rest is recommended.[7] Although there is no agreement on how many days the athlete should be symptom-free before beginning the return-to-play stepwise protocol, most in practice consider at least 7 to 10 days of rest for adolescent athletes before beginning the protocol.[76,77] The Zurich conference consensus statement recommends the following stepwise approach of management[7]:

(1) No activity; complete physical and cognitive rest
(2) Light aerobic exercise (walking, stationary cycling, keeping intensity <70% maximal predicted heart rate, and no resistance training
(3) Sport-specific exercise (skating in hockey, running in soccer)
(4) Noncontact training drills (progression to more complex training drills, eg, passing drills in football; may start resistance training)
(5) Full-contact practice following medical clearance
(6) Return to unrestricted sport participation.

With the stepwise progression, the athlete should continue to proceed to the next level if asymptomatic at the current level. If symptoms recur, the athlete should go back to the previous asymptomatic step and try to progress after 24 hours of rest.[7] Before the athlete is allowed to return to play, they must be asymptomatic at rest as well as on exertion, and the examination must be normal.[3,7,77] The athlete should be monitored for recurrence of any symptoms or signs on physical exertion.

Cognitive Rest

Adolescents should return to increasing levels of school work gradually.[6,7] They need cognitive rest until full cognitive recovery.[7,75,77–79] The school should be informed of the athlete's need for special accommodations (**Box 4**) during the recovery phase.[78] Although most student athletes recover fully from concussion within a few days or weeks, some may need to use special accommodations, which can be accomplished by implementing a Section 504 plan or Individualized Education Plan as necessary.[1,2,78] Cognitive rest also implies limiting such activities as playing video games, texting, and watching television during the recovery period.

Athletes with Multiple Concussions

It is generally believed that the adverse effects of repeated concussions on the brain are cumulative and greater as the interval between successive concussions gets shorter.[3,80–85] However, Bruce and Echemendia[86] reported no significant association between self-reported concussion history and performance on computerized or traditional NP tests, suggesting a need for prospective studies to delineate long-term neurocognitive outcomes of concussion. An athlete may sustain multiple concussions during the same day, during the same season, or during their career.

There is no agreement as to how many concussions in a given period of time (some have suggested 3) should disqualify the athlete from further participation in high-risk sports.[4,5,83,84] Given this lack of clarity, most in practice take a more conservative approach for young athletes. The risks of repeated concussions on the developing brain should be discussed with the young athlete and the parents to allow them to make an informed decision as to whether to return to high-risk sports.

RECOVERY AND OUTCOME

Most young athletes recover fully from concussion. Thirty percent of high-school and collegiate athletes return to play the same day, and 70% after 4 days.[4,7] Same-day return to sports is generally not recommended for adolescents. Based

---

Box 4
Educational accommodations for athletes recovering from concussion

Reduce the number of work assignments

Allow more time to complete class work

Allow more time for tests

Outline and break complex tasks into simple steps

Provide written instructions for student athletes

Provide distraction-free areas for work

Provide a note taker

Incorporate less stressful course work

on NP testing data, correlation between NP testing and clinical findings indicate that most athletes with mild concussion recover cognitive function within 7 to 10 days, and those with severe concussion show recovery in a period of 1 to 3 months.[1-4,7,10,54] Athletes who have recovered in terms of their neurocognitive deficits may still have persistent emotional or behavioral symptoms.

Studies suggest that children and adolescents tend to have a more prolonged recovery phase than adults following a concussion, and have a higher risk of having a subsequent concussion.[14,79,87-100] Adverse effects of concussion on neurocognitive functions can be cumulative and modified by proximity of successive concussions, their severity, and individual susceptibility.[7] Children and adolescents can have life-long implications as a result of concussion, in terms of poor academic achievement, emotional symptoms, and psychosocial difficulties.[1]

Second impact syndrome (SIS) is characterized by rapidly progressive brain edema, brain stem herniation, and high mortality within minutes of a second concussion in an athlete who still has persistent symptoms (or has not clinically fully recovered) from a previous concussion has been described in adolescent male athletes.[101] Although some reports have debated whether SIS represents a new brain injury or is a complication of the initial injury, its exact etiopathogenesis remains unclear. Given this lack of clarity about the occurrence and significance of SIS, and the increased neuronal vulnerability to injury within few days after a concussion, it is recommended not to allow the symptomatic athlete return to sport.[102-113]

PREVENTION

Increased public awareness of various aspects of sport-related concussion is the most essential element of prevention strategy.[1-7] The Centers for Disease Control and Prevention has developed an excellent program called Heads Up for public education about concussion in sport (http://www.cdc.gov/concussion/headsup). The physician should incorporate education about sport-related concussion in the anticipatory guidance during injury-free visits as well as during the evaluation and management of athletes who present with concussion. Such a discussion with the athlete and the parents should include how to recognize concussion (signs and symptoms), potential complications, importance of seeking timely medical attention, physical and cognitive rest during recovery, and return-to-play criteria.[1]

Enforcement of rules of the sport plays an important role in prevention of head and neck injuries. Use of helmets in American football has reduced the likelihood of severe skull injury; however, helmet use has not been shown to be effective in prevention of brain concussion.[2,7,104,109-111] Research to develop helmets that can prevent or reduce the effects of concussion is actively being pursued. Appropriate use of mouth guards has been shown to reduce the incidence of orofacial injuries; their efficacy in prevention of concussion has not been established.[105-107,112,113] It has been suggested that strong neck muscles may allow the athlete to tense these muscles and maintain the head and neck in a fixed position just before impact and help dissipate the forces, theoretically reducing the impact on the brain; however, research results are equivocal.[3,7,52] Also, in practical terms, there is little time to anticipate the event and fix the head and neck before the impact during a game or practice.

ACKNOWLEDGMENTS

The authors thank Kim Douglas, Kalamazoo Center for Medical Studies, for assisting in the preparation of this manuscript.

REFERENCES

1. Patel DR. Managing concussion in a young athlete. Contemp Pediatr 2006; 23(11):62–9.
2. Patel DR. Concussions, in Patel DR, Greydanus DE, Baker RJ. Pediatric practice: sport medicine. New York: McGraw-Hill; 2009. p. 110–118.
3. Patel DR, Shivdasani V, Baker RJ. Management of sport-related concussion in young athletes. Sports Med 2005;35(8):671–84.
4. Guskiewicz KM, Bruce SL, Cantu RC, et al. National Athletic Trainers Association position statement: management of sport-related concussion. J Athl Train 2004;39:280–97.
5. Landry GL. Central nervous system trauma: management of concussions in athletes. Pediatr Clin North Am 2002;49(4):723–42.
6. Kirkwood MW, Yeats KO, Wilson PE. Pediatric sport-related concussions: a review of the clinical management of an oft-neglected population. Pediatrics 2006;117(4):1359–71.
7. McCrory P, Meeuwisse W, Johnston K, et al. Consensus statement on concussion in sport, 3rd International Conference on Concussion in Sport held in Zurich, November 2008. Clin J Sport Med 2009;19:185–200.
8. Meehan WP, Bachur RG. Sport-related concussion. Pediatrics 2009;123: 114–23.
9. Quality Standards Subcommittee of the American Academy of Neurology. The management of concussion in sports (summary statement). Neurology 1997; 48:581–5.
10. MCrory P, Johnson K, Meeuwisse W, et al. Summary and agreement statement of the 2nd International Conference on Concussion in Sport, Prague, 2004. Clin J Sport Med 2005;15(2):48–55.
11. Wojtys EM, Hovda D, Landry G, et al. Concussion in sports. Am J Sports Med 1999;27(5):676–87.
12. American College of Sports Medicine. Concussion (mild traumatic brain injury) and the team physician: a consensus statement. Med Sci Sports Exerc 2005; 37(11):2012–6.
13. Gessel LM, Fields SK, Collins CL, et al. Concussions among United States high school and collegiate athletes. J Athl Train 2007;42(4):495–503.
14. Browne GJ, Lam LT. Concussive head injury in children and adolescents related to sports and other leisure physical activities. Br J Sports Med 2006;40(2):163–8.
15. Cusimano MD. Canadian minor hockey participants' knowledge about concussion. Can J Neurol Sci 2009;36(3):315–20.
16. Delaney JS, Abuzeyad F, Correa JA, et al. Recognition and characteristics of concussions in the emergency department population. J Emerg Med 2005; 29(2):189–97.
17. Dvorak J, McCrory P, Kirkendall DT. Head injuries in the female football player: incidence, mechanisms, risk factors and management. Br J Sports Med 2007; 41(Suppl 1):i44–6.
18. Dyson R, Buchanan M, Hale T. Incidence of sports injuries in elite competitive and recreational windsurfers. Br J Sports Med 2006;40(4):346–50.
19. Sullivan SJ, Bourne L, Choie S, et al. Understanding of sport concussion by the parents of young rugby players: a pilot study. Clin J Sport Med 2009;19(3): 228–30.
20. Sye G, Sullivan SJ, McCrory P. High school rugby players' understanding of concussion and return to play guidelines. Br J Sports Med 2006;40(12):1003–5.

21. Valovich McLeod TC, Bay RC, Heil J, et al. Identification of sport and recreational activity concussion history through the preparticipation screening and a symptom survey in young athletes. Clin J Sport Med 2008;18(3):235–40.

22. Williamson IJ, Goodman D. Converging evidence for the under-reporting of concussions in youth ice hockey. Br J Sports Med 2006;40(2):128–32.

23. Yang J, Phillips G, Xiang H, et al. Hospitalisations for sport-related concussions in US children aged 5 to 18 years during 2000–2004. Br J Sports Med 2008; 42(8):664–9.

24. Powel JW, Barber-Foss KD. Traumatic brain injury in high school athletes. JAMA 1999;282:958–63.

25. Emery CA, Meeuwisse WH. Injury rates, risk factors, and mechanisms of injury in minor hockey. Am J Sports Med 2006;34(12):1960–9.

26. Guskiewicz KM, Mihalik JP, Shankar V, et al. Measurement of head impacts in collegiate football players: relationship between head impact biomechanics and acute clinical outcome after concussion. Neurosurgery 2007;61(6):1244–52.

27. Mori T, Katayama Y, Kawamata T. Acute hemispheric swelling associated with thin subdural hematomas: pathophysiology of repetitive head injury in sports. Acta Neurochir Suppl 2006;96:40–3.

28. Hunt T, Asplund C. Concussion assessment and management. Clin Sports Med 2010;29:5–17.

29. McCrory P. Preparticipation assessment for head-injury. Clin J Sport Med 2004; 14:139–44.

30. American Academy of Pediatrics. American Academy of Family Medicine, American Medical Society for Sports Medicine, American College of Sports Medicine, American Orthopedic Society for Sports Medicine: Preparticipation physical evaluation monograph. 3rd edition. New York: McGraw-Hill; 2005.

31. Randolph C, Barr WB, McCrea M, et al. Concussion symptom inventory (CSI): an empirically-derived scale for monitoring resolution of symptoms following sport-related concussion. Arch Clin Neuropsychol 2009;24:219–29.

32. Alla S, Sullivan SJ, Hale L, et al. Self-reports/checklists for the measurement of concussion symptoms: a systematic review. Br J Sports Med 2009;43(Suppl 1): i3–i12.

33. Cavanaugh JT, Guskiewicz KM, Giuliani C, et al. Detecting altered postural control after cerebral concussion in athletes with normal postural stability. Br J Sports Med 2005;39(11):805–11.

34. Davis GA, Iverson GL, Guskiewicz KM, et al. Contributions of neuroimaging, balance testing, electrophysiology and blood markers to the assessment of sport-related concussion. Br J Sports Med 2009;43(Suppl 1):i36–45.

35. Ellemberg D, Henry LC, Macciocchi SN, et al. Advances in sport concussion assessment: from behavioral to brain imaging measures. J Neurotrauma 2009;26:2365–82.

36. Fox ZG, Mihalik JP, Blackburn JT, et al. Return of postural control to baseline after anaerobic and aerobic exercise protocols. J Athl Train 2008;43(5):456–63.

37. Hayden MG, Jandial R, Duenas HA, et al. Pediatric concussions in sports; a simple and rapid assessment tool for concussive injury in children and adults. Childs Nerv Syst 2007;23(4):431–5.

38. Hutchison M, Mainwaring LM, Comper P, et al. Differential emotional responses of varsity athletes to concussion and musculoskeletal injuries. Clin J Sport Med 2009;19(1):13–9.

39. LaBotz M, Martin MR, Kimura IF, et al. A comparison of a preparticipation evaluation history form and a symptom-based concussion survey in the

identification of previous head injury in collegiate athletes. Clin J Sport Med 2005;15(2):73–8.

40. Lovell MR, Iverson GL, Collins MW, et al. Measurement of symptoms following sports-related concussion: reliability and normative data for the post-concussion scale. Appl Neuropsychol 2006;13(3):166–74.

41. Piland SG, Motl RW, Guskiewicz KM, et al. Structural validity of a self-report concussion-related symptom scale. Med Sci Sports Exerc 2006;38(1):27–32.

42. Patel DR, Greydanus DE, Pratt HD. Youth sports: more than sprains and strains. Contemp Pediatr 2001;18(3):45–76.

43. Kelly JP, Rosenberg JH. The diagnosis and management of concussion in sports. Neurology 1997;48:575–80.

44. Maroon JC, Field M, Lovell M, et al. The evaluation of athletes with cerebral concussion. Clin Neurosurg 2002;49:319–32.

45. Van Kampen DA, Lovell MR, Pardini JE, et al. The "value added" of neurocognitive testing after sports-related concussion. Am J Sports Med 2006;34(10): 1630–5.

46. Grindel SH, Lovell MR, Collins MW. The assessment of sport-related concussion: the evidence behind neuropsychological testing and management. Clin J Sport Med 2001;11:134–43.

47. Schatz P, Zillmer EA. Computer-based assessment of sports-related concussion. Appl Neuropsychol 2003;10(1):42–7.

48. Maddocks D, Dicker G. An objective measure of recovery from concussion in Australian rules footballers. Sport Health 1989;7(Suppl):6–7.

49. Maddocks DL, Dicker G, Saling MM. The assessment of orientation following concussion in athletes. Clin J Sport Med 1995;5(1):32–5.

50. Bickley LS. Bates' guides to physical examination and history taking. 9th edition. Baltimore (MD): Lippincott Williams & Wilkins; 2006.

51. McCrea M, Kelly JP, Randolph C. Standardized Assessment of Concussion (SAC): on-site mental status evaluation of the athlete. J Head Trauma Rehabil 1998;13(2):27–35.

52. Cantu RC. Work-up of the athlete with concussion. Am J Sports Med 2002;4: 152–4.

53. Randolph C, McCrea M, Barr WB. Is neuropsychological testing useful in the management of sport-related concussion? J Athl Train 2005;40(3):139–54.

54. Lovell MR. The relevance of neuropsychological testing in sports-related head injuries. Curr Sports Med Rep 2002;1(1):7–11.

55. Collie A, Darby D, Maruff P. Computerised cognitive assessment of athletes with sports related head injury. Br J Sports Med 2001;35:297–302.

56. Collie A, Maruff P, McStephen M, et al. Psychometric issues associated with computerized neuropsychological assessment of concussed athletes. Br J Sports Med 2003;37(6):556–9.

57. Erlanger D, Kaushik T, Cantu RC, et al. Symptom-based assessment of the severity of a concussion. J Neurosurg 2003;98:477–84.

58. Erlanger D, Saliba E, Barth J, et al. Monitoring resolution of postconcussion symptoms in athletes: preliminary results of a web-based neuropsychological test protocol. J Athl Train 2001;36:280.

59. Cernich A, Reeves D, Sun W, et al. Automated Neuropsychological Assessment Metrics sports medicine battery. Arch Clin Neuropsychol 1997;22:S101.

60. Reeves DL, Winter KP, Bleiberg J, et al. ANAM(R) Genogram: historical perspectives, description, and current endeavors. Arch Clin Neuropsychol 2007;22:S15.

61. Segalowitz SJ, Mahaney P, Santesso DL, et al. Retest reliability in adolescents of a computerized neuropsychological battery used to assess recovery from concussion. NeuroRehabilitation 2007;22:243.

62. Collie A, Maruff P, Makdissi M, et al. CogSport: reliability and correlation with conventional cognitive tests used in postconcussion medical evaluations. Clin J Sport Med 2003;13:28.

63. Erlanger D, Feldman D, Kutner K, et al. Development and validation of a web-based neuropsychological test protocol for sports-related return-to-play decision-making. Arch Clin Neuropsychol 2003;18:293.

64. Makdissi M, Collie A, Maruff P, et al. Computerised cognitive assessment of concussed Australian Rules footballers. Br J Sports Med 2001;35:354.

65. Collie A, Maruff P. Computerised neuropsychological testing. Br J Sports Med 2003;37:2.

66. Macciocchi SN, Barth JT, Alves W, et al. Neuropsychological functioning and recovery after mild head injury in collegiate athletes. Neurosurgery 1996;39:510.

67. Covassin T, Elbin R III, Stiller-Ostrowski JL, et al. Immediate Post-Concussion Assessment and Cognitive Testing (ImPACT) practices of sports medicine professionals. J Athl Train 2009;44:639.

68. Maroon JC, Lovell MR, Norwig J, et al. Cerebral concussion in athletes: evaluation and neuropsychological testing. Neurosurgery 2000;47:659.

69. McCrea M. Standardized mental status testing on the sideline after sport-related concussion. J Athl Train 2001;36:274.

70. McCrea M, Kelly JP, Kluge J, et al. Standardized Assessment of Concussion in football players. Neurology 1997;48:586.

71. Valovich TC, Perrin DH, Gansneder BM. Repeat administration elicits a practice effect with the Balance Error Scoring System but not with the standardized assessment of concussion in high school athletes. J Athl Train 2003;38:51.

72. Broglio SP, Ferrara MS, Macciochi SN, et al. Test-retest reliability of computerized concussion assess programs. J Athl Train 2007;42:509.

73. Schatz P. Long-term test-retest reliability of baseline cognitive assessments using impact. Am J Sports Med 2010;38:47.

74. Schatz P, Putz B. Cross-validation of measures used for computer-based assessment of concussion. Appl Neuropsychol 2006;13:151.

75. Bruce JM, Echemendia RJ. History of multiple self-reported concussions is not associated with reduced cognitive abilities. Neurosurgery 2009;64(1):100–6.

76. McCrea M, Guskiewicz K, Randolph C, et al. Effects of a symptom-free waiting period on clinical outcome and risk of reinjury after sport-related concussion. Neurosurgery 2009;65(5):876–82.

77. Purcell L. What are the most appropriate return-to-play guidelines for concussed child athletes? Br J Sports Med 2009;43(Suppl 1):i51–5.

78. Piebes SK, Gourley M, McLeod TCV. Caring for student-athletes following a concussion. J Sch Nurs 2009;25(4):270–80.

79. Iverson GL, Brooks BL, Lovell MR, et al. No cumulative effects for one or two previous concussions. Br J Sports Med 2006;40(1):72–5.

80. Collins MW, Lovell MR, Iverson GL, et al. Cumulative effects of concussion in high school athletes. Neurosurgery 2002;51(5):1175–81.

81. McCrory P. What advice should we give to athletes postconcussion? Br J Sports Med 2002;36(5):316–8.

82. Kuehl MD, Snyder AR, Erickson SE, et al. Impact of prior concussions on health-related quality of life in collegiate athletes. Clin J Sport Med 2010;20(2):86–91.

83. McCrory P. Treatment of recurrent concussion. Curr Sports Med Rep 2002;1(1): 28–32.
84. Cantu RC. Recurrent athletic head injury: risks and when to retire. Clin Sports Med 2003;22(3):593–603.
85. Guskiewicz KM, McCrea M, Marshall SW, et al. Cumulative effects associated with recurrent concussion in collegiate football players: the NCAA Concussion Study. JAMA 2003;290:2549–55.
86. Bruce JM, Echemendia RJ. Concussion history predicts self-reported symptoms before and following a concussive event. Neurology 2004;63:1516–8.
87. Pellman EJ, Lovell MR, Viano DC, et al. Concussion in professional football: recovery of NFL and high-school athletes assessed by computerized neuropsychological testing, Part 12. Neurosurgery 2006;58(2):263–72.
88. Moser RS, Schatz P, Jordan BD. Prolonged effects of concussion in high-school athletes. Neurosurgery 2005;57(2):300–6.
89. Bleiberg J, Cernich AN, Cameron K, et al. Duration of cognitive impairment after sports concussion. Neurosurgery 2004;54(5):1073–80.
90. McClincy MP, Lovell MR, Pardini J, et al. Recovery from sport concussion in high-school and collegiate athletes. Brain Inj 2006;20(1):33–9.
91. Sterr A, Herron K, Hayward C, et al. Are mild head injuries as mild as we think? Neurobehavioral concomitants of chronic post-concussive syndrome. BMC Neurol 2006;6:7–17.
92. Field M, Collins MW, Lovell MR, et al. Does age play a role in recovery from sports-related concussion? A comparison of high school and collegiate athletes. J Pediatr 2003;142:546–53.
93. Reddy CC, Collins MW. Sports concussion: management and predictors of outcome. Curr Sports Med Rep 2009;8(1):10–5.
94. Lovell MR, Collins MW, Iverson GL, et al. Recovery from mild concussion in high school athletes. J Neurosurg 2003;98:296–301.
95. Iverson G. Predicting slow recovery from sport-related concussion: the new simple-complex distinction. Clin J Sport Med 2007;17(1):31–7.
96. Iverson GL, Brooks BL, Collins MW, et al. Tracking neuropsychological recovery following concussion in sport. Brain Inj 2006;20(3):245–52.
97. Lau B, Lovell MR, Collins MW, et al. Neurocognitive and symptom predictors of recovery in high school athletes. Clin J Sport Med 2009;19(3):216–21.
98. Sim A, Terryberry-Spohr L, Wilson KR. Prolonged recovery of memory functioning after mild traumatic brain injury in adolescent athletes. J Neurosurg 2008;108(3):511–6.
99. Slobounov S, Cao C, Sebastianelli W, et al. Residual deficits from concussion as revealed by virtual time-to-contact measures of postural stability. Clin Neurophysiol 2008;119(2):281–9.
100. Slobounov S, Slobounov E, Sebastianelli W, et al. Differential rate of recovery in athletes after first and second concussion episodes. Neurosurgery 2007;61(2): 338–44.
101. McCrory PR, Berkovic SF. Second impact syndrome. Neurology 1998;50(3): 677–83.
102. Kelly JP, Nichols JS, Filley CM, et al. Concussion in sports: guidelines for the prevention of catastrophic outcome. JAMA 1991;266(20):2867–9.
103. McCrea M, Hammeke T, Olsen G, et al. Unreported concussion in high school football players: implications for prevention. Clin J Sport Med 2004;14(1):13–7.
104. McIntosh AS, McCrory P. Effectiveness of headgear in a pilot study of under 15 rugby union football. Br J Sports Med 2001;35(3):167–9.

105. Wisniewski JF, Guskiewicz K, Trope M, et al. Incidence of cerebral concussions associated with type of mouthguard used in college football. Dent Traumatol 2004;20(3):143–9.
106. Labella CR, Smith BW, Sigurdsson A. Effect of mouthguards on dental injuries and concussions in college basketball. Med Sci Sports Exerc 2002;34(1):41–4.
107. Barbic D, Pater J, Brison RJ. Comparison of mouth guard designs and concussion prevention in contact sports: a multicenter randomized controlled trial. Clin J Sport Med 2005;15(5):294–8.
108. Benson BW, Hamilton GM, Meeuwisse WH, et al. Is protective equipment useful in preventing concussion? A systematic review of the literature. Br J Sports Med 2009;43(Suppl 1):i56–67.
109. Collins M, Lovell MR, Iverson GL, et al. Examining concussion rates and return to play in high school football players wearing newer helmet technology: a three-year prospective cohort study. Neurosurgery 2006;58(2):275–86.
110. Delaney JS, Al-Kashmiri A, Drummond R, et al. The effect of protective headgear on head injuries and concussions in adolescent football (soccer) players. Br J Sports Med 2008;42(2):110–5.
111. McIntosh AS, McCrory P, Finch CF, et al. Does padded headgear prevent head injury in rugby union football? Med Sci Sports Exerc 2009;41(2):306–13.
112. Mihalik JP, McCaffrey MA, Rivera EM, et al. Effectiveness of mouthguards in reducing neurocognitive deficits following sports-related cerebral concussion. Dent Traumatol 2007;23(1):14–20.
113. Singh GD, Maher GJ, Padilla RR. Customized mandibular orthotics in the prevention of concussion/mild traumatic brain injury in football players: a preliminary study. Dent Traumatol 2009;25(5):515–21.

APPENDIX 1: SPORT CONCUSSION ASSESSMENT TOOL 2 [SCAT2]

SCAT2
  FIFA®

Sport Concussion Assessment Tool 2

Name

Sport/team

Date/time of injury

Date/time of assessment

Age   Gender   ☐ M   ☐ F

Years of education completed

Examiner

What is the SCAT2?[1]

This tool represents a standardized method of evaluating injured athletes for concussion and can be used in athletes aged from 10 years and older. It supersedes the original SCAT published in 2005[2]. This tool also enables the calculation of the Standardized Assessment of Concussion (SAC)[3,4] score and the Maddocks questions[5] for sideline concussion assessment.

Instructions for using the SCAT2

The SCAT2 is designed for the use of medical and health professionals. Preseason baseline testing with the SCAT2 can be helpful for interpreting post-injury test scores. Words in Italics throughout the SCAT2 are the instructions given to the athlete by the tester.

This tool may be freely copied for distribtion to individuals, teams, groups and organizations.

What is a concussion?

A concussion is a disturbance in brain function caused by a direct or indirect force to the head. It results in a variety of non-specific symptoms (like those listed below) and often does not involve loss of consciousness. Concussion should be suspected in the presence of **any one or more** of the following:

- Symptoms (such as headache), or
- Physical signs (such as unsteadiness), or
- Impaired brain function (e.g. confusion) or
- Abnormal behaviour.

Any athlete with a suspected concussion should be REMOVED FROM PLAY, medically assessed, monitored for deterioration (i.e., should not be left alone) and should not drive a motor vehicle.

Symptom Evaluation

How do you feel?

You should score yourself on the following symptoms, based on how you feel now.

	none	mild		moderate		severe	
Headache	0	1	2	3	4	5	6
"Pressure in head"	0	1	2	3	4	5	6
Neck Pain	0	1	2	3	4	5	6
Nausea or vomiting	0	1	2	3	4	5	6
Dizziness	0	1	2	3	4	5	6
Blurred vision	0	1	2	3	4	5	6
Balance problems	0	1	2	3	4	5	6
Sensitivity to light	0	1	2	3	4	5	6
Sensitivity to noise	0	1	2	3	4	5	6
Feeling slowed down	0	1	2	3	4	5	6
Feeling like "in a fog"	0	1	2	3	4	5	6
"Don't feel right"	0	1	2	3	4	5	6
Difficulty concentrating	0	1	2	3	4	5	6
Difficulty remembering	0	1	2	3	4	5	6
Fatigue or low energy	0	1	2	3	4	5	6
Confusion	0	1	2	3	4	5	6
Drowsiness	0	1	2	3	4	5	6
Trouble falling asleep (if applicable)	0	1	2	3	4	5	6
More emotional	0	1	2	3	4	5	6
Irritability	0	1	2	3	4	5	6
Sadness	0	1	2	3	4	5	6
Nervous or Anxious	0	1	2	3	4	5	6

Total number of symptoms (Maximum possible 22)

Symptom severity score
(Add all scores in table, maximum possible: 22 x 6 = 132)

Do the symptoms get worse with physical activity?   ☐ Y   ☐ N
Do the symptoms get worse with mental activity?   ☐ Y   ☐ N

Overall rating

If you know the athlete well prior to the injury, how different is the athlete acting compared to his / her usual self? Please circle one response.

no different	very different	unsure

Cognitive & Physical Evaluation

1 **Symptom score** (from page 1)
22 **minus** number of symptoms   of 22

2 **Physical signs score**
Was there loss of consciousness or unresponsiveness?   ☐ Y   ☐ N
If yes, how long? _____ minutes
Was there a balance problem/unsteadiness?   ☐ Y   ☐ N

Physical signs score (1 point for each negative response)   of 2

3 **Glasgow coma scale (GCS)**

Best eye response (E)
No eye opening 1
Eye opening in response to pain 2
Eye opening to speech 3
Eyes opening spontaneously 4

Best verbal response (V)
No verbal response 1
Incomprehensible sounds 2
Inappropriate words 3
Confused 4
Oriented 5

Best motor response (M)
No motor response 1
Extension to pain 2
Abnormal flexion to pain 3
Flexion/Withdrawal to pain 4
Localizes to pain 5
Obeys commands 6

Glasgow Coma score (E + V + M)   of 15
GCS should be recorded for all athletes in case of subsequent deterioration.

4 **Sideline Assessment – Maddocks Score**
*"I am going to ask you a few questions, please listen carefully
and give your best effort."*

Modified Maddocks questions (1 point for each correct answer)

	0	1
At what venue are we at today?	0	1
Which half is it now?	0	1
Who scored last in this match?	0	1
What team did you play last week/game?	0	1
Did your team win the last game?	0	1

Maddocks score   of 5
Maddocks score is validated for sideline diagnosis of concussion only and is not
included in SCAT 2 summary score for serial testing.

5 **Cognitive assessment**
Standardized Assessment of Concussion (SAC)
Orientation (1 point for each correct answer)

	0	1
What month is it?	0	1
What is the date today?	0	1
What is the day of the week?	0	1
What year is it?	0	1
What time is it right now? (within 1 hour)	0	1

Orientation score   of 5

Immediate memory
*"I am going to test your memory. I will read you a list of words
and when I am done, repeat back as many words as you can
remember, in any order."*

Trials 2 & 3:
*"I am going to repeat the same list again. Repeat back as many
words as you can remember in any order, even if you said the
word before."*

Complete all 3 trials regardless of score on trial 1 & 2. Read the words at a rate
of one per second. Score 1 pt. for each correct response. Total score equals sum
across all 3 trials. Do not inform the athlete that delayed recall will be tested.

List	Trial 1	Trial 2	Trial 3	Alternative word list		
elbow	0 1	0 1	0 1	candle	baby	finger
apple	0 1	0 1	0 1	paper	monkey	penny
carpet	0 1	0 1	0 1	sugar	perfume	blanket
saddle	0 1	0 1	0 1	sandwich	sunset	lemon
bubble	0 1	0 1	0 1	wagon	iron	insect
Total						

Immediate memory score   of 15

Concentration
Digits Backward:
*"I am going to read you a string of numbers and when I am done,
you repeat them back to me backwards, in reverse order of how I
read them to you. For example, if I say 7-1-9, you would say 9-1-7."*

If correct, go to next string length. If incorrect, read trial 2. One point possible for
each string length. Stop after incorrect on both trials. The digits should be read at
the rate of one per second.

Alternative digit lists

	0	1			
4-9-3	0	1	6-2-9	5-2-6	4-1-5
3-8-1-4	0	1	3-2-7-9	1-7-9-5	4-9-6-8
6-2-9-7-1	0	1	1-5-2-8-6	3-8-5-2-7	6-1-8-4-3
7-1-8-4-6-2	0	1	5-3-9-1-4-8	8-3-1-9-6-4	7-2-4-8-5-6

Months in Reverse Order:
*"Now tell me the months of the year in reverse order. Start
with the last month and go backward. So you'll say December,
November ... Go ahead"*

1 pt. for entire sequence correct

	0	1
Dec-Nov-Oct-Sept-Aug-Jul-Jun-May-Apr-Mar-Feb-Jan	0	1

Concentration score   of 5

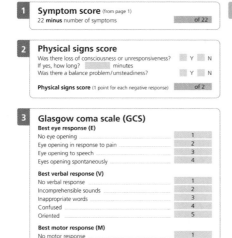

[1] This tool has been developed by a group of international experts at the 3rd
International Consensus meeting on Concussion in Sport held in Zurich,
Switzerland in November 2008. The full details of the conference outcomes
and the authors of the tool are published in British Journal of Sports
Medicine, 2009, volume 43, supplement 1.
The outcome paper will also be simultaneously co-published in the May
2009 issues of Clinical Journal of Sports Medicine, Physical Medicine &
Rehabilitation, Journal of Athletic Training, Journal of Clinical Neuroscience,
Journal of Science & Medicine in Sport, Neurosurgery, Scandinavian Journal
of Science & Medicine in Sport and the Journal of Clinical Sports Medicine.

[2] McCrory P et al. Summary and agreement statement of the 2nd International
Conference on Concussion in Sport, Prague 2004. British Journal of Sports
Medicine. 2005; 39: 196-204

[3] McCrea M. Standardized mental status testing of acute concussion. Clinical
Journal of Sports Medicine. 2001; 11: 176-181

[4] McCrea M, Randolph C, Kelly J. Standardized Assessment of Concussion:
Manual for administration, scoring and interpretation. Waukesha,
Wisconsin, USA.

[5] Maddocks, DL; Dicker, GD; Saling, MM. The assessment of orientation
following concussion in athletes. Clin J Sport Med. 1995;5(1):32-3

[6] Guskiewicz KM. Assessment of postural stability following sport-related
concussion. Current Sports Medicine Reports. 2003; 2: 24-30

6 Balance examination

This balance testing is based on a modified version of the Balance Error Scoring System (BESS)*. A stopwatch or watch with a second hand is required for this testing.

Balance testing
"I am now going to test your balance. Please take your shoes off, roll up your pant legs above ankle (if applicable), and remove any ankle taping (if applicable). This test will consist of three twenty second tests with different stances."

(a) Double leg stance:
"The first stance is standing with your feet together with your hands on your hips and with your eyes closed. You should try to maintain stability in that position for 20 seconds. I will be counting the number of times you move out of this position. I will start timing when you are set and have closed your eyes."

(b) Single leg stance:
"If you were to kick a ball, which foot would you use? [This will be the dominant foot] Now stand on your non-dominant foot. The dominant leg should be held in approximately 30 degrees of hip flexion and 45 degrees of knee flexion. Again, you should try to maintain stability for 20 seconds with your hands on your hips and your eyes closed. I will be counting the number of times you move out of this position. If you stumble out of this position, open your eyes and return to the start position and continue balancing. I will start timing when you are set and have closed your eyes."

(c) Tandem stance:
*"Now stand heel-to-toe with your **non-dominant foot** in back. Your weight should be evenly distributed across both feet. Again, you should try to maintain stability for 20 seconds with your hands on your hips and your eyes closed. I will be counting the number of times you move out of this position. If you stumble out of this position, open your eyes and return to the start position and continue balancing. I will start timing when you are set and have closed your eyes."*

Balance testing – types of errors
1. Hands lifted off iliac crest
2. Opening eyes
3. Step, stumble, or fall
4. Moving hip into > 30 degrees abduction
5. Lifting forefoot or heel
6. Remaining out of test position > 5 sec

Each of the 20-second trials is scored by counting the errors, or deviations from the proper stance, accumulated by the athlete. The examiner will begin counting errors only after the individual has assumed the proper start position. **The modified BESS is calculated by adding one error point for each error during the three 20-second tests. The maximum total number of errors for any single condition is 10.** If an athlete commits multiple errors simultaneously, only one error is recorded but the athlete should quickly return to the testing position, and counting should resume once subject is set. Subjects that are unable to maintain the testing procedure for a minimum of **five seconds** at the start are assigned the highest possible score, ten, for that testing condition.

Which foot was tested: ☐ Left   ☐ Right
(i.e. which is the **non-dominant** foot)

Condition	Total errors
Double Leg Stance (feet together)	of 10
Single leg stance (non-dominant foot)	of 10
Tandem stance (non-dominant foot at back)	of 10
Balance examination score (30 **minus** total errors)	of 30

7 Coordination examination

Upper limb coordination
Finger-to-nose (FTN) task: *"I am going to test your coordination now. Please sit comfortably on the chair with your eyes open and your arm (either right or left) outstretched (shoulder flexed to 90 degrees and elbow and fingers extended). When I give a start signal, I would like you to perform five successive finger to nose repetitions using your index finger to touch the tip of the nose as quickly and as accurately as possible."*

Which arm was tested: ☐ Left   ☐ Right

Scoring: 5 correct repetitions in < 4 seconds = 1
Note for testers: Athletes fail the test if they do not touch their nose, do not fully
extend their elbow or do not perform five repetitions. Failure
should be scored as 0.

Coordination score	of 1

8 Cognitive assessment
Standardized Assessment of Concussion (SAC)
Delayed recall
"Do you remember that list of words I read a few times earlier? Tell me as many words from the list as you can remember in any order."

Circle each word correctly recalled. Total score equals number of words recalled.

List		Alternative word list		
elbow	candle	baby	finger
apple	paper	monkey	penny
carpet	sugar	perfume	blanket
saddle	sandwich	sunset	lemon
bubble	wagon	iron	insect

Delayed recall score	of 5

Overall score

Test domain	Score
Symptom score	of 22
Physical signs score	of 2
Glasgow Coma score (E + V + M)	of 15
Balance examination score	of 30
Coordination score	of 1
Subtotal	**of 70**
Orientation score	of 5
Immediate memory score	of 5
Concentration score	of 15
Delayed recall score	of 5
SAC subtotal	**of 30**
SCAT2 total	**of 100**
Maddocks Score	**of 5**

Definitive normative data for a SCAT2 "cut-off" score is not available at this time and will be developed in prospective studies. Embedded within the SCAT2 is the SAC score that can be utilized separately in concussion management. The scoring system also takes on particular clinical significance during serial assessment where it can be used to document either a decline or an improvement in neurological functioning.

Scoring data from the SCAT2 or SAC should not be used as a stand alone method to diagnose concussion, measure recovery or make decisions about an athlete's readiness to return to competition after concussion.

Athlete Information

Any athlete suspected of having a concussion should be removed from play, and then seek medical evaluation.

Signs to watch for

Problems could arise over the first 24-48 hours. You should not be left alone and must go to a hospital at once if you:

- Have a headache that gets worse
- Are very drowsy or can't be awakened (woken up)
- Can't recognize people or places
- Have repeated vomiting
- Behave unusually or seem confused; are very irritable
- Have seizures (arms and legs jerk uncontrollably)
- Have weak or numb arms or legs
- Are unsteady on your feet; have slurred speech

Remember, it is better to be safe.
Consult your doctor after a suspected concussion.

Return to play

Athletes should not be returned to play the same day of injury. When returning athletes to play, they should follow a stepwise symptom-limited program, with stages of progression. For example:
1. rest until asymptomatic (physical and mental rest)
2. light aerobic exercise (e.g. stationary cycle)
3. sport-specific exercise
4. non-contact training drills (start light resistance training)
5. full contact training after medical clearance
6. return to competition (game play)

There should be approximately 24 hours (or longer) for each stage and the athlete should return to stage 1 if symptoms recur. Resistance training should only be added in the later stages.
Medical clearance should be given before return to play.

Tool	Test domain	Time	Score			
		Date tested				
		Days post injury				
SCAT2	Symptom score					
	Physical signs score					
	Glasgow Coma score (E + V + M)					
	Balance examination score					
	Coordination score					
SAC	Orientation score					
	Immediate memory score					
	Concentration score					
	Delayed recall score					
	SAC Score					
Total	SCAT2					
Symptom severity score (max possible 132)						
Return to play			Y N	Y N	Y N	Y N

Additional comments

✂---

Concussion injury advice (To be given to concussed athlete)

This patient has received an injury to the head. A careful medical examination has been carried out and no sign of any serious complications has been found. It is expected that recovery will be rapid, but the patient will need monitoring for a further period by a responsible adult. Your treating physician will provide guidance as to this timeframe.

If you notice any change in behaviour, vomiting, dizziness, worsening headache, double vision or excessive drowsiness, please telephone the clinic or the nearest hospital emergency department immediately.

Other important points:
- Rest and avoid strenuous activity for at least 24 hours
- No alcohol
- No sleeping tablets
- Use paracetamol or codeine for headache. Do **not** use aspirin or anti-inflammatory medication
- Do **not** drive until medically cleared
- Do **not** train or play sport until medically cleared

Clinic phone number

Patient's name

Date/time of injury

Date/time of medical review

Treating physician

Contact details or stamp

Resistance Training for Adolescents

Michael G. Miller, EdD[a],*,
Christopher C. Cheatham, PhD[a], Neil D. Patel[b]

KEYWORDS

- Resistance training • Strength training • Periodization
- Load • Repetitions • Sets

The term resistance training (RT) refers to a method of physical conditioning that uses progressively increasing resistive loads and various training techniques to achieve desired muscle strength, power, muscle hypertrophy, local muscular endurance, or a combination thereof (**Table 1**).[1–8] Various techniques are used in RT to increase work demands of the muscles (**Table 2**).[5–8] Often, the terms resistance training, strength training, weight training, and weight lifting are used interchangeably and inappropriately. Strength training is one of the specific goals achievable through various RT techniques. Weight lifting is a competitive sport that includes the snatch and clean and jerk lifts, not recommended for adolescents.[7] Similarly, participation in competitive power lifting and body building is not recommended for adolescents.[7]

RT is recommended as an integral component of any regular exercise program. The design of a RT program depends up on the specific goals of RT. The goal of a RT program can be to improve muscle strength, increase power, increase muscle bulk or size, enhance muscle endurance, or a combination of any of these goals. A RT program that is specifically designed as part of sport-specific training and conditioning takes into consideration the relative aerobic and anaerobic demands of the sport, and relative importance of achieving muscle strength, power, muscle hypertrophy, or local muscular endurance.[5] Therefore, sport-specific training and conditioning is more complex, and the training program should be designed and supervised by appropriately qualified professionals. This article reviews the general recommendations for RT for health-related physical fitness. Health-related physical fitness generally consists of various aspects of regularly recommended exercises that result in good health. In addition to RT, other components of health-related physical fitness exercises include aerobic exercise, flexibility exercises, and stretching. The discussion

[a] HPER Department, Western Michigan University, 1903 West Michigan Avenue, Kalamazoo, MI 49008, USA
[b] Human Resuscitation Learning Laboratory, Department of Emergency Medicine, Michigan State University Kalamazoo Center for Medical Studies, 1000 Oakland Drive, Kalamazoo, MI 49008, USA
* Corresponding author.
E-mail address: Michael.g.miller@wmich.edu

Pediatr Clin N Am 57 (2010) 671–682
doi:10.1016/j.pcl.2010.02.009
0031-3955/10/$ – see front matter © 2010 Elsevier Inc. All rights reserved.
pediatric.theclinics.com

Table 1 RT goals	
Strength	Maximal force that a muscle or muscle group generates at a specific velocity of movement
Power	The rate (how fast) a muscle or group of muscles can perform a given task. (Power = work/time; work = force exerted on an object × the distance the object moves in the direction in which the force is exerted)
Hypertrophy	Increase in the size (cross-sectional area) of the muscle; primarily results from hypertrophy of muscle fibers
Local muscular endurance	The ability of a muscles or muscle group to continue to perform contractions against a submaximal resistance

Data from Refs.[1,2,4,5]

here focuses on adolescents aged 13 to 18 years who have reached Tanner stage 3 and above.[1]

SAFETY OF RESISTANCE TRAINING

If appropriate for the emotional and developmental stage, RT poses minimal risk of injury to adolescents. Some studies have reported injuries resulting from RT; however, these are minor or occurred as a result of improper load or exercise technique.[9–12] Although there are acknowledged risks with RT for adolescents, these risks are no greater than the risks of participation in sport and recreational activities.[1] Injuries reported in RT do not occur any more frequently in youth than in adults.[13,14] Zaricznyj and colleagues[14] reported that RT accounted for less than 1% of all injuries, while football and basketball accounted for 19% and 15% of injuries, respectively.

Injuries from RT to growth plates, articular cartilage, and apophysis remain a concern in children and adolescents, because these areas are relatively weaker and therefore more susceptible to injuries from excess stress. The likelihood of growth plate or cartilage damage may be higher in adolescents than in preadolescents, because the growth cartilage is more resilient to shearing forces in preadolescents.[15] Although the potential risk of injury to growth cartilage may exist, RT has not been shown to adversely affect skeletal growth or maturation in adolescents.[16,17]

The potential for soft-tissue overuse injuries is also a concern in adolescents. Overuse injuries associated with RT in adolescents are not adequately documented; however, the incidence of lower back pain in adolescents is significant enough to warrant concern.[1] A properly designed RT program that focuses on strength and flexibility may help alleviate lower back pain.[1]

Most published reports suggest that the benefits of RT in adolescents far outweigh any concerns for potential injuries.[18,19] The use of weight machines, elastic bands, or

Table 2 Examples of techniques used in RT	
Techniques	**Examples**
Load-bearing exercises	Climbing
Specific bodyweight exercises	Curl-ups, press-ups, jumping, hoping
Use of resistive materials	Stretch or elastic bands of various resistance, weight machines, free weights

body weight all have been shown to be effective in RT.[17,20–26] Resistance training in children and adolescents has been shown to increase strength by 13% to 30%.[27,28] In addition to improved physical fitness, a well-designed RT program can contribute to improved psychosocial well-being and help establish and promote beneficial exercise habits at an early age.[1]

Properly supervised RT is an integral component of health-related and sport specific training and conditioning.[1,29] RT can be initiated at almost any age for children as long as they are emotionally and physically ready to undertake such a program—generally 7 to 8 years of age.[1,7] Supervision and instructions should be provided by qualified professionals who have training and background in RT techniques and an understanding of the unique needs, both physical and psychological, of children and adolescents.[1,7] Supervision should include feedback about form, speed of movement, breathing techniques, and proper lifting or performing the movements. Instructions in developing correct resistance training techniques will assist adolescents in achieving RT goals, limit the potential for injury, and promote program adherence.[1,30] In instances where instruction in complex techniques is included, more than one supervisor may be needed, thereby increasing the supervisor-to-adolescent ratio in the weight room. Supervisor or instructor to adolescent ratios of 1:10 to 1:25 can be appropriate, depending upon the complexity of exercises and the maturity of the adolescents being supervised.

EVALUATION BEFORE STARTING RT

Before starting RT, the adolescent should be evaluated to identify any medical conditions that may require appropriate modification of the RT program. History should include information about nutrition and use of supplements such as creatine and drugs such as anabolic–androgenic steroids.

It is important to assess the physical, cognitive, and psychosocial developmental status of the adolescent. The adolescent should have realistic expectations from RT. The adolescent should understand that to achieve the desired goals of RT, exercises need to be done on a regular basis for a long period of time. The adolescent should understand the importance of correct form and techniques of RT exercises and appropriate supervision and guidance by qualified professionals should be provided to reduce the risk of injury and to progress toward desired goals.

Before beginning an RT program, it is essential to ascertain the adolescent's RT status, so as to design a program that matches the adolescent's experience and current physical fitness. Adolescents can be placed into one of three groups based on their previous level of RT experience: novice or beginner, intermediate, and advanced. Novices or beginners are adolescents with limited (<2 to 3 months) to no resistance training experience; adolescents in the intermediate group are those who have had approximately 3 to 12 months of training experience. Adolescents with 12 or more months training experience are considered advanced.[1,5] When determining the exercises for the RT program, it is imperative that the exercises are appropriate for the adolescent's physical development, fitness level, and RT status.[1]

COMPONENTS OF AN RT PROGRAM

Proper warm-up and cool-down periods, level of intensity, frequency of training sessions, order of exercises, volume of exercise, and rest periods are main considerations in designing a RT program.[1,4,5,29,30] RT programs for adolescents also should include specific educational objectives, instructions in weight room etiquette, and desired performance outcomes.[1,29]

Warm-up

Warm-up consists of movements that prepare the body before the desired activity. A warm-up period is recommended to increase the range of joint motion, raise body temperature, and enhance awareness of body position. The warm-up period usually consists of two phases: general and specific. The general phase consists of 5 to 10 minutes of general activities to increase the heart rate, muscle temperature, and respiratory rate, and decrease joint viscosity.[31] The specific warm-up consists of activities similar to the movements performed during the resistance training exercises, lasting for approximately 8 to 12 minutes.[32] Dynamic activities during the warm-up period have been shown to assist in enhancing power performance for youth.[1,33–35]

Cool-down

The cool-down period occurs after the exercise session and consists of dynamic exercises similar to the warm-up period. The aims of the cool-down period are to facilitate the elimination of waste products from the muscles, and to return the heart rate and respirations to preactivity levels. In addition, a cool-down period should include a flexibility component that includes static stretching. Stretching exercises after activity can increase flexibility while increasing performance and reducing the risk of injury over the long term.[36,37] Typically, the cool-down period lasts approximately 5 minutes and is also an appropriate time to reflect on the day's activities and focus on training objectives for future exercise sessions.[33–35]

Order of Exercises

Generally, the exercises selected should start with single-joint, simple movements and progress to multijoint and complex movements. Progression to the complex exercises should be based upon demonstration of proper exercise technique, confidence, and attainment of goals and objectives. In more experienced adolescents, multijoint exercises, performed using proper techniques and lower weights, can be initiated in early exercise sessions. Within a training session, large muscle groups typically should be exercised before small muscle groups, while multijoint exercises should be performed before single-joint exercises.[1,4,5] This pattern helps reduce the risk of injury by stressing neuromuscularly demanding exercises at the beginning of a session when fatigue is minimal.[1]

Load or Intensity

The training load refers to the amount of weight lifted for that specific resistance exercise.[5] As the load becomes heavier, the number of repetitions decreases. Conversely, more repetitions can be accomplished with lighter loads. The load usually is described as a percentage of 1 repetition maximum (1 RM) or as the maximum weight lifted in 1 repetition.[5,32] The weight should be lifted through the entire joint range of motion. The use of a 1 RM to determine the load is more appropriate for experienced resistance trained individuals, whereas, a 5 RM or up to 10 RM method is preferred for less experienced individuals and adolescents.[1,5,6] Determining the RM depends upon the goals and demands of the sport.[32]

Another method used to determine the percent of maximum load lifted during an exercise session is the RM equivalent. The RM equivalent is calculated as[38–41]: RM equivalent = (weight lifted × number of reps × 0.03) + weight lifted. For example, an RM equivalent for an adolescent who lifted 125 lb during an inclined bench press exercise a total of 8 times would be calculated as: (125 × 8 × 0.03) + 125 = 155. Although not as accurate, the RM equivalent procedure may be best suited for inexperienced adolescents.

The relationship between possible RM and percentages of 1 RM varies with the amount of muscle mass needed to perform the exercise (eg, a leg press requires more muscle mass than a knee extension). Because different muscles or muscle groups exert different amounts of force depending up on their mass and strength, the load for a given number of repetitions can vary depending upon the muscles or muscle group involved in a particular exercise.[5] The velocity of muscle contraction, that is how fast or slow a muscle contraction is achieved, during dynamic muscle action is inversely related to the exercise load during maximal muscle contraction.[4] The velocity of muscle contraction affects the neural, hypertrophic, and metabolic adaptations to RT exercises.[4]

Sets and Repetitions

Repetitions refer to the number of times a weight is lifted in a set; conversely, a set consists of the number of repetitions performed between rest periods.[5] In RT programs, the number of repetitions and sets are manipulated according to the goal of the RT and desired outcomes for the adolescent. The number of sets and repetitions may vary for different muscles or muscle groups. For example, it generally is recommended that adolescents perform three sets of six to eight repetitions for multijoint exercises, and two sets of 10 to 12 repetitions for single joint exercises.[1] Generally, multiple sets of RT exercises have been shown to be more effective than single-set exercises. The number of sets and repetitions do not have to be the same for all muscle groups or exercises.[1,4,5]

Frequency

The term training frequency refers to the number of training sessions completed in a given time period. Training frequency depends upon the experience, maturity, and training status of the adolescent, and sport or outcome requirements. Adolescents should begin RT with one to three sessions a week on nonconsecutive days. As the adolescent becomes more experienced, sessions can increase up to three times per week, but the load and rest periods may need to be manipulated for optimal recovery between sessions.[1]

Rest between two RT sessions should not exceed more than 3 days.[1–4] A split-routine regime allows for more frequent RT sessions. In a split routine, exercises involving different muscles or muscle groups are performed on different days. Exercises can be divided, for example, into upper body and lower body, in which upper body exercises are done on days 1 and 3, and lower body exercises are done on days 2 and 4. Similarly, exercises can be divided as push exercises (bench press, triceps extension) or pull exercises (lat pull down, biceps curl) and done on different days of the week.

Factors such as training volume, exercise intensity, exercise selection, nutrition, and sleep habits should be taken into consideration when determining the optimal recovery period between RT sessions.[1,4] As the number of training sessions increases, attention should be given to maintaining appropriate training habits, with less intense workouts interspersed throughout the week.

Rest Periods

The duration of rest periods between sets varies according to the specific goal of the RT, load lifted, and training status of the adolescent. For adults, the duration of rest periods between sets varies from 2 to 5 minutes for multijoint exercises, depending upon the goal of the training. The duration of rest periods in adults may not be applicable to adolescents, however, because of differences in maturity, growth, and development. Studies have shown that adolescents may recover more quickly than adults for high-intensity, short-duration exercises.[42,43] Rest periods of approximately 1 to 3 minutes may suffice in adolescents for moderate-intensity RT depending upon the goal of resistance training.[1]

Volume of Exercise

The volume of exercise refers to the total amount of weight lifted during an exercise session.[4,5] Volume or load volume equals the total number of sets multiplied by the number of repetitions per set multiplied by the weight lifted per repetition.[2,4,5,32] If each set is performed using a different weight or load, the volume is calculated for each set, and then the volume for each set is added to obtain the total volume of the exercise session. Thus, the volume of the exercise session can be manipulated by altering number of sets, number of repetitions per set, or weight lifted per repetition. Variation in training volume is essential during long-term training for those who are more advanced in their training. Constant-volume exercise sessions may result in staleness and decreased adherence to training.

TYPES OF EXERCISES AND MUSCLE ACTIONS

Exercises can be considered core or assistance type based on the extent of the muscle areas involved.[5] Core exercises involve large muscle areas such the chest, shoulder, or back, whereas assistance exercises involves smaller muscle groups, such as the neck, upper arms, or lower legs. Core exercises involve two or more primary joints, whereas assistance exercises involve only one primary joint. In general, core exercises are relatively more important for sport-specific training.

The main types of muscle actions are summarized in **Table 3**.[2,4,5] RT programs should include both eccentric and concentric muscle actions.[1] Multiple joint exercises, such as the bench press or squat, allow for a greater amount of load to be lifted; therefore they are considered more effective for overall improvement in muscle strength. On the other hand, single-joint exercises such as knee extensions or knee curls allow for a relatively smaller amount of load to be lifted and are more useful for targeting specific muscles or muscle groups. In general, weight machines are considered relatively safer to use for adolescents. Use of weight machines allows one to perform multijoint exercises more easily than using free weights. Because machines stabilize the body, they limit movements about specific joints. This results in less neural activation compared to free weights, allowing for more free movement of specific joints.

Specific exercises should be designed to avoid imbalances in muscle strength between opposing muscle groups. While performing bilateral exercises, for example using a machine for chest press, the relative weakness of one side may be compensated for by the stronger side, resulting in muscle strength imbalance. Therefore, both unilateral and bilateral exercises should be included in the RT program.[4,5]

PRINCIPLES OF TRAINING PROGRESSION

Progressive overload, specificity, and program variation or periodization are the main principles of resistance training progression.[1-5]

Table 3 Types of muscle actions	
Concentric	Muscle fibers shorten as the joint is moved through the range of motion For example lifting the weight during biceps curl Swimming and cycling involve predominantly concentric muscle actions
Eccentric	Muscle fibers lengthen as the joint is moved through the range of motion For example lowering the weight during biceps curl
Isometric	Muscle fiber length remains constant as the joint is moved through the range of motion
Isokinetic	Typically performed using isokinetic device or equipment Isokinetic device allows only single-joint movements Speed of movement through the range of joint motion is kept constant by the isokinetic device Because most sport and other activities require varying speed of movements, application of isokinetic training limited in sports training
Isotonic	Isontonic muscle action involves both concentric and eccentric components Muscle tension or muscle mass remains constant during the movement For example, lifting free weights or moving a person's body weight; the free weight or person's body weight remains the same, while the force needed to move the weight varies depending up on the joint angle and velocity of movement Tension generated in the muscle varies depending up on weight lifted, velocity of joint movement, strength of muscles involved, and type of muscle action

Data from Refs.[1–9,32]

Progressive Overload

Progressive overload refers to the gradual increase of load during RT. General guidelines for RT exercises are summarized in **Table 4**, and an example of a strength training program for beginners is outlined in **Table 5**.[1–8] It is necessary to progressively increase the load to continue to gain benefits from RT. Overall demands of RT on the body can be increased or decreased gradually by manipulating exercise load or intensity, number of repetitions, number of sets, velocity of muscle action, duration of rest periods, or total volume of exercise, depending upon the specific goals of RT.[1–8]

How an adolescent progresses through RT depends on the primary goal of the training. Intensity should increase progressively as the adolescent gains experience. A novice might start between 50% and 70% of a RM and eventually progress to 70% to 85% of a RM at the advanced level.[1] As experience is gained, the number

Table 4 Resistance training guidelines[a]				
Goal	Load (% 1 RM)[b]	Sets	Repetitions	Rest Period
Strength	Moderate (75–85)	2–6	≤10	2–5 min
Power	Moderate (75–85)	2–5	3–8	2–5 min
Hypertrophy	Heavy (≥85)	3–6	6–12	30–90 s
Endurance	Light (≤70)	6–8	≥12	≤30 sec

[a] Range in values for different parameters reflect individual differences.
[b] Start with lighter loads, higher repetitions, and sets, and progress to heavier loads and fewer repetitions and sets.
Data from Refs.[1–9,29,32]

Table 5
Example of an adolescent strength training program for the beginner

Goal Sets	Primarily to increase muscle strength 1–3
Repetitions	10–15, depending upon experience
Load	Use a load that the adolescent can lift for the desired number of repetitions
Frequency	2–3 nonconsecutive days per week
Exercises	Involve all major muscle groups: chin-ups, bench press, lat pulldown, leg press, leg flexion and extensions, abdominal crunches, biceps and triceps curls, calf raises, stability or ball exercises, rowing

Data from Vaughn J, Micheli L. Strength training recommendations for the young athlete. Phys Med and Rehabil Clin N Am 2008;19(2):235–45; and Miller MG, Michael TJ. Strength training and conditioning. In: Patel DR, Greydanus DE, Baker RJ, editors. Pediatric practice sports medicine. New York: McGraw Hill; 2009. p. 46–55.

of sets is increased, while the number of repetitions per set is decreased. Concurrent with the increase in number of sets and the decrease in repetitions, the duration of rest periods should increase. If the goal of RT is to increase strength, adolescents should begin with one to two sets of 6 to 15 repetitions involving all major muscle groups using lighter loads.[1] If the goal of RT is to increase muscle power, three to six repetitions should be performed because of increased muscle fatigue associated with power exercises.[1]

Although there are individual variations, generally it takes at least 8 or more weeks of consistent exercises before training effects from RT are realized.[1–8] The load, number of sets, and number of repetitions per set can all be altered to accommodate for exercise adaptations and to maintain or gain training effects. The exact methods of determining the amount and timing of load increase are not defined clearly. One simple way suggested is to increase the weight lifted or number of repetitions per set, when the current weight lifted or the number of repetitions can be accomplished with relative ease. One method to judge when to increase the weight or load lifted during an exercise is called the "two for two rule." The weight or load is increased when the adolescent can perform two or more repetitions over the current number of repetitions for that particular exercise over two consecutive exercise sessions.[32]

In general, the load is initially increased keeping the number of sets and repetitions per set the same. How much to increase load may vary depending upon the individual response, capability, and goal of training. If the primary goal is to increase muscle strength, a general guideline to work with is to increase the load by 5% to 10% with a relatively smaller increase for upper body exercises, and a larger increase for lower body exercises.[1,4] For most adolescents, in practical terms, the load or weight lifted can be increased by 1 to 4 kg for upper body exercises and by 4 to 7 kg for lower body exercises.[1,4]

The recommended progression for focused training for power shares some similarities with the progression for focused training for strength. There are some key differences, however, that must be considered. Adolescents training for power should use multijoint exercises rather than single-joint exercises. Like the progression for strength, when training for power, intensity should be increased progressively as experience is gained. Similarly, the number of sets should be increased while the number of repetitions per set decreases. Rest intervals, the velocity of muscle action, and the frequency of training sessions should also increase as the adolescent progresses from the novice to advanced level.

Specificity

Adaptations of muscles to RT are specific to the stimulus applied. This is known as the specific adaptations to imposed demands (SAID) principle.[4] Factors that determine the specific physiologic adaptations resulting from RT include the type of muscle actions involved, the velocity or speed of movement with which a muscle action is performed, range of motion, muscle groups trained, energy system involved, and the intensity and volume of training.[4,5]

Periodization

For long-term RT, different program variables are manipulated to maintain or continue to gain training effects. Variation in RT throughout the training period is called periodization, and is especially important for sports-specific training.[4] Periodization usually is divided into different phases based on the time of year or desired training outcomes to increase performance, minimize overtraining, or decrease the likelihood of training effect plateaus.[5,32] Periodization also may reduce boredom and encourage adolescents to adhere to their resistance training programs throughout the year. Different types of exercises, intensity, duration of rest periods, and overall volume of exercise session are manipulated based upon the RT experience and goal of the adolescent.

Box 1
General guidelines for an adolescent RT program

Establish a training program that is both challenging and exciting for participation

Qualified strength and conditioning professionals such as those certified by the National Strength and Conditioning Association or American College of Sports Medicine should develop training programs for adolescents

A preparticipation screening by qualified physicians or allied health professionals is essential to screen for pre-existing conditions or injuries

If the preparticipation screening detects physical limitations or strength deficits, a comprehensive program to correct these deficiencies should be implemented when beginning a RT program

RT programs for adolescents should emphasize submaximal efforts, using their body weight or bars with no added weights. Improving muscular strength and endurance are preferred goals initially; power exercises are included as the adolescent becomes more experienced

The RT program should focus first on mastery of technique and motor skills using light weights before progressing to heavier resistance training and more complex multijoint exercises

Avoid maximum load lifts. The multiple-repetition maximum method is preferred to determine load

Perform all exercises through the entire range of joint motion and with proper form

Instruct on the proper methods to breathe during exercise and make sure participants do not hold their breath

Have adequate supervision in the facility, including the use of spotters if necessary

Make sure the facility is safe, well-ventilated, and illuminated properly

Resistance training should be performed only 2 to 3 nonconsecutive days a week with adequate rest and recovery between sessions. Each session should comprise a general warm-up period, flexibility, resistance training exercises, and a cool-down period.

Data from Refs.[1,29,32]

SUMMARY

A RT program can benefit adolescents significantly by increasing physical fitness, sports performance, and psychosocial well-being. Any potential risks are minimal and primarily related to inadequate supervision and incorrect training techniques. Therefore, most risks can be alleviated significantly through the use of proper supervision and appropriately designed training programs that emphasize proper techniques. Although differences exist between levels of experience, all participants should follow basic recommended resistance training guidelines (**Box 1**).[1,29] To achieve, maintain, and gain training effects, resistance exercises must be done consistently and regularly over time. It takes several weeks to gain training effects, and the adolescent begins to lose the gains after complete cessation of exercises for 2 weeks. The longer the RT experience, the longer it takes to lose the training effects. RT exercises constitute one component of training and conditioning; other aspects such proper nutrition, rest, and healthy lifestyle choices are equally important. Adolescents must be advised against use of any performance-enhancing drugs or nutritional supplements to gain muscle mass and strength.

REFERENCES

1. Faigenbaum A, Kraemer W, Blimkie CJR, et al. Youth resistance training: updated position statement paper from the national strength and conditioning association. J Strength Cond Res 2009;23(Suppl 5):S60–79.
2. Kraemer WJ, Fleck SJ. Strength training for young athletes. 2nd edition. Champaign (IL): Human Kinetics; 2005.
3. Kraemer WJ, Vingren JL, Hatfield DL, et al. Resistance training program. In: Thompson WR, Baldwin KE, Pire NI, et al, editors. ACSM's resources for the personal trainer. 2nd edition. Philadelphia: Lippincott Williams and Wilkins; 2007. p. 372–403.
4. Ratamess NA, Alvar BA, Evetoch TK, et al. Progression models in resistance training for healthy adults. American College of Sports Medicine Position Stand; 2009. Available at: http://www.acsm-msse.org. Accessed February 22, 2010.
5. Baechle TR, Earle RW, Wathen MS. Resistance training. In: Baechle TR, Earle RW, editors. National Strength and Conditioning Association Essentials for resistance training. 3rd edition. Champaign (IL): Human Kinetics; 2008. p. 381–412.
6. Stratton G, Jones M, Fox KR, et al. British Association of Exercise and Sport Sciences position statement on guidelines for resistance exercise in young people. J Sports Sci 2004;22:383–90.
7. American Academy of Pediatrics Council of Sports Medicine and Fitness. Strength training by children and adolescents. Pediatrics 2008;121(4):835–40.
8. Behm DG, Faigenbaum AD, Falk B, et al. Canadian Society for Exercise Physiology position paper: resistance training in children and adolescents. Appl Physiol Nutr Metab 2008;33:547–61.
9. Brenner J, Brenner J. Overuse injuries, overtraining, and burnout in child and adolescent athletes. Pediatrics 2007;119(6):1242–5.
10. Lillegard WA, Brown EW, Wilson DJ, et al. Efficacy of strength training in prepubescent to early postpubescent males and females: effects of gender and maturity. Pediatr Rehabil 1997;1(3):147–57.
11. Brown E, Kimball R. Medical history associated with adolescent power lifting. Pediatrics 1983;72(5):636–44.
12. Gumbs V, Segal D, Halligan J, et al. Bilateral distal radius and ulnar fractures in adolescent weight lifters. Am J Sports Med 1982;10(6):375–9.

13. Myer G, Quatman C, Khoury J, et al. Youth versus adult weightlifting injuries presenting to United States emergency rooms: accidental versus nonaccidental injury mechanisms. J Strength Cond Res 2009;23(7):2054–60.

14. Zaricznyj B, Shattuck L, Mast T, et al. Sports-related injuries in school-aged children. Am J Sports Med 1980;8(5):318–24.

15. Micheli L. Strength training in the young athlete. In: Brown E, Branta C, editors. Competitive sports for children and youth. Champaign (IL): Human Kinetics Books; 1988. p. 99–105.

16. Falk B, Eliakim A. Resistance training, skeletal muscle and growth. Pediatr Endocrinol Rev 2003;1:120–7.

17. Malina R. Weight training in youth-growth, maturation, and safety: an evidence-based review. Clin J Sport Med 2006;16(6):478–87.

18. Davis J, Tung A, Chak S, et al. Aerobic and strength training reduces adiposity in overweight Latina adolescents. Med Sci Sports Exerc 2009; 41(7):1494–503.

19. Dorgo S, King G, Candelaria N, et al. Effects of manual resistance training on fitness in adolescents. J Strength Cond Res 2009;23(8):2287–94.

20. Faigenbaum A, Milliken L, Loud R, et al. Comparison of 1 and 2 days per week of strength training in children. Res Q Exerc Sport 2002;73(4):416–24.

21. Faigenbaum A, Milliken L, Moulton L, et al. Early muscular fitness adaptations in children in response to two different resistance training regimens. Pediatr Exerc Sci 2005;17(3):237–48.

22. Faigenbaum AD, Loud RL, O'Connell J, et al. Effects of different resistance training protocols on upper body strength and endurance development in children. J Strength Cond Res 2001;15:459–65.

23. McGuigan MR, Tatasciore M, Newton RU, et al. Eight weeks of resistance training can significantly alter body composition in children who are overweight or obese. J Strength Cond Res 2009;23(1):80–5.

24. Annesi J, Westcott W, Faigenbaum A, et al. Effects of a 12-week physical activity protocol delivered by YMCA after-school counselors (youth fit for life) on fitness and self-efficacy changes in 5–12–year-old boys and girls. Res Q Exerc Sport 2005;76(4):468–76.

25. Falk B, Mor G. The effects of resistance and martial arts training in 6 to 8 year old boys. Pediatr Exerc Sci 1996;8:48–65.

26. Siegal J, Camaione D, Manfredi T. Upper body strength training and prepubescent children. Med Sci Sports Exerc 1988;20:S53.

27. Andersen LB, Henckel P. Maximal voluntary isometric strength in Danish adolescents 16–19 years of age. Eur J Appl Physiol 1987;56:83–9.

28. Gilliam RB, Villanacci JF, Freedson PS, et al. Isokinetic torque in boys and girls ages 7–13: Effect of age, height, and weight. Res Q 1979;50(4): 599–609.

29. Vaughn J, Micheli L. Strength training recommendations for the young athlete. Phys Med Rehabil Clin N Am 2008;19(2):235–45.

30. Coutts A, Murphy A, Dascombe B. Effect of direct supervision of a strength coach on measures of muscular strength and power in young rugby league players. J Strength Cond Res 2004;18(2):316–23.

31. deVries HA. Physiology of exercise for physical education and athletics. Dubuque (IA): Brown; 1974.

32. Miller MG, Michael TJ. Strength training and conditioning. In: Patel DR, Greydanus DE, Baker RJ, editors. Pediatric practice sports medicine. New York: McGraw Hill; 2009. p. 46–55.

33. Faigenbaum A, Bellucci M, Bernieri A, et al. Acute effects of different warm-up protocols on fitness performance in children. J Strength Cond Res 2005;19(2): 376–81.
34. Faigenbaum A, Kang J, McFarland J, et al. Acute effects of different warm-up protocols on anaerobic performance in teenage athletes. Pediatr Exerc Sci 2006;18(1):64–75.
35. Siatras T, Papadopoulos G, Mameletzi D, et al. Static and dynamic acute stretching effect on gymnasts' speed in vaulting. Pediatr Exerc Sci 2003;15(4):383–91.
36. Shrier I. Does stretching improve performance? A systematic and critical review of the literature. Clin J Sport Med 2004;14:267–73.
37. Stone M, Ramsay M, Kinser A, et al. Stretching: acute and chronic? The potential consequences. Strength Cond J 2006;28:66–74.
38. Landers J. Maximum based on reps. NSCA J 1985;6:60–1.
39. Rhea MR, Alvar BA, Burkett LN. Single versus multiple sets for strength: a meta-analysis to address the controversy. Res Q Exerc Sport 2002;73:485–8.
40. Rhea MR, Alvar BA, Burkett LN, et al. A meta-analysis to determine the dose response for strength development. Med Sci Sports Exerc 2003;35:456–64.
41. Hedrick A. Training for hypertrophy. Strength and Conditioning 1985;17(3):22–9.
42. Faigenbaum A, Ratamess N, McFarland J, et al. Effect of rest interval length on bench press performance in boys, teens, and men. Pediatr Exerc Sci 2008; 20(4):457–69.
43. Falk B, Dotan R. Child-adult differences in the recovery from high-intensity exercise. Exerc Sport Sci Rev 2006;34(3):107–12.

Preventing Injuries and Illnesses in the Wilderness

David Angert, BS[a], Eric A. Schaff, MD[b],*

KEYWORDS

- Wilderness • Injury • Travel • Review
- Adolescents • Prevention

Getting away for the weekend, summer wilderness trips, and organized outdoor outings are becoming increasingly popular. These outings provide a way to decompress from the stresses of routine family life, school, and work while enjoying the benefits of exercise and experiencing the beauty of nature. It allows families, friends, and peer groups to spend time together, often in challenging and educational settings. The wilderness also can be fraught with dangers under the best of circumstances. Trouble is foreseeable when teenagers are placed in this setting who have the drive to explore and test their limits while pushing their physical capabilities at a developmental time when they are both impulsive and have a sense of invulnerability.

Some of the concerns for the practitioner to consider include potential injuries and illnesses that occur during various wilderness experiences and the frequency with which they occur, as well as the age, gender, medical or psychological conditions that place youth at greater risk. This article focuses on common injuries and illnesses as well as dangerous scenarios encountered in the outdoors. The authors emphasize the need for greater understanding, education, and preventive measures regarding youth trips into the wilderness.

EPIDEMIOLOGY

The 2000 National Survey on Recreation and the Environment surveyed over 57,000 individuals who were 16 years of age or older across the United States.[1] It found that 97% of Americans had participated in outdoor recreation activities in the past year. Hiking, backpacking, and developed (family or group campgrounds) camping

a Department of Physiology, Cardiovascular Research Center, Temple University School of Medicine, Medical Education and Research Building, 3500 North Broad Street, 10th Floor, Philadelphia, PA 19140, USA
b Department of Pediatrics, Temple University School of Medicine, Kresge Building West, Room 222, 3440 North Broad Street, Philadelphia, PA 19140, USA
* Corresponding author.
E-mail address: eric.schaff@tuhs.temple.edu

Pediatr Clin N Am 57 (2010) 683–695
doi:10.1016/j.pcl.2010.02.001
0031-3955/10/$ – see front matter © 2010 Elsevier Inc. All rights reserved.

experiences had increased significantly, with an estimated 72 million people hiking in 2002 and 24 million backpackers spending an average of 17 days per year in the woods.

There are limited data about the morbidity and mortality associated with such activities. Most data in the United States comes from the National Parks Services, organized outfitters such as the National Outdoor Leadership School (NOLS), and surveys of hikers on major trails. Because research on wilderness injuries is limited to descriptive studies, determining accurate injury rates are difficult.[2] The literature is also limited in children and teens. Many of the studies in adults are consistent, however, and some data can be extrapolated to youth.

In a 1987 to 1988 study of 224 hikers who successfully hiked the entire 2100-mile Appalachian Trail,[3] 82% responded to a 3-page survey regarding their experience. Eighty-two percent of the respondents reported an injury or illness, with the most common injuries being extremity or joint related. The loss of at least one day of hiking from an illness or injury occurred in 52% of hikers, diarrhea in 63% (only 7% drank exclusively from protected water), and foot blisters in 7%. Hypothermia or frostbite was reported in four hikers, hospitalization in three hikers, and one hiker reported being struck by lightning. The most frequent allergic reaction was caused by insect bites.

Ten years later, in a 1997 prospective study of 334 hikers on the Appalachian Trail who had planned to hike at least 7 days or longer, complete data were obtained from 280 respondents.[4] The most common medical complaints included feet blisters in 180 (64%), diarrhea in 156 (56%), skin irritation in 143 (51%), acute joint pain in 102 (36%), sunburn in 72 (26%), tick bites in 68 (24%), dehydration in 55 (20%), heat exhaustion in 13 (5%), and hypothermia in 13 (5%) of the participants. The risk of diarrhea was significantly greater in those who reported that they frequently drank untreated water from the streams or ponds (odds ratio [OR] = 7.7; 95% confidence interval [CI]: 2.7 to 23; $P<.0001$). In contrast, routine washing of cooking utensils and hands after bowel movements was associated with a significantly decreased risk of diarrhea (OR = 0.46; 95% CI: 0.22 to 0.97; $P = .04$). Eighty-eight hikers (31%) did not complete the hike as expected, with reported reasons of injury, time limitations, and psychosocial problems.

In the NOLS study (1999 to 2002), involving 1679 students and 233 staff, 678 injuries were reported, of which 50% were from sprains and strains of knees, ankles, and back (most commonly caused by falls, slips, and overuse factors). Thirty-one percent were from soft tissue injuries including burns, blisters, wound infections, and stings. There were 549 illnesses reported, of which 26% were gastrointestinal and 17% were respiratory.[5]

In a 2-year US National Parks study, children and adolescents ($\leq$19 years of age) accounted for 13% of the 356 deaths.[6] Adolescents made up 23% of search-and-rescue operations in Alaska's National Park Service units that resulted in a death.[7] In a study of the California-based National Parks Service, children and adolescents suffered disproportionately more with hypothermia, diarrhea, and noninsect anaphylaxis.[8] In a 5-year study in five contiguous counties in western Washington State, there were 40 wilderness recreational deaths among children and adolescents aged 12 months to 19 years, of which 34 occurred in teens 13 to 19 years of age.[9] Most deaths were associated with hiking, swimming, and river rafting, with the youngest children experiencing drowning and closed head injury as the most frequent cause of death. In 27 of the 40 deaths, youth were lacking in basic preparedness including inadequate clothing layers and the absence of life vests. In another study of wilderness injuries in Mount Rainier and Olympic National Parks in Washington State over a 5-year period, there were no youth deaths, but almost 25% of those injured were under the age of 18 years. Children sustained more injuries during the winter months compared with adults, emphasizing the importance of cold weather preventive measures.[10]

In a study from a nationally representative sample of emergency department visits for outdoor recreational injuries over a 2-year period, 52% of 212,700 injuries per year were in 10- to 24-year-olds, and 68% were males. Fractures and sprains were the most common injuries.[11] The epidemiology shows that illness and injuries in the wilderness are prevalent among children and adolescents and that this population is at a greater risk for certain types of injuries compared with adults. Education, preparedness, and prevention efforts will be necessary to help minimize these events as the popularity of wilderness activities grows.

PREVENTION OF INJURIES AND ILLNESSES

Injury prevention has the potential to make a significant difference in decreasing the number of child and adolescent wilderness-related incidents, although more rigorous study is needed. The NOLS has introduced significant programmatic changes that include providing fitness information to their students in their enrollment packets; reducing backpack weights; carefully planning wilderness courses; and stressing the importance of good camp hygiene, hand washing, and disinfecting drinking water. NOLS was able to document a decrease in injury rate from 2.3 incidents per 1000 program days from 1984 to 1989 to 1.07 incidents per 1000 program days from 1999 to 2002, and an illness rate dropping from 1.50 to 0.87 incidents per 1000 program days during the same time period.[5]

Preparticipation Evaluation and Anticipatory Guidance

Many youth seek a medical visit before a wilderness experience to make sure their immunization status is up to date or to obtain travel medications such as antidiarrheals, antibiotics, or analgesics. Often a preparticipation evaluation is required by sponsoring organizations to decrease liability. While the benefits of such a preparticipation evaluation are being further evaluated,[12] physicians should take this opportunity to question children, adolescents, and parents, about their wilderness plans, to assess their preparedness, and to provide anticipatory guidance to help youth and their families avoid preventable injuries and illness.

Although most teens will have no significant medical conditions, one cannot assume this for all. Identifying risk factors or pre-existing medical and mental health conditions or a lack of physical fitness is important for their safety and for the group with which they may travel. It is important for youth to be able to accurately assess and have realistic expectations regarding their physical abilities and experience level when preparing for a wilderness trip. Gender and age, periods of rapid growth, poor coaching, poor dynamic balance, and previous injury are associated with an increased risk for sports injury.[13] There is some evidence in the sports literature that life stress can be a strong predictor of injury.[14] Fears such as that of heights or claustrophobia are better addressed before confronting these dilemmas on mountains or in caves, where the situation could become frightening or dangerous.

Educating youth about the need for certain protective equipment and the signs and symptoms of dehydration, altitude sickness, hypothermia, and other risks potentially can prevent injury and illnesses. There is evidence in the sports injury literature that supports preseason conditioning, functional training, and strength and balance programs.[15] There is sufficient evidence that health care providers should be recommending clean drinkable water by filtering, chemicals, or boiling. Lack of adequate protection from the sun and lack of clean water can lead to sunburn, heat exhaustion, and heat stroke. It seems prudent to recommend appropriate clothing and attention to weather conditions, because cool temperatures, winds, rain, and exhaustion can lead to hypothermia. A suggestion for a first aid kit that includes simple dressings, Band-Aids and analgesics seems reasonable. Because of the high incidence of gastrointestinal distress, hikers may benefit from carrying antacids and antidiarrheals. International trips may require additional vaccinations, medications, and water purification supplies. It is imperative to have information available regarding necessary travel medications and informational brochures for commonly visited international destinations.

Basic Survival Skills

Safety starts with having a well thought out plan regarding the trip, necessary gear, and potential problems. The type of trip, including location, length of travel time, risk of illness or injury, and distance from rescue or medical access, have a major impact on and should dictate the type of equipment and supplies that are necessary for a wilderness trip (**Table 1**). Having extra food and a plan for bringing or accessing water will help if delays occur. Getting lost is always possible and so it is safer to travel with at least one buddy and inform friends or family of detailed travel plans. Basic wilderness skills include knowing how to read a contour map[16] and how to align it with a compass' north direction to find one's way.[17] More recent rescue tools include cellular phones (if cell towers are available) and global positioning satellite (GPS) units. New technology, however, can lead to a false sense of security, and basic map reading and survival skills are essential for anyone venturing into the wilderness.

PREVENTION OF SPECIFIC CONDITIONS
Hypothermia, Trench Foot, and Frostbite

Hypothermia is the number one killer in the wilderness, with over 700 people dying each year in the United States.[18,19] It results from the lowering of body temperature at a rate faster than the body can generate heat that interferes with the body's ability to regulate basic functions. It is often caused by a lack of warm clothes or rain gear given weather conditions. Additive factors include the sudden wetting of the body by rain or falling into water with aggravation by wind and exhaustion. Hypothermia starts with core temperatures dropping to 35.5°C (96°F) when shivering is apparent and progresses to mental status changes with core temperatures from 35° to 32°C (95 to 90°F). Muscle rigidity with the loss of fine motor skills, physical collapse, and unconsciousness occurs at 32° to 30°C (90° to 86°F), and death occurs from cardiac arrhythmias at temperatures less than 25°C (77°F).

Trench foot is caused by many hours of wet or damp conditions at a temperature just above freezing and can cause difficulty walking, numbness, and eventually, gangrene. Severe frostbite of exposed fingers, toes, ears, and the nose results from tissue necrosis caused by vasoconstriction and venous thrombosis.[20]

Prevention measures include following weather reports and avoiding bad weather conditions. It is important to stay dry, because wet clothes, in particular cotton and down feathers, lose up to 90% of their insulation properties when wet, and it can be nearly impossible to dry these items if the weather does not cooperate. When it is getting cold, avoid wind, because it rapidly carries away body heat and can result in hypothermia. It is best to remove wet clothing when possible, because it pulls heat away from the body.

Winter brings special challenges, and appropriate clothing becomes critical for survival. Layering of clothing provides better temperature control, because air

Table 1
Equipment: packing considerations for a wilderness trip[a]

Upper body	T-shirts (cotton, synthetic), long sleeved shirts (light/medium weight), jackets (fleece, waterproof shell, goose down/synthetic down)
Lower body	Underwear (short/long, light/midweight), shorts, pants (hiking, fleece, waterproof shell, snow, goose down/synthetic down)
Head	Hats (synthetic, baseball cap, warm, windproof), balaclava, face mask, glasses (sun, prescription), ski goggles, bandanas
Hands	Lightweight gloves/liners, heavyweight gloves or mittens, chemical hand-warming packets
Feet	Socks (liner, wool, light/heavyweight), shoes (walking, trail), hiking/climbing/mountaineering boots, vapor barrier socks, down booties, chemical foot-warming packets
Sleeping	Sleeping bags (light/heavyweight), tents and camping related gear, foam mats: comfort/warmth, lightweight air mattress: comfort/warmth
Climbing gear	Shoes, harness, trekking poles, snow shoes, crampons, ice axe/tools, technical climbing equipment
Food	Water purification, meals (fresh, dehydrated), energy bars/gels/drinks, Gatorade/electrolyte replacement powder, snack food
Accessories	Backpack/travel bags, tent/camping equipment, padlocks, waterproof stuff sacks, duct tape, maps, compass, headlamp/flashlight/lanterns, multipurpose knife/tool, watch/alarm clock, repair kits (sewing, gear), lighter, matches (flint), water bottles, cooking equipment, sunscreen, bug spray, plastic/zip-lock bags, binoculars, trash bags, books, playing cards, ear plugs, camera, first aid kit, medications, international travel accessories

[a] Dependent on the extent of the trip and expected weather conditions.

between layers provides insulation. Additionally, layers are easy to add and remove when weather conditions change. There are four clothing layers to consider: inner layer, middle layer, insulation layer, and outer layer. The preferred inner layer is light or midweight short or long underwear that wicks sweat from skin during high aerobic activity to stay comfortable without being damp. It also provides extra insulation. Unfortunately, while cotton is comfortable when dry, it absorbs and holds sweat and takes a long time to dry. The preferred underwear is polypropylene, other new synthetic fabrics, or silk, with silk being the least durable. Midlayer clothing includes protection in moderate-to-warm conditions and includes long pants, long-sleeved shirts, shorts, and T-shirts. They should be lightweight, comfortable, and durable. The next insulation layer includes clothing (vests, jackets, pullovers, and sweaters) that provides additional warmth when conditions warrant. Ideally, they should be warm, lightweight, not too bulky, and breathable (ie, allow sweat and excess body heat to escape). Wool, pile, and fleece are common insulation layers that retain some insulation capabilities even when wet. The outer layer of clothing protects from wind, rain, and snow. This clothing should not be too bulky, heavy, or interfere with outdoor activities. Ideally, waist, cuffs, underarm, and neck region with a hood for the head can be sealed to keep out elements or opened for additional ventilation. Lots of pockets help for storage. These items should be breathable to keep the user dry and warm. Rain gear made of polyvinylchloride (PVC) is inexpensive and waterproof but not breathable. Fabrics like GORE-TEX are more expensive but do a good job at being both waterproof and breathable.[21] Nearly all waterproof material is less breathable than other fabrics. It is important to notice excessive sweating and over-heating while wearing waterproof clothing and understand that if the weather suddenly turns cold, hypothermia is a serious risk if additional clothing is not available.

Boots should be insulated and waterproof to keep feet dry. Wearing two pairs of socks, one a liner sock and the other an outer, wool sock, will help provide insulation and wick perspiration away from the feet. Simply pulling trouser legs or using gaiters over the top of boots will block water, snow and rocks from getting into boots. Mittens are warmer than fingered gloves, although they decrease dexterity. Chemical hand and foot warmers are inexpensive and should be considered for winter outings. Wearing a warm hat, scarf around the neck, and ski mask over the face will reduce heat loss significantly.

The treatment of hypothermia is to reverse the process and rewarm the entire body when the hypothermic person is in a safe place. This can include a warm bath of 38° to 43°C (100° to 110°F) or wrapping the victim in a warmed sleeping bag with another person. If conscious, it is critical to give hot, sweetened drinks.

Lightning Safety

There are over 2000 thunderstorms in progress above the earth's surface at any given time, which amounts to approximately 8 million lightning strikes each day. Lightning travels as fast as 100,000 miles a second and lasts from .01 to .0001 second. There are approximately 500 human lightening strikes per year in the United States, resulting in 50 deaths. Although uncommon, these events are severe, and survivors often experience significant disabilities.[22] To estimate the distance from a lightning strike, count seconds from lightning to thunder, and then divide the number of seconds by five to get the distance in miles. Seek shelter when lightning is separated from thunder by 30 seconds or less, or approximately 5 to 6 miles away. Resume activities 30 minutes after lightning has passed.

Always monitor the weather, and if lightning is predicted or a storm is approaching, avoid mountain ridges, summits, drainages, shallow caves, open fields, isolated trees, and rappelling down mountainsides. Remove and avoid metal objects like fences, posts, bikes, and small boats that can conduct electricity. Run to the nearest safe building, vehicle, or lower stand of trees or scuba dive if on the water.

Sunburn

Natural sunlight contains ultraviolet (UV) photons UVB and UVA. These photons strike the skin and generate free radicals that damage DNA. Damaged DNA releases prostaglandins and cytokines, which lead to dilation of cutaneous blood vessels and recruitment of inflammatory cells. Sunburn is an acute toxic reaction to UV radiation that causes cutaneous edema, redness, swelling, pain, and peeling of the skin. It can cause systemic symptoms including itching, fever, and nausea. UV radiation in excess can cause first- or second-degree burns. It often takes 4 to 6 hours after excessive sun exposure for symptoms to develop.

Certain antibiotics, oral contraceptives, and tranquilizers sensitize some people to sunburn. Those with fair skin or freckles have a greater risk. Sunburn can occur at all temperatures, and it occurs significantly faster at higher altitudes. The sunlight also reflects off of snow, ice, and water. It is necessary to put sunscreen on parts of the body where the reflections of the sunlight hit, such as in the nostrils, under the chin and on the palms of the hands. The DNA damage caused by UV light is irreversible and increases the risk for skin cancer and premature aging of the skin. Melanoma is 20 times more common in whites than in African Americans and four times more common in whites than in Hispanics.[23]

Eyes are sensitive to sun exposure, and over time this can lead to cortical cataracts and pteryglum. Pteryglum is a fleshy tissue that grows in a triangular shape over the cornea and may interfere with vision. It is common throughout the world, with highest rates seen in tropical countries near the equator. Sunglasses should block out 99% to 100% of UVA and UVB radiation.[24]

The best protection against sunburn is to use long-sleeved clothing and hats, avoid sun exposure between 10 AM and 4 PM, and use sunscreen. Sun tanning can prevent sunburn, as it increases melanin, a photoprotectant pigment. Unfortunately, tanning beds have less UVB and more UVA, and excessive tanning has been associated with an increased risk of melanoma.[25] Using sunscreen prevents squamous cell skin cancer, while the evidence for preventing melanoma is mixed.[26] Sunscreens contain organic molecules and pigments that absorb, scatter, and reflect UV radiation. It is best to use broad-spectrum sunscreens against both UVA and UVB. Sun blocks differ from sunscreens in that they block all sun exposure and contain either zinc oxide or titanium dioxide but can be irritating to the skin. Sun Protection Factor (SPF) is the time needed for UVB radiation to cause minimal erythema with sunscreen versus no sunscreen based on 1 oz of sunscreen lotion applied to an average adult's entire body surface; SPF 10 blocks out 90% UVB and SPF 20 blocks out 95%. In general, one does not need more than SPF 20. It is best to apply sunscreen 15 to 30 minutes before exposure, reapply 15 to 30 minutes after exposure, and then every 2 to 3 hours. Use waterproof formulations for water-based activities and plan on reapplying after 80 minutes in the water. When at higher elevations or on snow or ice, sunscreen should be reapplied every hour. Lip balm with SPF 15 or greater should be used to prevent sunburned and chapped lips.

Most first-degree sunburns resolve with time and may only need symptomatic relief. Lidocaine or benzocaine spray or ointment can help with pain. Hydrating the skin with aloe vera or vitamin E, which also reduces inflammation, improves comfort. Hydrocortisone cream may reduce inflammation and itching.

Dehydration, Heat Exhaustion, and Heat Stroke

Maintenance fluids are needed to replace approximately 1.5 L of urine per day and additional 1 L of water loss from respiration, perspiration, and stool. In a typical day, one needs about 2 to 2.5 L (or eight 8 oz drinks) of fluids to maintain adequate body fluid levels. Fruits and vegetables contain significant water and count toward maintenance fluids. Extreme weather conditions and high levels of exertion lead to significant on-going water and electrolyte losses from perspiration and breathing. At high levels of activity and extreme hot or cold temperatures, it may be necessary to drink up to 1 L of fluid/h, often a difficult task.

Usually, the body is able to cool itself by sweating. When unable to replace fluids, heat exhaustion can progress to life-threatening heat stroke as core temperature rises. In 2001, there were 300 deaths in the United States related to excessive heat exposure.[27] Preventive measures include scheduling activities before 10 AM or after 4 PM, when it is cooler outside. Young children and some adolescents will be more sensitive to heat, and care must be taken to avoid heat-related illness. It is best to wear loose-fitting clothes, drink sufficient fluids, and be aware of the first signs of dehydration including thirst, muscle cramps, fatigue, and lightheadedness.

Treatment measures for heat-related illnesses include reducing the body temperature by washing with cool water, taking sips of water, finding cooler or shaded areas, and evacuation, when possible. Having packets of oral rehydration salts or powdered sports drinks on hand will help to replace electrolyte losses, as long as clean water is available.

Traveler's Diarrhea

Traveler's diarrhea is commonly experienced in the wilderness. Having access to potable water is critical. Two liters of water only cover maintenance fluids, so additional water must be carried or be available along the route while hiking or traveling. Unfortunately, streams and lakes can have debris, dirt, and infectious agents such as *Giardia, Cryptosporidium, Shigella, Salmonella,* and *Entamoeba.*

There are four ways to avoid contaminated water:

1. Bring sufficient potable water
2. Use a commercial lightweight hiker's water filtering system that will significantly reduce particles, organisms, and sediment and make water taste better
3. Boil water for 1 minute to kill all microorganisms (although this does not neutralize chemical pollutants, and water needs to cool before it can be used)
4. Use chemical tablets, typically chlorine purification tablets; 1 tablet per liter or 32 oz bottle (kills microorganisms in 30 minutes).

Good hygiene, including hand washing with soap and water, and using antiseptic alcohol spray or gels, also reduces the risk for infection and should be practiced after going to the bathroom and before drinking and eating.

Blisters

Hiking on hard, rough terrain for miles is hard on the feet. Blisters can occur randomly, in any season, and with most activities. Early hot spots should not be ignored. Significant blisters can derail a trip.

The skin has three layers: the epidermis, subdermis, and subcutaneous tissue. The epidermis, which is avascular, has five layers: stratum corneum, stratum lucidum, stratum granulosum, stratum spinosa, and stratum germinativum (or basale). Most blisters form between the stratum germinativum and stratum spinosa of the epidermis due to horizontal shear forces that cause delamination and fluid leaking into the space.

To prevent blisters, feet should be kept dry and clean. Feet can be conditioned by walking barefoot to toughen the skin. New hiking shoes or boots should be well broken in, ideally for at least 3 months, before any long hikes or hiking trips. Toenails should be trimmed. Synthetic socks wick excess moisture away from the surface. The goal is to create weaker shear layers between the skin and sock, between multiple socks, or between the sock and footwear. Two socks are recommended.

Once blisters have formed, collagen, the principal protein of connective tissue, is necessary for healing. If the top layer of the blister is left intact, the damaged area remains moist and heals. If the top skin is removed, the damaged area must be kept moist. If the blister is left unbroken and pressure continues, pain and more delamination continue. If the blister is punctured, in most cases it will refill with fluid, and the risk of infection is increased.

If a blister has occurred and the trip is over, it may be best to leave the blister intact. To complete a day hike, the blister can be drained with a sterile needle and the skin around the blister can be padded with moleskin or similar fabric. To complete a multiple-day hike, the blister can be drained, covered with Second Skin (Spenco Medical Corporation, Waco, TX, USA) or a petroleum-based ointment and gauze, and secured in place with a porous cloth tape.

Sprains, Strains, and Fractures

Injuries can usually be traced to:

Bad judgment about using (or not using) equipment
Bad judgment about one's performance or ability
Weather-related hazards
Equipment failure.

Lower extremity injuries such as knee or ankle sprains most often result from falling and tripping in the wilderness. The 175,000 anterior cruciate ligament (ACL) knee injuries per year are usually sports related and occur frequently in active, healthy 15- to 24-year-olds. The cost of ACL reconstructive surgery, not including initial evaluation or rehabilitation, is just under $1 billion per year in the United States.[28] More serious injuries can lead to concussions and even death.

It is important to match the necessary physical conditioning for the planned activity. Training and physical conditioning techniques are numerous, with both resources, as well as methods that lack scientific evidence, available in bookstores and online. The training process ideally should be accomplished gradually over a longer period of time. Time to train is not always available. Shorter training periods are typically adequate to get into shape for so weekend trips. More extensive training should be undertaken for long wilderness trips (more than a week) or expeditions. Consultation with a nutritionist and personal trainer can help when working toward reaching specific training goals. The necessary gear depends on the wilderness endeavor, but needs to be available, in working order, and fit appropriately, well in advance of the planned trip. Examples of necessary gear include life jackets for water activities and helmets for biking or rappelling (see **Table 1**). Fortunately, gear has gotten lighter, more durable, and accessible locally or on the Internet.

Bites and Stings

Most insect, bee, and wasp bites cause a localized reaction and can become infected from scratching. If there has been previous exposure, anaphylactic shock is possible and can be life threatening. Mosquitoes also are known to carry arboviral encephalitides such as West Nile virus and equine encephalitis, malaria, dengue fever, and yellow fever. Ticks can carry Lyme disease, Rocky Mountain spotted fever, and tularemia. Fleas can harbor plague.[29]

Netting and long-sleeved clothing help to prevent insect bites. Avoid going outdoors during dawn and dusk when mosquitoes are most active and use an insect repellent such as 30% to 50% DEET (N,N-Diethyl-meta-toluamide) or 15% picaridin. DEET provides longer protection and needs to be applied less often. Clothing also can be sprayed with repellent. Permethrin can be applied to clothing and bed netting to repel insects. Avoid walking around barefoot. If stung and the stinger is still present, it can be removed by scraping. Apply cold to reduce swelling.

The best way to remove ticks is to grasp them as close to the skin as possible and pull out with steady pressure. An antiseptic (>60% alcohol) should be used afterwards on the hands and bite area. Do not use petroleum jelly or burn the tick.

All vaccinations should be up to date. If traveling outside the United States, check the Centers for Disease Control and Prevention Web site and make health care appointments in sufficient time to allow immunizations to produce antibodies to become effective.[30]

Teenage boys have a perilous attraction to snakes (and small rodents). Fortunately, the risk of being bitten by a snake is small. There are an estimated 45,000 snakebites yearly in the United States (about 40% occurring from people handling snakes), although only about 6680 persons require treatment for snake venom poisoning. The four poisonous snakes in the United States are rattlesnakes, cottonmouth moccasin, copperhead, and coral snakes. The number of deaths from snake bites in the United States typically ranges from 9 to 14 per year.[30] Most deaths are attributed to rattlesnakes and occur in children, in the elderly, in untreated, or undertreated patients, or in cases complicated by other serious disease states.[31]

Be familiar with venomous snakes in the area to be traveled. Avoid rocky areas, heavy vegetation and where heavy rodent infestations exist. Prevent rodents from getting into camp areas by keeping these areas clean. Snakebites can be avoided by simply moving away from a snake after a snake is encountered. If a bite should occur, it is important to keep calm. The wound should be cleaned. The limb should be immobilized below the heart and the person evacuated. There should not be an attempt to cut the skin, suck out the venom or use a tourniquet.

Wilderness Stress

While many seek a wilderness experience to avoid the stresses of daily life, they often confront a unique set of stressors in the wilderness that can challenge one's coping mechanisms. Because it is an uncontrolled environment in terms of terrain, weather, insects, and wildlife, the outdoors can lead to uncertainty. Many people experience a loss of privacy, and some experience a sense of isolation. Physical activity can lead to exhaustion. Injuries and illnesses such as those described, can lead to pain and discomfort and contribute to distress. The need to have adequate food and water increases significantly on multiple-day trips and adds additional stress. Although some may thrive in wilderness, others experience distress, regardless of one's prior experience or expertise.

Symptoms of distress include anxiety, angry outbursts, doubts about one's abilities, inability to make judgments or take action, nausea, fatigue, dizziness, decreased appetite, fear, restlessness, and headache. It is common for high-altitude endeavors to magnify the extent of these symptoms. Long-term effects after the incident can include difficulty sleeping, dreams or mental images about the incident, depression, anger or grief, feelings of isolation, and anxiety.

Ideally, identifying stress-inducing situations in advance and then planning accordingly will help to reduce levels of distress when in the wilderness. Practice sessions can include discussions of how to cope with severe weather conditions, equipment failure or deficiencies, injuries or illnesses, and difficult group dynamics.

Altitude Illness

High-altitude areas are becoming popular tourist destinations, and it is common for children and adolescents to be included in these trips. The benefits from such travel must be weighed against the environmental concerns of hypoxia and cold. Altitude sickness occurs when there is a lack of sufficient time for acclimatization. The oxygen level decreases with altitude at a time when the demand for oxygen due to physical activity increases. Hypoxia occurs at greater than 2000 m (6560 ft), and above 5500 m (18,045 ft) supplemental oxygen is sometimes used to help prevent altitude illness or to treat people with severe acute mountain sickness (AMS), high-altitude pulmonary edema (HAPE), or high altitude cerebral edema (HACE). Serious complications begin at 3000 m (9840 ft). The initial symptoms of altitude sickness include headache, lassitude, drowsiness, dizziness, chilliness, nausea and vomiting, facial pallor, dyspnea, and cyanosis. These are followed by high-altitude pulmonary edema and cerebral edema that can be fatal.[32]

AMS can be difficult to assess in children, because the signs and symptoms may be expressed differently than in adults. AMS, however, is becoming increasingly recognized in young children and often results from the rapid ascent to altitudes above 2500 m.[33] AMS may manifest as fussiness, a lack of playfulness, change in stool pattern, vomiting, and appetite and sleep disturbances.[34] There is some evidence that children are more susceptible to AMS than adults. In a study of high-altitude illness in the mountain regions of Chile, compared at the same elevation, all of the children, 50% of the teenagers, and 27% of the adults developed AMS.[35] A recent study in the Himalayas followed 36 children between 3 and 15 years of age, who underwent a rapid ascent from 1950 to 4380 m, during a pilgrimage trip to Gosaikunda Lake in the Langstang National Park Region of Nepal.[36] AMS was diagnosed in 17 of 36 (47.2%) of the children. AMS was seen in only 25% of the children who took 2 or more days (and 2 or more nights) to ascend, compared with 75% of the children who rested only one night before completing the same ascent. The study concluded that the risk of AMS and its severity in children, like adults, is increased by the rapidity of ascent.

The prevention measures for altitude illness include optimal physical conditioning and gradual ascent. Sleeping elevation should not be greater than 300 to 500 m/d. There should be a period of rest and inactivity for 1 to 2 days after arrival at high altitudes. The use of supplemental oxygen and medications such as bronchodilators, steroids, and acetazolamide have a role in prevention and treatment of altitude illness, but many of these therapies have not been tested in children at altitude and should be used with caution. The most important treatment of altitude illness is to safely return to lower altitudes as quickly as possible.

SUMMARY

Participating in wilderness experiences is increasing significantly in the pediatric population and is associated with minor and sometimes catastrophic injury causing lifelong disability or death. There is a need to move away from descriptive studies to an analytic etiologic approach that seeks to explain why and how injuries and illnesses occur in the wilderness and then to develop and introduce injury prevention strategies in a controlled way.[37] There is also a need for large-scale injury surveillance programs.

Preventing injuries and illnesses in the wilderness is an important endeavor in keeping children and adolescents healthy as well as making outdoor activities enjoyable. Prevention is well within the skill set of pediatricians.

REFERENCES

1. National survey on recreation and the environmental: 2000–2002. Available at: http://www.srs.fs.usda.gov/trends/. Accessed January 15, 2010.
2. Heggie TW. Pediatric and adolescent sport injury in the wilderness. Br J Sports Med 2010;44:50–5.
3. Crouse BJ, Josephs D. Health care needs of Appalachian trail hikers. J Fam Pract 1993;36:521–5.
4. Boulware DR, Forgey WW, Martin WJ II. Medical risks of wilderness hiking. Am J Med 2003;114:288–93.
5. Leemon D, Schiemelpfenig T. Wilderness injury, illness, and evacuation: National Outdoor Leadership School's incident profile, 1999–2002. Wilderness Environ Med 2003;14:174–82.
6. Heggie TW, Heggie TM, Kliewer C. Recreational travel fatalities in US national parks. J Travel Med 2008;15:404–11.
7. Heggie TW. Search and rescue in Alaska's national parks. Travel Med Infect Dis 2008;6:355–61.
8. Montalvo R, Wingard DL, Bracker M, et al. Morbidity and mortality in the wilderness. West J Med 1998;168:248–54.
9. Newman LM, Diekema DS, Shubkin CD, et al. Pediatric wilderness recreational deaths in western Washington State. Ann Emerg Med 1998;32:687–92.
10. Stephens BD, Diekema DS, Klein EJ. Recreational injuries in Washington State national parks. Wilderness Environ Med 2005;16:192–7.
11. Flores AH, Haileyesus T, Greenspan AI. National estimates of outdoor recreational injuries treated in emergency departments, United States, 2004–2005. Wilderness Environ Med 2008;19:91–8.
12. Wingfield K, Matheson GO, Meeuwisse WH. Preparticipation evaluation: an evidence-based review. Clin J Sport Med 2004;14:109–22.
13. Caine D, Maffuli N, Caine C. Epidemiology of injury in child and adolescent sports: injury rates, risk factors and prevention. Clin Sports Med 2008;27:19–50.
14. Anderson MB, Williams JM. Psychosocial antecedents of sport injury: review and critique of the stress and injury model. J Appl Sport Psychol 1998;10:5–25.
15. Abernethy L, Bleakley C. Strategies to prevent injury in adolescent sport: a systematic review. Br J Sports Med 2007;41:627–38.
16. Available at: http://www.map-reading.com/ch10-3.php. Accessed September 24, 2009.
17. Available at: http://www.wilderness-backpacking.com/how-to-use-a-compass.html. Accessed September 24, 2009.
18. Jurkovich GJ. Environmental cold-induced injury. Surg Clin North Am 2007;87:247–67.
19. Fritz RL, Perrin DH. Cold exposure injuries: prevention and treatment. Clin Sports Med 1989;8:111–28.
20. Golant A, Nord RM, Paksima N, et al. Cold exposure injuries to the extremities. J Am Acad Orthop Surg 2008;16:704–14.
21. Available at: http://www.gore-tex.com/remote/Satellite/content/customer-service/faq#faq11. Accessed September 21, 2009.

22. Ritenour AE, Morton MJ, McManus JG, et al. Lightning injury: a review. Burns 2008;34:585–94.
23. National Cancer Institute. Surveillance epidemiology and end results cancer statistics review, 1975–2004. Available at: http://seer.cancer.gov/csr/1975_2004/. Accessed September 24, 2009.
24. Available at: http://www.skincancer.org/understanding-uva-and-uvb.html. Accessed September 24, 2009.
25. Available at: http://www.aad.org/Public/sun/toolkit/index.html. Accessed September 24, 2009.
26. Available at: http://www.ahrq.gov/clinic/3rduspstf/skcacoun//skcarr.htm. Accessed September 24, 2009.
27. Available at: http://emergency.cdc.gov/disasters/extremeheat/heat_guide.asp. Accessed September 25, 2009.
28. Gottloab CA, Baker CL, Pellissier JM, et al. Cost effectiveness of anterior cruciate ligament reconstruction in young adults. Clin Orthop Relat Res 1999;367:272–82.
29. Available at: http://www.cdc.gov/ncidod/diseases/insects/index.htm. Accessed March 21, 2010.
30. Available at: http://gorp.away.com/gorp/health/snakefaq13.htm. Accessed September 20, 2009.
31. Curry SC, Horning D, Brady P, et al. The legitimacy of rattlesnake bites in central Arizona. Ann Emerg Med 1989;18(6):658–63.
32. Firth PG, Zheng H, Windsor JS, et al. Mortality on Mount Everest, 1921–2006: descriptive study. BMJ 2008;337:a2654.
33. Yaron M, Waldman N, Niermeyer S, et al. The diagnosis of acute mountain sickness in preverbal children. Arch Pediatr Adolesc Med 1998;152:683–7.
34. Yaron M, Niermeyer S, Lindgren KN, et al. Evaluation of diagnostic criteria and incidence of acute mountain sickness in preverbal children. Wilderness Environ Med 2002;13:1–4.
35. Moraga FA, Osoriao JD, Vargas ME. Acute mountain sickness in tourists with children at Lake Chungara (4400 m) in Northern Chile. Wilderness Environ Med 2002;13:31–5.
36. Pradhan S, Yadav S, Neupane P, et al. Acute mountain sickness in children at 4380 meters in the Himalayas. Wilderness Environ Med 2009;20:359–63.
37. Shanmugam C, Maffuli N. Sports injuries in children. Br Med Bull 2008;86:33–57.

The Adolescent Female Athlete: Current Concepts and Conundrums

Donald E. Greydanus, MD, FAAP, FSAM, FIAP (H)[a,b,*],
Hatim Omar, MD[c,d], Helen D. Pratt, PhD[a,e]

KEYWORDS

• Adolescent females • Athletes • Physiology

The adolescent female athlete has become a common part of the sports environment at all levels from childhood play to professional adult sports.[1–16] This article reviews basic sports physiology and then considers specific conditions, including iron deficiency anemia (IDA), stress urinary incontinence (SUI), breast issues (ie, pain, asymmetry, galactorrhea, injury), the female athlete triad (ie, menstrual dysfunction, abnormal eating patterns, and osteopenia or osteoporosis), and injuries. Various clinical conundrums are reviewed, including working with an athlete whose intense exercise patterns can lead to menstrual dysfunction and compromise of bone health.

PHYSIOLOGY
The Role of Gender

Children of both genders have basically the same physical condition with respect to such parameters as weight, height, injury risks, motor skills, percent body fat, endurance, strength, and hemoglobin levels.[1,8,9,11,12,14,15] Once the activation of the hypothalamic-pituitary-gonadal axis called puberty occurs, these specific parameters are altered;

[a] Department of Pediatrics & Human Development, Michigan State University College of Human Medicine, 1000 Oakland Drive, Kalamazoo, MI 49008-1284, USA
[b] Pediatrics Program, Kalamazoo Center for Medical Studies, 1000 Oakland Drive, Kalamazoo, MI 49008, USA
[c] Division of Adolescent Medicine, Department of Pediatrics, KY Clinic, Room J422, University of Kentucky, Lexington, KY 40536-0284, USA
[d] Department of Obstetrics & Gynecology, KY Clinic, Room J422, University of Kentucky, Lexington, KY 40536-0284, USA
[e] Behavioral-Developmental Pediatrics, MSU/Kalamazoo Center for Medical Studies, 1000 Oakland Drive, Kalamazoo, MI 49008, USA
* Corresponding author. Pediatrics Program, MSU/Kalamazoo Center for Medical Studies, 1000 Oakland Drive, Kalamazoo, MI 49008.
E-mail address: Greydanus@kcms.msu.edu

Pediatr Clin N Am 57 (2010) 697–718
doi:10.1016/j.pcl.2010.02.005
0031-3955/10/$ – see front matter © 2010 Elsevier Inc. All rights reserved.
pediatric.theclinics.com

changes in ability in sports competition are observable. Despite these differences, exercise training results are different for specific athletes depending on intensity of training and genetic traits rather than on gender alone. In the past, the female athlete was limited by inadequate equipment and limited training. As these factors have been corrected, the results in female athlete achievements have exponentially increased as well.[1,4]

Effect of Puberty

The phenomenal process of puberty affects the female in various ways (**Table 1**).

For example, the body fat percentage is particularly affected in the female, and the final result is an average body percentage in adult females of 23% to 27% versus a range of 13% to 15% in adult males.[1,4] As a result of intense and prolonged training, the elite female athlete can lower these levels to 12% to 16% (in distance runners) and 8% to 10% (in sprinters) versus 4% to 8% in highly trained male gymnasts.[1,4,14,15]

The thermoregulatory capacity is similar between genders; having fewer sweat glands in the female is offset by producing less heat because of reduced body mass, reduced muscle bulk, and large body surface area. There is a higher risk for heatstroke in athletes of both genders if they are late maturing, are obese, or are exercising in hot climates. Females tend to have better balancing and flexibility abilities, which initiate in childhood and peak at 14 or 15 years of age; in contrast, males improve in flexibility from midadolescence until the end of puberty.[1,4,7]

After puberty, females develop less strength than males, as noted in **Table 2**. Although the proportion of muscle fiber type is similar, the muscle fiber size is less in the female.[1,4] Females develop a small increase in muscle strength after menarche (onset of menstruation), whereas the male continues to increase muscle strength throughout the process of puberty.[1,4,11–14] Trained female athletes can achieve about 70% body strength compared with males of similar training, whereas the upper body strength is 30% to 50% that of males.[1,4,7,11–14]

In the adolescent male, maximal speed peak occurs before peak height velocity (PHV) whereas power and strength peaks occur after PHV; a similar pattern is not observed in adolescent females, who typically have the most weight gain rate 12 to 14 months after maximum growth velocity in Tanner stage (sexual maturity rating [SMR]) 2 or 3.[7,8,14–16] In the female, there is a small muscle mass increase in contrast to a large increase in body fat. Research notes a heightened response to training (strength and endurance) 12 to 24 months after PHV at an SMR of 4 or 5. Intense weight training in females results in only a small increase in observable muscle and perhaps some measurable strength increase; intensive exercise may lead to less adipose tissue and more muscle definition. The progression of puberty allows males to grow into their chosen sport because they get closer to their physical optimum and thus, potentially reach their optimum sports performance. However, the process of puberty in females impedes their best sports performance by lowering their physical optimum.[1,4]

Table 1
Changes in females induced by puberty
Size of heart, volume of cardiac stroke and size of left ventricle are smaller
Lung volume and aerobic capacity are less
Hemoglobin levels are reduced
Female is smaller and has shoulders that are more narrow and reduced articular surface
Female has greater flexibility and increased balance

Table 2
Strength comparison between equal or similar size females and males
Ages birth to 10 years (before puberty): same strength
Ages 11–12 years: female strength is 90% of males of same age
Ages 13–14 years: female strength is 85%
Ages 15–16 years: female strength is 75%

Normal weight and height gains from childhood to puberty allow improved performance in various sports (including basketball, volleyball and swimming), depending on genetic potential and training. Females have shorter extremities and a lower center of gravity, which may have a potential competitive advantage in sports that emphasize balancing abilities, such as gymnastics. However, research tends to note that the center of gravity is influenced by the athlete's specific weight as well as height and not by gender itself.[1,4]

A delay in puberty can be an advantage for the athletically gifted female, who may be attracted to sports that place a priority on a thin or lean physique, such as synchronized swimming, gymnastics, dance, and figure skating. Society has not encouraged the female adolescent athlete to become involved in American football; she does not face the risks for concussion, brain damage, and spinal injury now faced by males in modern football teams at all levels because of the emphasis on winning.[1]

However, the pressure to win may result in parents and society failing to notice and prevent the sexual advances of a predatory coach or trainer, who may promise to take the female adolescent athlete to high levels of victory.[1]

IDA

IDA (**Table 3**) is the most common cause of anemia in adolescents and research reports a prevalence of up to 24%, with frank anemia noted in 10% of 14- to 18-year-olds.[17,18] Iron deficiency (ID) and IDA are seen more commonly in females versus males and a similar prevalence is reported in female athletes versus nonathletes, except for long-distance runners, who have a higher prevalence of IDA.[3,19–21] In contrast to males, the adolescent female has 6% reduced red blood cells, reduced

Table 3	
Laboratory parameters of IDA in adolescent females	
Hematocrit	<35%; 12-year-old females <36%; 12–18-year-old females
Hemoglobin	<11.5 g/dL; 12-year-old females <12.0 g/dL; 12–18-year-old females
Serum ferritin	<10 mg/L (normal, 15–200 mg/L)
Mean corpuscular volume (MCV)	<76 fl in 12-year-old <78 fl in mid- and older adolescents
Serum iron	<40 mg/dL (normal, 50–140 mg/dL)
Serum transferrin saturation (Fe/TIBC ratio)	<16% (normal, 35%–40%)
TIBC	350–500 mg/dL (normal, 250–380 mg/dL)
FEP	> or = 150–200 mg/dL RBCs (normal, 54 ± 20)

Abbreviations: Fe, iron; FEP, free erythrocyte protoporphyrin; TIBC, total iron-binding capacity.

Reprinted from Greydanus DE, Patel DR. The female athlete: before and beyond puberty. Pediatr Clin North Am 2002;49:572; with permission.

(up to 19%) lower hemoglobin levels, lower iron stores, and increased iron levels.[17] Those individuals dedicated to optimum performance in their sports are concerned about IDA, because even mild IDA may result in lowered sports performance.

Various issues can lead to IDA, including limited oral intake of dietary iron, menstruation, iron loss in sweat and urine resulting from exercise, gastrointestinal bleeding, and intravascular hemolysis, which can be precipitated by exercise.[17,22] Routine screening for IDA is not recommended for adolescent athletes unless they are at risk because of such issues as heavy menstruation, history of anemia, being a long-distance runner, or having a vegetarian diet.[17,19,23]

There are 3 stages of developing IDA: first there is a lowering of iron stores as well as serum ferritin, followed by a lowering of serum iron along with an increase in total iron-binding capacity; the third step is development of microcytic hypochromic anemia.[17] The IDA that occurs is typically mild and basically asymptomatic. Most research concludes that there is no overt impairment of sports performance in those with non-anemic ID (ie, those with normal hemoglobin as well as hematocrit levels and low levels of serum ferritin). However, athletes with low to normal hemoglobin and low ferritin levels may report enhanced sports performance with iron supplementation; more research is needed in this area.[1,4,24] Athletes who develop sports anemia or pseudoanemia do not require iron supplementation because this is a normal reaction to intense and prolonged exercise. The plasma volume may expand up to 20%, although iron supplementation is not needed as long as the red blood cell mass remains normal. When the intense exercise is stopped, plasma volume returns to normal pre-exercise levels.

IDA management involves educating the young people about proper nutrition, including foods with iron (such as fortified cereals and breads), fish, meat, and eggs. If iron supplementation is required because of overt ID, elemental iron is prescribed at a dose of 3 to 6 mg/kg/d. This strategy results in an increase in hemoglobin and hematocrit levels typically in 1 to 3 weeks, whereas normal ferritin levels may not develop for several months, indicating the development of normal body iron content.[1,4]

SUI

SUI, the involuntary loss of urine during exercise, is reported in approximately one-quarter of nulliparous female athletes with a mean age of 20 years.[1,4] SUI is particularly noted in activities referred to as impact sports such as gymnastics, basketball, jumping, and running (ie, track and field events); less commonly implicated sports include skiing, tennis, skating, and jogging.[23,25–27] Risk factors are noted in **Table 4** and the basic cause is usually linked to an increase in intra-abdominal pressure caused by exercise that leads to urethral sphincteric unit alterations. A medical history of the

Table 4
Risk factors for exercise-induced SUI
↑ age
Female gender
Hypoestrogenic amenorrhea
Involvement in high-impact sports activity
Heavy exertion
Parity that is increased
Possibly obesity

female athlete may reveal the presence of SUI, with further identification of known risk factors (see **Table 4**). A general medical examination may be performed, including a pelvic examination to assess for anatomic pelvic floor integrity and dysfunction of the posterior urethrovesical angle.[1]

Because SUI is normally a self-limiting, benign condition in the adolescent female athlete, basic education about the nature of this condition is usually all that is needed. The athlete can be given information about the need to take enough fluid for the exercise event but not so much as to induce SUI; sanitary napkins placed before exercise are also helpful. If the female feels that more treatment options are needed, a variety of approaches are available, including behavior management, Kegal exercises, pharmacologic management, biofeedback counseling, vaginal cones, and electrical stimulation.[1] Imipramine and pseudoephedrine hydrochloride have been used to prevent or reduce exercise-induced SUI. Phenylpropolamine was withdrawn from the market in the United States because of an increase in reported cerebrovascular accidents in women less than age 50 years. Use of anticholinergic medications is not recommended because they may induce abnormal sweating and overt heat disorders.

BREAST ISSUES
Effect of Exercise

Exercise does not alter the breast size by changing muscle tissue, because there is only a small amount of muscle in the areolar area and none in the rest of the breast structure. However, exercise can alter the appearance of breast size by changes in the underlying pectoralis muscle. In addition, intense exercise can reduce mammary adipose tissue, with a resultant smaller breast.[1,4,28,29] The size of the breast is also affected by factors that enlarge or reduce breast size as noted with various dietary regimens.[2,9,30] Exercise provides a protective effect with regard to breast cancer in the adult years.[28,31–34]

Pain

Exercise-induced breast pain may be a hidden concern of the adolescent female athlete, especially in the individual with large breasts, and may prevent some of these athletes from participating in sports.[28,30] Breast soreness or tenderness induced by exercise was noted in 31% of female athletes in 1 report, and 52% of the women with breast discomfort also noted exercise-induced injury to breast tissue.[1,4,35,36] Research reveals that breast motion in exercise can be considerable, particularly in gymnastics, soccer, volleyball, basketball, running, and other sports.[35–37] Excessive breast movement can result in overt strain of the fascial attachments of the underlying pectoralis muscle in addition to intense shoulder pain.[1,35,37] Breast discomfort can also be increased from menstrual cycle-induced breast fluid retention, as noted by some individuals during the premenstrual phase of menses and with overt premenstrual syndrome (PMS).[37,38] Excessive perspiration can cause local excoriation, abscess development, and even intrabreast-fold cellulitis. If the female adolescent presents with breast pain, various underlying causes should be considered, including those already mentioned in addition to overt breast masses, such as a fibroadenoma.[1,35,38,39]

Breast discomfort and pain in female athletes may be reduced or prevented by having the individual wear a properly fitted sports brassiere that allows maximum support to the mammary tissue and minimizes exercise-induced breast movement.[39–46] A sports brassiere should consist of breathable (ie, minimizing sweating) material that is nonabrasive and is manufactured to have proper cups (soft, firm), few seams, and hooks that are few in number and padded in quality. Selected women may also benefit from brassieres with shoulder straps that are properly padded. A properly fitted sports brassiere lifts and carefully separates the mammary glands in a way that reduces or minimizes overt breast motion. As noted with sports equipment in general, sports bras should be changed often (eg, every 6 months). Guidelines for sports brassieres have been published by researchers and manufacturers.[28,36,45,46]

Asymmetry

Asymmetry of breasts is a common situation in growing adolescent females that resolves over time in most, although visible asymmetry remains in 1 in 4 adult women.[35,39] Examination should look for other causes, including a breast mass, although asymmetry is usually a normal variant in growth.[1,39] Injury to the breast may occur without proper protection, and padded brassiere and foam inserts should be used as needed; female swimmers with breast asymmetry can wear a swimming suit with breast supports. The athlete may find help at places that work with or specialize in patients who have had a mastectomy.

Galactorrhea

Females who present with nipple discharge not associated with pregnancy (galactorrhea) need a medical evaluation to look for a variety of causes, such as mental health concerns (eg, anxiety, depression), effect of medications (eg, phenothiazines, oral contraceptives), hypothyroidism, pituitary neoplasms, and hypothalamic injury (eg, infection, surgery).[1,39] Most cases are idiopathic and management depends on the underlying cause. For example, hypothyroidism can be corrected, neoplasm removed, implicated medication withdrawn, and counseling provided to stop self-manipulation if appropriate.

MENSTRUATION AND SPORTS
Menstrual Physiology

Under the influence of an activated hypothalamic-pituitary-ovarian-uterine axis, the adolescent female begins to have menstrual periods that are controlled by changes in pubertal hormones (ie, estrogen and progesterone), resulting in 3 menstrual phases: follicular, ovulatory, and luteal.[1,39,47] Estrogen is produced by the ovaries and its increase leads to the follicular menstrual phase, in which there is endometrial growth characterized by endometrial gland growth (number and length) within a compact, proliferative stroma. When ovulation occurs, at some point after menarche, estrogen and progesterone are produced by the corpus luteum, which induces a secretory endometrium because of progesterone effects. The last part of the normal menstrual cycle is the luteal phase, with development of an endometrium with an edematous stroma containing dilated, tortuous glands. If conception does not occur, the corpus luteum becomes atretic, with a resultant precipitous decrease in the pubertal hormones and eventual menstruation.

It may take 1 to several years to proceed from menarche to menstrual periods that are regular, and this complex phenomenon is subject to a wide variety of factors, many of which can be found in the sports-minded female. An adult female (or mature adolescent female) has a menstrual cycle that occurs every 28 days ($\pm$7 days); the median blood loss per cycle is 30 mL, with an upper normal limit of 60 to 90 mL of blood.[1,39,47]

Irregular (infrequent) menstruation that occur at intervals of more than 45 days is called oligomenorrhea. The absence of menstrual cycles (amenorrhea) can be identified as primary or secondary amenorrhea, in which primary amenorrhea refers to absence of menstrual cycles by age 14 years with no pubertal development (SMR or Tanner stage of 1) or absence of menses by age 16 years without respect to SMR rating. The absence of menses after menarche has occurred for a total of 3 previous periods or for 6 months without any periods after menarche is called secondary amenorrhea. Normal young females may have no menstrual periods for 3 to 6 months during years 1 and 2 after menarche. However, if an adolescent female presents with oligomenorrhea, primary amenorrhea, or secondary amenorrhea, the clinician should launch an investigation into potential causes (**Table 5**).[1,39,47]

Menstrual Cycles and Athletic Performance

Conflicting research results have been published regarding the effect of menstruation on female athletic performance.[16,47–49] One investigation of 86 female soccer players noted athletes reporting more injuries when having premenstrual symptoms than at any other menstrual phase, and anecdotal reports exist of exercise leading to increased menstrual bleeding or dysmenorrheal.[1,49] However, research tends to note fewer menstrual symptoms (ie, bleeding, pain, premenstrual symptoms) with exercise and no overt menstrual cycle-related differences in lactate levels, exertion efforts, or overall sports performance.[1]

Amenorrhea

Menstrual dysfunction is well known in female athletes and includes oligomenorrhea, amenorrhea (primary or secondary), and luteal phase dysfunction; this includes 10% to 15% of female athletes and two-thirds of elite athletes.[2,5,7,16,30,50–67] A delay of menarche can be seen at a level of 5 months for each year of intense training before the onset of puberty; if the athlete lowers her level of exercise training, menarche or return of menstrual cycles usually results.[1] Secondary amenorrhea is commonly seen in females engaging in such sports as distance running, ballet, gymnastics,

Table 5 Causes of amenorrhea in adolescents	
Primary amenorrhea	Physiologic delay
	Pseudoamenorrhea
	Imperforate hymen
	Transverse septum
	Rare: agenesis of vagina, cervix, uterus
	Mayer-Rokitansky-Kuster-Hauser syndrome
	Turner syndrome
	Chronic illness
	Hypothalmic-induced
	Such as weight loss, eating disorders, exercise, stress, others
	Pituitary disorders
	Polycystic ovary syndrome (hyperandrogenemia syndromes)
	Thyroid disorders
	Others
Secondary amenorrhea	Pregnancy
	Hypothalamic-induced
	Such as weight loss, eating disorders, exercise, stress
	Polycystic ovary syndrome (hyperandrogenemia syndromes)
	Thyroid disorders
	Pituitary disorders (pituitary adenoma)
	Chronic illness
	Others

Reprinted from Greydanus DE, Patel DR. The female athlete: before and beyond puberty. Pediatr Clin North Am 2002;49:563; with permission.

and cycling. Menstrual dysfunction is reported in 12% of swimmers as well as cyclists, up to 20% in females reporting vigorous exercise, 44% of ballet dancers, 50% of female triathletes, and 51% of endurance runners.[1,16]

Multiple issues underpin athletic amenorrhea, including genetics, percent body fat, intensity of exercise, age, weight, nutritional deficits, and stress.[68] The type of sport chosen can influence menstrual dysfunction as well. For example, dance and gymnastics support or encourage a female athlete with a thin body habitus. However, specific weight alone does not lead to absence of menstruation because those with the same weight can be amenorrheic or have a normal menstrual pattern. Specific body fat is not the sole factor and earlier research suggesting that menstruation does not occur in females with body fat less than 17% has not been verified by research.[1,4] The precise role of leptin in this complex process of menstruation is not clear.[69,70]

A wide variety of causes must be considered when a clinician evaluates an adolescent female with amenorrhea or other menstrual dysfunction.[1,39,47] Often, amenorrhea in such athletes is classified as hypothalamic amenorrhea, with gonadotropin-releasing hormone and luteinizing hormone pulsivity abnormality. One theory suggests that menstrual dysfunction in athletes results from an energy drain because of the intense exercise level associated with a caloric intake that is not sufficient to maintain normal menstruation.[16,71,72] Such an energy drain can be compounded by other issues, such as having a previous history for menstrual problems, positive family history for menstrual dysfunction, and chronic illness. Thus, any athlete with abnormal menses (ie, oligomenorrhea or amenorrhea) should receive a comprehensive evaluation.[1,39,47,52,54,66] The evaluation should investigate such positive findings as congenital anomalies, short stature, galactorrhea, virilization, hypoestrogenemia, and other endocrine findings or disorders (see **Table 5**).[1,39,47] Some suggested laboratory testing is listed in **Table 6**.

The specific causes of amenorrhea in an adolescent female determine precise management plans; if the menstrual dysfunction is related to her intense exercise patterns, advice should be given to decrease exercise intensity and increase nutritional intake along with providing calcium supplements (see later discussion).[16,73–79] Improvement in the amenorrhea or oligomenorrhea will occur if this advice is followed and if there are no other underlying causes.

Table 6
Laboratory testing for amenorrhea in adolescents
Pregnancy test
Thyroid hormone levels
Bone age
Antiovarian antibodies
Chromosome evaluation
Head CT/MRI
LH and FSH: ↓ in ovarian failure/dysgenesis; normal or ↑ in others
Pelvic/abdominal MRI
Pelvic ultrasound to define anatomy
Prolactin levels
Renal ultrasound/IVP
Vaginal smear to evaluate for epithelial cell estrogenization virilization/hirsutism: DHEAS, LH/FSH ratio (normal <2.5:1), testosterone (total and free)

Abbreviations: CT, computed tomography; DHEAS, dehydroepiandrosterone sulfate; FSH, follicle-stimulating hormone; IVP, intravenous pyelogram; MRI, magnetic resonance imaging.

However, the experienced clinician quickly learns that many if not most committed athletes do not want to reduce their exercise intensity for fear of decreasing their sports performance. They often continue in this sports pattern even when informed that their menstrual problems may be related to a pattern of chronic hypoestrogenemia that may lead to reduced bone mineral density (BMD), osteopenia, and eventual osteoporosis (see later discussion).[1,4] The research in this area is complex and more is needed. However, studies in recent decades note that females with chronic amenorrhea and low BMD may never acquire healthy BMD, even if the menstrual pattern eventually becomes normal.[1,80] Some female dancers and other athletes who have delayed menstruation progress into a state of low BMD and have an increased risk for stress fractures that can limit their sports performance.[1,4]

Experts generally recommend daily supplementation with calcium (1200–1500 mg) and vitamin D (400–800 IU) for the adolescent athlete with menstrual abnormalities or overt eating pattern dysfunction.[1,16] The literature remains conflicted about the use of estrogen supplementation (ie, conjugated estrogen or oral contraceptives) for those with exercise-induced low BMD in attempts to prevent lowering of the BMD. If the athlete has low BMD, estrogen supplementation (oral contraceptive or conjugated estrogen) may help in some cases to preserve some bone loss.[1,4,39,47]

One well-known approach is to avoid prescribing such hormonal treatments for amenorrheic athletes who are within 3 years of menarche, and clinicians should emphasize the need to lower the intensity of exercise workouts and the need for improved nutritional intake along with calcium supplementation.[81] Oral contraceptives are suggested if the athlete is 3 years after menarche, is more than 16 years of age, and is amenorrheic; earlier hormonal intervention is acceptable with a history of stress fracture.[81]

Clinical judgment is needed because there is no clear research-supported consensus on managing these young people and there is no proven benefit to providing such hormonal intervention to improve or preserve BMD with or without weight gain.[1,4] Use of combined oral contraceptives (COCs) does not correct the underlying physiologic dysfunction of this abnormal menstrual pattern and the amenorrhea or oligomenorrhea typically resumes once the COC is withdrawn. Side effects of the oral contraceptive can be distressing to some females; these include breast congestion, headache, and nausea.[1,47] Even with the past few decades of research and observation, it is not clear what the acute and long-term implications are for the female adolescent athlete with chronic amenorrhea and potential estrogen deficiency.[1,80]

Adolescents who are thin and inactive tend to have the lowest BMD. Also complicating this picture is that intense exercise with weight bearing may neutralize the low BMD effect of having a thin body habitus because of enhanced bone accretion. Thus, athletes in some sports (ie, tennis players, ice skaters, runners, gymnasts) who are amenorrheic may still have normal or even increased bone density because of exercise-induced high mechanical forces.[1] Some research has observed an enhanced bone density effect in some athletes if they are taking oral contraceptives; however, osteoporosis may not be prevented if the pill has less than 50 µg of ethinyl estradiol.[82] COCs more than 50 µg are not recommended for adolescent females because of the increased risks for adverse effects. Complicating this picture is the observation that the female acquires an increased risk for osteoporosis if she never acquires normal BMD.[1,83] More research is needed in this arena.

Oral Contraceptives and Athletic Performance

There is no evidence from research studies that athletic performance is reduced for females taking oral contraceptives.[51,84,85] COCs can provide a positive influence because of their beneficial effect on improving dysfunctional uterine bleeding (DUB), anemia related to DUB, dysmenorrhea, PMS, absence of pregnancy, possibly reduced injury risk in those with dysmenorrheal or PMS, possibly reduced bone mineral loss (see earlier discussion), and possibly less risk for stress fractures.[1,39,47,86–90]

Manipulation of COCs can be used to the athlete's advantage by allowing few menstrual cycles when she stays on active hormone pills for longer than usual.[1,4,39,47] For example, she can remain on a 21-day pack or not take the inactive pill that is part of the 28-day pack to prolong the interval between menstrual periods and thus avoid menstruation during an important sports event. Monophasic pills are less confusing to the female athlete than triphasic pills and provide more consistent hormone blood levels. However, concerns about potential adverse effects of COCs may prevent some athletes from going on or staying on these pills.[1,39,47] Also, pharmaceutical companies have now produced continuous pills to allow reduced menses. For example, current extended cycle hormonal contraceptive pills in the US market include Seasonale, Quasense, and Seasonique, which allow a menstrual period once every 3 months. Lybrel is an extended cycle hormonal formulation that is taken every day and prevents any menstrual period.

EXERCISE AND PREGNANCY

Sexually active women who do not take contraception or use contraceptives ineffectively are at risk for pregnancy. The pregnancy certainly affects their overall sports performance. However, if a woman becomes pregnant, she may wish to continue to exercise to some degree.[1,91–95] Concern has been expressed that excessive exercise induces diversion of blood away from the fetus to the mother's exercising muscles, with possible fetal hypoxia as a result, or that fetal hyperthermia may occur because of increased core temperature in the exercising pregnant woman. The fetus is well insulated from these potential adverse effects of exercise and studies have not found these theories to be valid; thus, some physical activity is acceptable to clinicians and guidelines in this regard have been published to offer advice for the pregnant woman.[95] Sensible exercise is recommended and includes swimming as perhaps the best form of exercise during pregnancy, but other forms of exercise are recommended, such as walking and cycling.

Table 7 lists specific contraindications to exercise in the pregnant woman and **Table 8** provides reasons for reduced sports performance during pregnancy. Exercise should be based on acceptable guidelines and common sense for each specific woman based on her prepregnancy exercise pattern. Workouts and physical exertion that were not included in exercise patterns before the pregnancy should not be attempted during pregnancy. Excessive exercise is limited to 15 minutes, although strenuous anaerobic activity is typically never recommended. In addition to avoidance

Table 7
Contraindications to exercise in pregnancy
Hypertension induced by pregnancy
Preterm membrane rupture
Second or third trimester bleeding that is persistent
Intrauterine growth retardation
Incompetent cervix or cerclage
History of preterm labor or presence of preterm labor in a current pregnancy

Data from Refs.[91–95]

Table 8
Pregnancy-induced factors that may negatively affect sports performance
Abdominal growth
Adipose tissue
Altered center of gravity
Breast ducts
Cardiac output
Fluid retention
Ligamentous laxity (caused by increased estrogen and relaxin levels)
Maternal blood volume
Overall expenditure of energy

or limitation of excessive exercise, physical exertion should be avoided in very hot weather and cease if the mother has a fever (ie, more than 38°C). Pregnancy increases breast congestion and nipple prominence; thus, a well-fitted, supportive brassiere is necessary. Physical exertion using the upper body is permitted but it should not subject the upper torso to overt or excessive mechanical stress.

The pregnant athlete who is exercising should always be well hydrated and should cease exertion under specific conditions, such as the occurrence of dizziness, shortness of breath, vaginal bleeding, severe headache, tachycardia (pulse more than 180 beats per minute), muscle weakness, or pain in the chest, hips, back, or elsewhere. Jumping may lead to relaxation and pelvic ligament stretching and is thus not recommended. Also avoided is exercising in the supine position, even if this was practiced before the pregnancy developed. Several sporting activities should be avoided during pregnancy, including horseback riding, weight lifting, and scuba diving and other water sports.

Engaging in competitive sporting activities is not recommended, especially when the risk of injury is substantial and the activity is classified as a contact sport. After delivery, exercise may resume in 4 to 6 weeks after a vaginal delivery and 6 to 8 weeks after a cesarean section.[95] Breastfeeding is not a contraindication for exercise in the mother.[96] Diabetes mellitus in the pregnant woman is not a contraindication to sensible exercise if approved by her clinician and if the metabolic state is stable and closely monitored.[97]

FEMALE ATHLETE TRIAD

The female athlete who becomes seriously engaged in her sports, especially sports that emphasize specific weight or body size, is at risk for what has been called the female athlete triad: amenorrhea, disordered eating, and osteoporosis (osteopenia).[5,7,52–54,58,60,66–68] Although not accepted by all researchers, the term is useful because it reminds clinicians of 3 important issues that may complicate the lives of adolescent athletes. It reminds clinicians that some sports may be more precarious for adolescent females than others, specifically those that focus on various weight categories, lean appearance, prepubertal appearance, or a lean body (**Table 9**). These athletes may struggle to attain an ideal sports body because their sport seems to demand goals that are difficult to achieve unless the athlete develops abnormal eating patterns that induce or promote nutritional deficiencies and abnormal exercise patterns. The result is a condition that may contain various components of this triad.[52–54,56]

Table 9 Sports that increase risks for the features of the female athlete triad	
Emphasis on various weight categories	Judo Rowing Taekwondo Weight lifting Wrestling
Emphasis on a prepubertal appearance	Ballet Figure skating Gymnastics
Emphasis on a lean body	Cross-country skiing Long-distance running Swimming
Emphasis on lean appearance	Dance Diving Figure skating Gymnastics Synchronized swimming

Disordered Eating

Dysfunctional eating schedules are noted in 15% to 75% of adolescent female athletes and are characterized by a combination of self-induced vomiting, fasting, skipping meals, and consumption of diet pills, laxatives, and/or diuretics.[1,73,75–77,98] Critical windows of time occur in the lives of these athletes when they become more vulnerable to developing such abnormal eating patters, such as the period of PHV, transition to high school or college (university), giving up sports competition, death (eg, member of the family, coach, trainer, friends), and postpartum depression.[1] Sports that insist on intense exercise patterns and/or low body weights (ie, < what is physiologically normal) are sports with athletes at increased risk for the development of poor eating habits; these sports include but are not limited to swimming, diving, track, distance running, and gymnastics (see **Table 9**).[1,54]

Anorexia Nervosa

The increased risk for eating dysfunction is found in dedicated adolescent athletes, although most do not develop overt bulimia nervosa or anorexia nervosa. However, 5% to 20% of ballet dancers may develop anorexia nervosa; the incidence is associated with the intensity of exercise as well as level of competition.[1,4] Hypothalamic amenorrhea occurs in these athletes with anorexia nervosa who develop disordered eating of a severe degree that leads to low bone density at a critical time of bone development, when they need to gain bone density not lose it.[1,98]

The presence of anorexia nervosa in athletes and nonathletes may lead to osteopenia because of starvation, deficiency of estrogen, lowered intake of calcium, low BMD, increased glucocorticoid levels, and other factors. Research notes that osteopenia develops early and often in the female with anorexia nervosa and depletes normal bone health so much that she never develops normal BMD even if management eventually allows a return to normal weight. Her risk for development of overt osteoporosis (see earlier discussion) as an adult has also been noted by research studies.

Prevention of reduced BMD and disordered eating patterns is the best management strategy; however, if this is not possible, intense management should be directed to allow return to a normal weight as soon as possible during the adolescent years while an increase in BMD is still possible. As noted earlier, prescribing conjugated estrogen formulations (such as the COC) have been used to increase BMD in those with anorexia nervosa and severe malnutrition. There is no overt proof that use of estrogen combinations restores normal bone density in adolescent athletes with anorexia nervosa. BMD may optimize in females with anorexia nervosa who resume normal menstruation.[1,4] Current research implies that BMD is not protected by such estrogen supplementation without weight gain and this becomes a major conundrum of sports participation for female adolescents and their caring clinicians.[1]

Osteoporosis and Adolescence

There are various factors critical to osteoporosis acquisition, such as genetics (70%), estrogen status, calcium intake, exercise patterns, and body weight (**Table 10**).[1,76,98–112] Studies reveal that 50% to 63% of peak bone mass (ie, BMD amount gained during growth) develops during childhood, whereas up to 50% accumulates during the adolescent years.[1] During growth it is critical that sufficient amounts of calcium are acquired into BMD to maximize bone mineralization and gains are greatest during early pubertal periods if sufficient estrogen and calcium are available. Classic studies on females in late adolescence (ie, ages 17 to 20 years) reveal that no significant BMD increase was found after age 17 years.[113] In general, BMD usually decreases in the middle of the fourth decade, with significant lowering when menopause starts in the fifth or sixth decade of life. In addition, weight resistance training can lead to a 4.5% increase in BMD for 1 year in females who are postmenopausal in contrast to those not exercising or training.[99]

Adolescent females with delayed menarche and thin body habitus tend to have the lowest BMD and as noted, suboptimal BMD is found in adolescents with menstrual dysfunction (ie, amenorrhea or oligomenorrhea) complicated by anorexia nervosa or other features of hypothalamic amenorrhea, such as found in athletes with intense exercise patterns and weight loss.[1,4] Estrogen facilitates calcium movement into bone, and thus those with chronic, hypoestrogenic amenorrhea (including postmenopausal states) develop significant risk for osteoporosis and stress fractures.[1] Thus, dancers, runners, and other female athletes as well as those with eating disorders have increased incidence of stress fractures during their careers, even as adolescents.

As noted with eating disorders, the best management for osteopenia (and osteoporosis) is prevention, by preventing the various factors noted in **Table 10** from taking

Table 10
Risk factors for osteoporosis
Limited calcium intake in childhood/adolescence
Positive family history (first-degree relatives) for osteoporosis
Low levels of physical (weight-bearing) activity
History of amenorrhea/irregular menses
Thin habitus (anorexia nervosa, others)
Alcoholism (toxic to bone-building cells and possibly induces decreased calcium absorption)
Cigarette smoking (decreases estrogen effectiveness)
Medications (glucocorticoids, phenytoin, others)
Various chronic diseases (primary hyperparathyroidism, Cushing syndrome, Addison disease, leukemia, celiac disease, Crohn disease, others)
Others[1,101]

Reprinted from Greydanus DE, Patel DR. The female athlete: before and beyond puberty. Pediatr Clin North Am 2002;49:565; with permission.

root in the adolescent athlete. Always advise the athlete to eschew low intake of calcium because this is a significant factor in later development of osteoporosis. The adolescent female accumulates up to 240 mg of calcium in the bone mass each day, whereas the male adds 400 mg per day; increased calcium amounts are added during periods of rapid growth. All children, adolescents, and their parents (guardians) should be taught that a major issue in later osteoporosis development is to ensure sufficient calcium intake during childhood and adolescence. Adolescents have a daily calcium requirement of 1200 to 1500 mg, and another 400 mg per day is added for pregnant or breastfeeding women.[1,78] There are many foods rich in calcium, such as canned sardines, salmon (with bones), tofu, skim milk, and yogurt (plain, nonfat). Calcium absorption can be enhanced with vitamin D, phosphorus, and citric acid, whereas inhibition of calcium absorption is noted with phytates, oxalates, and iron.

Other factors in osteoporosis development include physical inactivity, drug abuse (particularly nicotine addiction), and estrogen deficiency. Individuals at increased risk for low BMD or osteopenia should be cautioned about use of depomedroxyprogesterone acetate (Depo-Provera) because research has revealed it leads to bone loss.[1,114–118] As noted earlier, weight-resistant exercising may be beneficial in the prevention of stress fractures.

INJURIES

Injuries in female and male adolescent athletes are generally the same for the same sports played, with the exception of an increase in anterior cruciate ligament (ACL) (noncontact) and patellofemoral disorders (PFD) in females.[9,10,119–126] The specific sport and intensity of play and not the gender of the athlete determine the prevalence and nature of injuries in most situations. Reduction of injuries in both genders is based on such basic and time-honored principles as appropriate sports equipment, proper training, and expert attention to exercise- or sports-related injuries before, during, and after the specific sport season. The athlete with low BMD, such as an amenorrheic female, is at increased risk for stress fractures with exercise, especially if the exertion is intense. Approximately half of all sports injuries in both genders are associated with overuse injuries characterized by microtrauma-induced damage to musculotendinous units. Lumbar spine and knee injures are common in female and male athletes involved in gymnastics, basketball, and volleyball.

The reasons for an increased prevalence of PFD in female athletes are not clear and remain unproven.[119–126] Cause is linked to such factors as the controversial concept of the female having an increased Q angle linked to a pelvis that is wider and a femoral notch that is narrower versus the male athlete; other cited factors include increased flexibility, muscles that are not so developed (eg, the vastus medialis obliquus), greater genu valgum, and increased external tibial tortion seen in the female.[13] Some research identifies neuromuscular reflex patterns specific to females as contributing to PFD and ACL injuries.[1,16]

Estrogen and progestin receptors are found in knee synovial tissues and this may be involved as well in injury tendencies of female athletes, although more research is needed.[1] Some research has suggested that there are increased ACL injuries during the ovulatory phase of the menstrual period versus other menstrual phases.[1] Studies note that foot problems in the female athlete are related to females often wearing sports shoes that were designed for the anatomy of males; these injuries include corns, bunions, calluses, and metatarsalgia.[1,16]

BREAST INJURIES
Nipple Injury

The nipple is often the breast part most injured in sports because it is the most prominent breast part. Jogging or other breast motion during exercise can lead to abrasive nipple injury (acute or chronic) as a result of constant or frequent nipple rubbing. It is sometimes called jogger's nipple in male and female runners, associated with shirts that are tight-fitting as well as brassieres or other irritating clothes in contact with the nipples.[127–130] Nipple abrasion and trauma worsens if the nipple(s) stay in contact with any irritating or abrasive clothing or object while the sports-related motion continues. In 1 report there was a 20:1 male/female ratio of such trauma to nipples in marathon runners.[129] Complicating this injury is the presence of cold air and/or direct stimulation, which can induce nipple musculature to produce a prominent nipple. Painful, raw, and even bleeding nipples in bicycle riders exposed to cold air or wind have led to the term bicyclist's nipple.[130]

To prevent this exercise-induced nipple injury, various steps of prevention are recommended, such as always using properly fitted sports brassieres and other measures as presented in **Table 11**. Always use good hygiene, reduce or prevent nipple trauma, and provide antibiotic management if secondary infection occurs. The clinician should also remember that a painful, bleeding nipple may also be suggestive of other diagnoses, such as nipple intraductal papilloma or carcinoma.[1,39,47]

Other Breast Injury

Direct trauma to breast tissue may also occur during sports play and although not common may result in breast contusion, abrasion, hematoma, or laceration.[1,39,47] The mechanism of such damage to mammary gland tissue may be from falls, seatbelt injuries, kicks, injuries from elbows, or abrasion injury from brassiere parts (ie, clips, straps, hooks, metal underwire).[1] Contusion of the breast is typically mild and caused by superficial capillary rupture, resulting in edema and ecchymosis that normally resolves within 21 days. A breast hematoma occurs because of a forceful hit, leading to deep blood vessel bleeding that may resolve into fat necrosis that has secondary induration, scarring, and even calcification for many years; this calcification may be misdiagnosed later as breast carcinoma. Breast trauma can also lead to mastitis or breast abscess. **Table 12** outlines basic management principles for such breast injuries. A laceration of the breast is typically closed surgically and then the athlete is followed for potential development of a painful breast abscess (see **Table 12**).

Thrombophlebitis of the superficial breast veins is called Mondor disease and may be a rare complication of breast trauma; however, history of breast injury is often not

Table 11
Prevention of exercise-induced nipple injury
Before and during the physical activity, use a plastic bandage or petroleum jelly
Females should always wear a properly fitted sports brassiere
Try to avoid exercising in cold weather
Wind-breaking clothes can be placed over the chest area
Remember that nipple prominence and injury risk are increased in pregnancy

Data from Greydanus DE, Patel DR. The female athlete: before and beyond puberty. Pediatr Clin North Am 2002;49:560.

Table 12 Management of trauma-related breast injuries	
Contusion	Application of cold every 15–20 minutes for several hours Appropriate analgesia Firm support
Abrasion	Direct pressure to control bleeding Suturing may be necessary
Laceration	Close with steri-strips or sutures Use good hygiene principles Apply a firm postclosure dressing She should wear a supportive brassiere (including at night) Pain and swelling can be reduced with a cold pack Provide a tetanus toxoid if warranted Antibiotics may be needed, depending on the situation
Hematoma	Most resolve without treatment Surgical aspiration may be necessary

Reprinted from Greydanus DE, Patel DR. The female athlete: before and beyond puberty. Pediatr Clin North Am 2002;49:560; with permission.

identified.[1,39,47] There is usually spontaneous and full resolution. Females with augmentation surgery with silicone breast implants may develop implant rupture, bleeding, and breast deformity if subjected to direct breast trauma.

SUMMARY

After centuries of being excluded from sports play, the female athlete has become a common part of competitive and noncompetitive sports activity in the twenty-first century around the world.[1,131] Male and female prepubertal athletes have basically the same physical potential in such parameters as weight, height, endurance, motor skills, strength (see **Table 2**), body fat percentages, hemoglobin levels, and injury risks. Puberty changes these dynamics in the female. Important issues for the female athlete include IDA, SUI, breast issues (eg, pain, asymmetry, injury), female athlete triad (menstrual dysfunction, abnormal eating patterns, osteopenia or osteoporosis), effects of oral contraception and menstruation on sports performance, and exercise during pregnancy.[1,131–137] Pediatricians can encourage the safe and rewarding sports play of adolescent females and help them prevent or manage such sports-related phenomena so they can stay in the game and prepare for a lifetime of exercise for their enhanced health and enjoyment.[1,3,4,137]

REFERENCES

1. Greydanus DE, Patel DR. The female athlete: before and beyond puberty. Pediatr Clin North Am 2002;49:553–80.
2. Joy EA, Van Hala S, Cooper L. Health-related concerns of the female athlete: a lifespan approach. Am Fam Physician 2009;79(6):79–84.
3. Greydanus DE, Tsitsika AK. Special considerations for the female athlete. In: Patel DR, Greydanus DE, Baker RJ, editors. Pediatric practice: sports medicine. New York: McGraw-Hill Medical Publishers; 2009. p. 86–101. Chapter 9.
4. Greydanus DE, Patel DR. Medical aspects of the female athlete at puberty. International Sportmed J 2004;5(1):1–25.

5. Griffin LY. The female athlete. In: DeLee JC, Drez D Jr, Miller MD, editors. DeLee & Drez's orthopaedic sports medicine. Principles and practice. Philadelphia: Elsevier/Saunders; 2003. p. 505–20. Chapter 13.

6. Piya-Anant M. Common gynecologic problems in female athletes. Siriraj Med J 2008;60(6):366–7.

7. Nattiv A, Arendt EA, Hecht SS. The female athlete. In: Garrett WE, Kirkendall DT, Squire DL, editors. Principles and practice of primary care sport medicine. Philadelphia: Lippincott Williams and Wilkins; 2001. p. 93–113. Chapter 8.

8. Beunen G, Malina RM. Growth and physical performance relative to the timing of the adolescent spurt. Exerc Sport Sci Rev 1988;16:503.

9. Greydanus DE, Patel DR, Luckstead EF. Office orthopedics and sports medicine symposium. Adolesc Med 1998;9:425–626.

10. Patel DR, Nelson TL. Sport injuries in adolescents. Pediatr Clin North Am 2000; 84:983–1007.

11. Wilmore JH. The application of science to sport: physiologic profiles of male and female athletes. Can J Appl Sport Sci 1979;4:103–15.

12. Komi PV, editor. Strength and power in sport. Oxford (UK): Blackwell Scientific; 1992. p. 404.

13. Ireland ML. Special concerns of the female athlete. In: Fu F, Stone R, editors. Sports injuries: mechanisms, prevention and treatment. 2nd edition. Baltimore (MD): Williams and Wilkins; 2000. p. 156–87.

14. Malina RM. Effects of physical activities on growth in stature and adolescent growth spurt. Med Sci Sports Exerc 1994;26:759.

15. Malina RM. Physical growth and biological maturation of young athletes. Exerc Sport Sci Rev 1994;22:389.

16. Yurko-Griffin L, Harris SS. Female athletes. In: Sullivan A, Anderson S, editors. Care of the young athlete. Rosemont (IL): American Academy of Orthopedic Surgery and American Academy of Pediatrics; 2000. p. 137–48. Chapter 15.

17. Kulkarni R, Gera R, Scott-Emuakpor AB. Adolescent hematology. In: Greydanus DE, Patel DR, Pratt HD, editors. Essential adolescent medicine. New York: McGraw-Hill Medical Publishers; 2006. p. 371–90. Chapter 17.

18. Patel DR. Hematologic conditions. In: Patel DR, Greydanus DE, Baker RJ, editors. Pediatric practice: sports medicine. New York: McGraw-Hill Medical Publishers; 2009. p. 167–80. Chapter 16.

19. Harris SS. Exercise-related anemia. In: Drinkwater BA, editor. Women in sport. Oxford (UK): Blackwell Scientific; 2000. p. 311–20. Chapter 21.

20. Risser WL, Risser JM. Iron deficiency in adolescent and young adults. Phys Sportsmed 1990;18:87–101.

21. Balaban E, Cox J, Snell P, et al. The frequency of anemia and iron deficiency in the runner. Med Sci Sports Exerc 1989;21:643–8.

22. Greydanus DE, Torres AD, Wan JH. Genitourinary and renal disorders. In: Greydanus DE, Patel DR, Pratt HD, editors. Essential adolescent medicine. New York: McGraw-Hill Medical Publishers; 2006. p. 329–70. Chapter 16.

23. Nattiv A. Track and field. In: Drinkwater BA, editor. Women in sport. Oxford (UK): Blackwell Scientific; 2000. p. 470–85. Chapter 32.

24. Gera T, Sachdev HP, Nestel P. Effect of iron supplementation on physical performance in children and adolescents: systemic review of randomized controls. Indian Pediatr 2007;44(1):15–24.

25. Bo K. Urinary incontinence, pelvic floor dysfunction, exercise, and sports. Sports Med 2004;34(7):451–64.

26. Fine PM. Urinary symptoms: incontinence. In: Hillard PJA, editor. The 5-minute obstetrics and gynecology consult. Philadelphia: Wolters Kluwer/Lippincott Williams & Wilkins; 2008. p. 46–7.

27. NIH Consensus Development Panel. Urinary incontinence in adults. JAMA 1989; 261:2685–90.

28. Hindle WH. The breast and exercise. In: Hale W, editor. Caring for the exercising woman. New York: Elsevier Science Publishers; 1991. p. 83–92. Chapter 8.

29. Kaul P, Beach RK. Breast disorders. In: Greydanus DE, Patel DR, Pratt HD, editors. Essential adolescent medicine. New York: McGraw-Hill Medical Publishers; 2006. p. 569–90. Chapter 27.

30. Shangold MM. Gynecologic concerns in the woman athlete. Clin Sports Med 1984;3:869–79.

31. Friedenreich CM, Rohan TE. A review of physical activity and beast cancer. Epidemiology 1995;6:311–7.

32. Thune I, Brenn T, Lund E, et al. Physical activity and the risk of breast cancer. N Engl J Med 1997;336:1269–75.

33. Hoffman-Goetz L, Husted J. Exercise and breast cancer: review and critical analysis of the literature. Can J Appl Physiol 1994;19:237–52.

34. Frisch RE, Wyshank G, Albright NL, et al. Lower prevalence of breast cancer and cancers of the reproductive system among former college athletes compared to nonathletes. Br J Cancer 1995;52:885–91.

35. Greydanus DE, Patel DR, Baxter TL. The breast and sports: issues for the clinician. Adolesc Med 1998;9:533–50.

36. Haycock CE. How I manage breast problems in athletes. Phys Sportsmed 1987; 15:89–95.

37. Gehlsen S, Stoner LJ. The female breast in sports and exercise. Med Sport Sci 1987;24:13–22.

38. Greydanus DE, Tsitsika AD, Gains MJ. The gynecology system and the adolescent. In: Greydanus DE, Feinberg AN, Patel DR, et al, editors. Pediatric physical diagnosis. New York: McGraw-Hill Medical Publishers; 2008. p. 701–50. Chapter 21.

39. Greydanus DE, Matytsina L. Breast disorders in children and adolescents. Prim Care Clin Office Pract 2006;33:455–502.

40. Gehlsen G, Albohm M. Evaluation of sports bras. Phys Sportsmed 1980;8: 88–97.

41. Lorentzen D, Lawson L. Selected sports bras: a biomechanical analysis for breast motion while jogging. Phys Sportsmed 1987;15:128.

42. Berger-Dumound J. Sports bras: everything you need to know from A to D. Women's Sports and Fitness 1986;8:31–49.

43. Cummins C. Sports bra round-up. Women's Sports Fitness 1989;4:66.

44. Lee J. Sport support. Women's Sports and Fitness 1995;17:72–3.

45. American Society for Testing and Materials (ASTM). Standard classification of brassieres. 1982 Yearbook Standard F753-82. Philadelphia: ASTM; 1982.

46. Sports bras. Women's Sports and Fitness 1995;17:72.

47. Greydanus DE, Omar HA, Tsitsika AK, et al. Menstrual disorders in adolescent females: current concepts. Dis Mon 2009;55(2):39–114.

48. Pfeifer S, Patrizio P. The female athlete: some gynecological considerations. Sports Med Athlet Rev 2002;10(1):2–9.

49. Moller-Nielson J, Hammar M. Women's soccer injuries in relation to the menstrual cycle and oral contraceptive use. Med Sci Sports Exerc 1989;21:152–60.

50. Redman LM, Loucks AB. Menstrual disorders in athletes. Sports Med 2005; 35(9):747–55.

51. Ireland ML, Ott SM. Special concerns of the female athlete. Clin Sports Med 2004;23:623–36.
52. Beals KA, Meyer NL. Female athlete triad update. Clin Sports Med 2007;26: 69–89.
53. Nattive A, Loucks AB, Manore MM, et al. American College of Sports Medicine Position Stand. The female athlete triad. Med Sci Sports Exerc 2007;39: 1867–82.
54. Brunet M II. Female athlete triad. Clin Sports Med 2005;24:623–36.
55. Constantini NW, Gubnov G, Lebrun CM. The menstrual cycle and sports performance. Clin Sports Med 2005;24:51–82.
56. American Academy of Pediatrics. Medical concerns in the female athlete. Pediatrics 2000;106:610–3.
57. Greenfield TP, Blythe M. Menstrual disorders in adolescents. In: Greydanus DE, Patel DR, Pratt HD, editors. Essential adolescent medicine. New York: McGraw-Hill Medical Publishers; 2006. p. 591–612. Chapter 28.
58. Gutterman DD, Hoffmann RG, Moraski L. Prevalence of the female athlete triad in high school athletes and sedentary students. Clin J Sport Med 2009;19(5): 421–8.
59. Callahan LR. The evolution of the female athlete: progress and problems. Pediatr Ann 2000;29:149–53.
60. Nichols JF, Rauh MJ, Lwson MJ, et al. Prevalence of female athlete triad among high school athletes. Pediatrics 2008;160(2):137–42.
61. Cobb KL, Bachrach LK, Greendale G, et al. Disordered eating, menstrual irregularity, and bone mineral density in female runners. Med Sci Sports Exerc 2003;35: 711–9.
62. Marshall LA. Amenorrhoea. In: Drinkwater BA, editor. Women in sport. Oxford (UK): Blackwell Scientific; 2000. p. 377–90. Chapter 26.
63. The Practice Committee of the American Society for Reproductive Medicine. Current evaluation of amenorrhea. Fertil Steril 2006;86(Suppl 4):S148–55.
64. Loucks AB, Vaitukaitis J, Cameron JL. The reproductive system and exercise in women. Med Sci Sports Exerc 1992;24(Suppl):S288–93.
65. Marshall LA. Clinical evaluation of amenorrhea in active and athletic women. Clin Sports Med 1994;13:371–89.
66. Hobart JA, Smucker DR. The female athlete triad. Am Fam Physician 2000;61: 357–64.
67. Yeager KK, Agostini R, Nattive A, et al. The female athlete triad: disordered eating, amenorrhea, osteoporosis. Med Sci Sports Exerc 1993;25:775–7.
68. DeSouza MJ, Williams NI, Alleyne J, et al. Correction of misinterpretations and misrepresentations of the female athlete triad. Br J Sports Med 2007;41(1): 58–9.
69. Laughlin GA, Yen SS. Hypoleptinemia in women athletes: absence of a diurnal rhythm with amenorrhea. J Clin Endocrinol Metab 1997;82:318–21.
70. Thong FS, McLean C, Graham TE. Plasma leptin in female athletics: relationship with body fat, reproductive, nutritional and endocrine factors. J Appl Physiol 2000;88:2037–44.
71. Loucks AB, Strachenfeld NS, DiPetro L. The female athlete triad: do female athletes need to take special care to avoid low energy availability? Med Sci Sports Exerc 2006;38:1694–700.
72. DeSouza MJ, Lee DK, Van Heest JL, et al. Severity of energy-related menstrual disturbances increases in proportion to indices of energy conservation in exercising women. Fertil Steril 2007;88(4):971–5.

73. Sundgot-Borgen J. Eating disorders. In: Drinkwater BA, editor. Women in sport. Oxford (UK): Blackwell Scientific; 2000. p. 364–76. Chapter 25.
74. American Psychiatric Association. Practice guideline for the treatment of patients with eating disorders, 3rd edition. Am J Psychiatry 2006;163(1 Suppl):4–54.
75. Sanborn CF, Horea M, Siemers BJ, et al. Disordered eating and the female athlete triad. Clin Sports Med 2000;19:1–11.
76. Mitan LAP. Diet, eating disorders: anorexia nervosa. In: Hillard PJA, editor. The 5-minute obstetrics and gynecology consult. Philadelphia: Wolters Kluwer/Lippincott Williams & Wilkins; 2008. p. 268–9.
77. Currie A, Morse ED. Eating disorders in athletes: managing the risks. Clin Sports Med 2005;24:871–83.
78. National Institutes of Health. Optimal calcium intake. NIH Consensus Statement 1994;12:1–31.
79. Teegarden D, Weaver CM. Calcium supplementation increases bone density in adolescent girls. Nutr Rev 1994;52:171.
80. Hergenroder AC, Smith EO, Shypailo R, et al. Bone mineral changes in young women with hypothalamic amenorrhea treated with oral contraceptives, medroxyprogesterone, or placebo over 12 months. Am J Obstet Gynecol 1997; 176(5):1017–25.
81. American Academy of Pediatrics. Amenorrhea in adolescent athletes. Pediatrics 1989;84:394–5.
82. Polatti F, Perotti F, Filippa N, et al. Bone mass and long-term monophasic oral contraceptive treatment in young women. Contraception 1995;51:221–4.
83. Rosen CJ, editor. Primer on the metabolic bone diseases and disorders of mineral metabolism. 6th edition. Hoboken (NJ): Wiley and Sons Publishers. American Society for Bone and Mineral Research; 2006.
84. Frankovich RJ, Lebrun CM. Muscle cycle, contraception and performance. Clin Sports Med 2000;19:1–6.
85. Labrun CM. Effects of the menstrual cycle and oral contraceptives on sports performance. In: Drinkwater BA, editor. Women in sport. Oxford (UK): Blackwell Scientific; 2000. p. 37–61. Chapter 3.
86. Greydanus DE, Patel DR, Rimsza ME. Contraception in the adolescent: an update. Pediatrics 2001;107:562–73.
87. Greydanus DE, Rimsza ME, Matytsina L. Contraception for college students. Pediatr Clin North Am 2005;52:135–61.
88. Kamboj MK. Metabolic bone disease in adolescents: recognition, evaluation, treatment, and prevention. Adolesc Med 2007;18:24–46.
89. Moller-Nielson J, Hammar M. Sports injuries and oral contraceptive use: is there a relationship? Sports Med 1991;12:152–60.
90. Paupoo A, Glass MLS. Osteoporosis and osteopenia. In: Hillard PJA, editor. The 5-minute obstetrics and gynecology consult. Philadelphia: Wolters Kluwer/Lippincott Williams & Wilkins; 2008. p. 130–1.
91. Morris SN. Exercise during pregnancy: a critical appraisal of the literature. J Reprod Med 2005;50:81–8.
92. Weiss Kelly AK. Practical exercise advice during pregnancy: guidelines for active and inactive women. Phys Sportsmed 2005;33(6):1–10.
93. Mottola MF, Wolfe LA. The pregnant athlete. In: Drinkwater BA, editor. Women in sport. Oxford (UK): Blackwell Science; 2000. p. 194–207. Chapter 14.
94. DeHoop TA. Exercise in normal pregnancy. In: Hillard PJA, editor. The 5-minute obstetrics and gynecology consult. Philadelphia: Wolters Kluwer/Lippincott Williams & Wilkins; 2008. p. 342–3.

95. American College of Obstetrics and Gynecology (ACOG) Committee on Obstetric Practice. Exercise and the postpartum period. ACOG Committee Opinion No. 267. Obstet Gynecol 2002;99(1):171–3.
96. Prentice A. Should lactating women exercise? Nutr Rev 1994;52:358–60.
97. Campaigne BN. Diabetes and sport. England. In: Drinkwater BA, editor. Women in sport. Oxford (UK): Blackwell Scientific; 2000. p. 265–79. Chapter 18.
98. Golden NH. Eating disorders: anorexia nervosa and bulimia nervosa in the adolescent. In: Greydanus DE, Patel DR, Pratt HD, editors. Essential adolescent medicine. New York: McGraw-Hill Medical Publishers; 2006. p. 635–50. Chapter 30.
99. Nelson ME, Fiatarone MA, Morganti CM, et al. Effects of high-intensity strength training on multiple risk factors for osteoporotic fractures. JAMA 1994;272:1909.
100. Gibson JH, Mitchell A, Harries MG, et al. Nutritional and exercise-related determinants of bone density in elite female runners. Osteoporos Int 2004;15:611–8.
101. Rutherford OM. Spine and total body bone mineral density in amenorrheic endurance athletes. J Appl Phys 1993;74:2904–8.
102. Nelson ME, Fisher EC, Catsos D, et al. Diet and bone status in amenorrheic runners. Am J Clin Nutr 1986;43:910–6.
103. Fruth SJ, Worrell TW. Factors associated with menstrual irregularities and decreased bone mineral density in female athletes. J Orthop Sports Phys Ther 1995;22:26–38.
104. Linnell ST, Stager JM, Blue PW, et al. Bone mineral content and menstrual regularity in female runners. Med Sci Sports Exerc 1984;16:343–8.
105. Snyder AC, Wenderoth MP, Johnston CC, et al. Bone mineral content of elite lightweight amenorrheic women. Hum Biol 1986;58:863–9.
106. Rosenthal DI, Mayo-Smith W, Hayes CW, et al. Age and bone mass in premenopausal women. J Bone Miner Res 1989;4:533–8.
107. Wolman RL, Clark P, McNally E, et al. Menstrual state and exercise as determinants of spinal trabecular bone density in female athletes. Br Med J 1990;301:516–8.
108. Harber VJ, Webber CE, Sutton JD, et al. The effect of amenorrhea on calcaneal bone density and total bone turnover in runners. Int J Sports Med 1991;12:505–8.
109. Warren MP, Brooks-Gunn J, Fox RP, et al. Lack of bone accretion and amenorrhea: evidence for a relative osteopenia in weight bearing bones. J Clin Endocrinol Metab 1991;72:847–53.
110. Wolman RL, Clark P, McNally E, et al. Dietary calcium as a statistical determinant of spinal trabecular bone density in amenorrheic and estrogen-replete athletes. Bone Miner 1992;17:415–23.
111. Lane JM, Riley EH, Wirganowicz PC. Osteoporosis: diagnosis and treatment. J Bone Joint Surg Am 1996;78:618.
112. Lloyd T, Meyers C, Buchanan JR, et al. Collegiate women athletes with irregular menses during adolescence have decreased bone density. Obstet Gynecol 1998;72:639–42.
113. Theintz G, Buchs B, Rizzoli R, et al. Longitudinal monitoring of bone mass accumulation in healthy adolescents: evidence from a marked reduction after 16 years of age at the levels of lumbar spine and femoral neck in female subjects. J Clin Endocrinol Metab 1992;75:1060–5.
114. American College of Obstetricians and Gynecologists. Use of hormonal contraception in women with coexisting medical conditions. ACOG Practice Bulletin, Number 73. Obstet Gynecol 2006;107:1453–72.
115. Emery-Cohen A, Kaunitz AM. Contraception: hormonal: injection. In: Hillard PJA, editor. The 5-minute obstetrics and gynecology consult. Philadelphia: Wolters Kluwer/Lippincott Williams & Wilkins; 2008. p. 250–1.

116. Schrager SB. DMPA's effect on bone mineral density: a particular concern for adolescents. J Fam Pract 2009;58(5):E1–8.

117. Cromer BA, Scholes D, Berenson A, et al. Depot medroxyprogesterone acetate and bone mineral density in adolescents. The black box warning: a position paper of the Society for Adolescent Medicine. J Adolesc Health 2006;39: 296–301.

118. Gibson J. Osteoporosis. In: Drinkwater BA, editor. Women in sport. Oxford (UK): Blackwell Scientific; 2000. p. 391–406. Chapter 27.

119. Cline S. Acute injuries of the knee. In: Patel DR, Greydanus DE, Baker RJ, editors. Pediatric practice: sports medicine. New York: McGraw-Hill Medical Publishers; 2009. p. 313–29. Chapter. 26.

120. Patel DR, Luckstead Sr EF, Greydanus DE. Sports injuries. In: Greydanus DE, Patel DR, Pratt HD, editors. Essential adolescent medicine. New York: McGraw-Hill Medical Publishers; 2006. p. 677–92. Chapter 33.

121. Loud K, Micheli L. Common athletic injuries in adolescent girls. Curr Opin Pediatr 2001;13:317–27.

122. Knowles SB. Is there an injury epidemic in girls sports? Br J Sports Med 2010; 44:38–45.

123. Hagglund M, Walden M, Atroshi I. Preventing knee injuries in adolescent female football players—design of a cluster randomized controlled trial. BMC Musculoskelet Disord 2009;10:75–82.

124. Sands WA, Shaltz BB, Newman AP. Women's gymnastics injuries: a five year study. Am J Sports Med 1993;21:271–6.

125. Liu SH, Al-Shaikh R, Panossian V, et al. Primary immunolocalization of estrogen and progesterone target cells in the human anterior cruciate ligament. J Orthop Res 1996;14:526–33.

126. Wojtys EM, Huston LG, Lindenfeld TN, et al. Association between the menstrual cycle and anterior cruciate ligament injuries in female athletes. Am J Sports Med 1998;26:614–9.

127. Otis CL. Women and sports: breast and nipple injuries. Sports Med Dig 1988; 10:7.

128. Rubin CJ. Sports injuries in the female athlete. N J Med 1991;88:643–5.

129. Nequin ND. More on jogger's ailments. N Engl J Med 1978;298:405–6.

130. Powell B. Bicyclist's nipples. JAMA 1983;249:2457.

131. Torstveit MK, Sungot-Borgen J. The female athlete triad: are elite athletes at increased risk? Med Sci Sports Exerc 2005;37:184–93.

132. Patel DR, Greydanus DE. The adolescent athlete. In: Hofmann AD, Greydanus DE, editors. Adolescent medicine. 3rd edition. Stamford (CT): Appleton and Lange; 1997. p. 612–4. Chapter 28.

133. Fulkerson J. Diagnosis and treatment of patients with patellofemoral pain. Am J Sports Med 2002;30:447–56.

134. Eliakim AB. Exercise training, menstrual irregularities, and bone development in children and adolescents. J Pediatr Adolesc Gynecol 2003;16(4):201–6.

135. Madd LM, Fornetti W, Pivarnik JM. Bone mineral density in college female athletes. J Athl Train 2007;43(3):403–8.

136. Barrack M, Rauh MJ, Barkai H-S, et al. Dietary restraint and low bone mass in female adolescent endurance runners. Am J Clin Nutr 2008;87(1):36–43.

137. Omar H, Greydanus DE, Patel DR, et al. Pediatric and adolescent sexuality and gynecology. New York: Nova Biomedical Books; 2010. 450 pages.

Gene Doping: The Hype and the Harm

Trudy A. McKanna, MS*, Helga V. Toriello, PhD

KEYWORDS

- Gene therapy • Mutations • Detection • Polymorphisms
- Athletic performance

As genetic technologies and breakthroughs continue to progress at a rapid pace, so does the potential misuse of these advancements. Although "conventional" doping technologies are also evolving over time, one of the most intriguing and potentially destructive performance-enhancing concepts has arisen in the form of "gene doping." Gene therapy has been established as a technique with the potential to correct nonworking genes that lead to disease, however, with only some success in human trials.[1] Adapting the principles of gene therapy to supply athletes with a competitive advantage is the (as of yet theoretical) goal of gene doping.

The World Anti-Doping Agency (WADA) categorizes gene doping as a "prohibited method" in its 2010 Prohibited List and defines it as "1 - The transfer of cells or genetic elements (eg, DNA, RNA); 2 - The use of pharmacologic or biologic agents that alter gene expression... with the potential to enhance athletic performance."[2] Although to date, confirmation of gene doping in competition has not occurred, WADA has acknowledged both the potential for misuse of gene therapy in this regard and the vigilance necessary to be ready to address this threat to fair play once gene doping moves from the realm of possibility to probability.[3] The allure of gene doping for an athlete looking to cheat is multifaceted but largely involves the inherent difficulty in detection.[4] However, although the unknowns associated with gene doping suggest detection difficulties, these same unknowns underscore the serious potential threat to the health and safety of the doping subjects.

METHODS OF GENE THERAPY OR DOPING

The general goal of gene therapy is to promote expression of a functional gene in an unhealthy individual to correct a disease caused by an underlying genetic mutation. The ideal gene therapy candidate is a monogenic condition caused by a nonfunctional or aberrant gene product, such as in Duchenne muscular dystrophy (DMD). In DMD, mutations in the dystrophin gene lead to absent, decreased, or dysfunctional

---

Spectrum Health Genetic Services, 25 Michigan Street NE, Suite 2000, Grand Rapids, MI 49503, USA
* Corresponding author.
E-mail address: trudy.mckanna@spectrum-health.org

Pediatr Clin N Am 57 (2010) 719–727
doi:10.1016/j.pcl.2010.02.006
0031-3955/10/$ – see front matter © 2010 Elsevier Inc. All rights reserved.

dystrophin protein production. "Classic" gene therapy in this case would be the mechanism to deliver the dystrophin gene to an affected individual to produce functional dystrophin. This is the most common approach to gene therapy for monogenic conditions. "Nonclassic" gene therapy is the term used to describe this procedure when the goal of treatment is to control the expression of genes or the effects of gene expression, such as in cancer. Gene therapy is a promising tool in the treatment of genetic disease as it establishes treatment at the source of the underlying defect, and if continuous cell expression is achieved, it allows for a more constant administration of the gene product.[5,6]

To facilitate the introduction of a gene into the cells of the recipient, a delivery vehicle is required. These delivery systems can be classified into 3 main types: biologic, physical, and chemical.[7] The use of a biologic vector is the most common delivery mode for gene therapy. Viral vectors such as retroviruses, adenoviruses, and adeno-associated viruses (AAVs) are commonly used as they function to integrate into host cells and use this cell to replicate their own genetic material.[6,8] In gene therapy, these viruses are modified to reduce the potential for viral infection while carrying the ability to be delivered to specific cells for expression. Plasmid DNA (pDNA) is an alternative biologic vector but differs from viral vectors in that they are synthetic and may be grown in bacteria, then purified. Although more inefficient than viral vectors, pDNA has the advantage of avoiding a possible immune response.[5,6] Liposomes can assist in the penetration of cell membranes. RNA interference is another method of manipulating and controlling gene expression to enhance or manage gene therapy techniques that are under investigation.[6]

Gene transfer can be accomplished by direct physical injection or enhanced by physical methods, such as electroporation, ultrasound, laser, and magnetic particles.[5]

Gene expression can occur in vivo or ex vivo.[5,7] Both techniques have pros and cons, inside and outside of the laboratory (**Table 1**).

Of importance is the difference between somatic and germline gene therapies. Somatic gene therapy is limited to adult cells, and the effects are not a permanent change to an individual's DNA. Germline gene therapy, or transgenesis, is the process used in many animal studies and involves changing the genetic makeup of the animal permanently, including gametes, thereby making this genetic change present in all body cells and also heritable. Many of the animal studies in gene therapy that report the most significant results have induced germline mutations.[5]

The fundamental difference, physically, biochemically, and ethically, between gene therapy and gene doping is that the goal of gene doping is not to replace an absent or dysfunctional protein in an unhealthy individual but rather to artificially alter gene expression in an otherwise healthy individual. The evolution of gene therapy from a strictly medical tool to a performance-enhancement mechanism has significant ramifications both in the competitive sports world and in the general population.

CANDIDATES FOR GENE DOPING

What makes a gene a good candidate for doping? Obviously, the targets for gene doping would depend on the desired effect. Overexpression or underexpression of the gene product should enhance traits that are desirable for peak athletic performance. For endurance sports, such as long distance running or swimming, genes that bolster oxygen production or usage and delay fatigue would be the likely candidates. For sports in which strength or agility provide the competitive advantage, genes involved in muscle mass stimulation and injury recovery are the more likely targets.

Table 1
Ex vivo versus in vivo approaches to inducing gene expression

	Method	Advantages	Disadvantages
Ex vivo	Cells from patient treated in culture, then administered to the patient	• Allows for sorting and screening of gene product before expo sure to patient	• Low efficiency • Specific to an individual, which leads to higher costs, and the need for more specialized laboratories
In vivo	Gene is delivered via vector or direct physical route in to patient	• Allows for mass production of gene product • Lower costs	• Presorting or screening not possible • May cause immune response, which can cause efficacy, safety, and detection issues • Allows for possible germline integration

Research into gene therapy for disease treatment has led to a bounty of information that could theoretically be incorporated into gene doping programs.

Genes for Endurance

- *Erythropoietin (EPO)*: EPO is a hormone produced in response to decreased oxygen levels in the blood that signals the body to increase hemoglobin production.[9] EPO-stimulating agents have long been a part of performance-enhancing doping.[10] Overexpression of EPO by gene doping would increase endogenous hemoglobin production and thereby oxygen distribution to muscles.
- *Peroxisome proliferator-activated receptor delta (PPAR-δ)*: PPAR-δ and its family of hormones are involved in changing type I (fast twitch) skeletal muscle fibers to type II (slow twitch) muscle fibers.[9] Upregulation of this gene could produce an increase in the number of type II muscle fibers desired for endurance sports, even in the absence of endurance training. The WADA 2010 Prohibited List bans PPAR-δ agonists (eg, GW1516) and PPAR-δ–adenosine monophosphate–activated protein kinase axis agonists (eg, AICAR),[2] the only genes specifically mentioned under the gene doping section.
- *Phosphoenolpyruvate carboxykinase (PEPCK)*: the role of PEPCK in skeletal muscle is somewhat unclear, but overexpression in mice increases endurance and longevity and leads to decreased body fat.[7]
- *Vascular endothelial growth factor*: this growth factor is instrumental in the development of new blood vessels and also appears to be important in some injury-healing molecular pathways.[11,12]

Genes for Strength

- *Insulinlike growth factor 1 (IGF-1)*: IGF-1 is the primary target of growth hormone action. Increased gene expression leads to increased muscle mass and power.[8,13] In addition to promoting muscle hypertrophy, IGF-1 also hastens muscle repair.[8]
- *Myostatin*: unlike many other candidate genes for gene doping, myostatin would be targeted to promote decreased expression of this gene. Myostatin is a negative regulator of muscle growth, and by impeding its actions, increased muscle mass would be expected.[11]

Genes for Tissue Repair/Other

- *Bone morphogenetic protein (BMP)*: the BMP family of growth factors enhance bone repair and would theoretically shorten recovery time from injury. In the absence of an injury, these growth factors have the potential to increase bone, cartilage, or tendon strength in an effort to stave off potential career-ending injuries.[12,13]
- *Endorphins*: Endorphins are important components of pain management, fatigue delay, and endurance.[11] Genes that increase endorphins would increase pain threshold both acutely during competition by reducing lactic acid–related pain and chronically by dulling the effects of prior injury.[11,14] These effects make genes related to endorphin production, expression, and release reasonable targets for gene doping.

This is by no means a complete list of gene doping targets but an overview of prime candidates due to their cellular function. As more genes are identified and characterized with regard to athletic potential, the list of potential gene doping candidates is sure to expand as well.

GENE DOPING IN PRACTICE—ANIMAL MODELS

Animal models of gene doping have provided a wealth of information on the positive and negative effects of this procedure. Methods of successful gene transfer to adult animal cells have been demonstrated, and the successes of these transfers have been documented.[15] For example, gene doping with IGF-1 has proven successful in mouse models, whereby a discernible increase in muscle mass and strength was noted even months after the treatment concluded. These same studies showed that combining gene doping with athletic training provided a significant advantage over nontreated controls.[16] PPAR-δ transgenic mice showed an increase in running time, longer endurance, and lower likelihood of obesity.[7] EPO gene doping in macaques has demonstrated systemic effects, including increased aerobic capacity, improved performance, and elevated hematocrit levels.[17] Follistatin, an inhibitor of myostatin, has been used in gene therapy trials with AAV vectors to create increased muscle bulk in a variety of animal models.[18]

However, in addition to shedding light on the potential enhancement effects of gene doping in humans, animal studies have also uncovered concerns that may directly affect human subjects. It is perhaps unsurprising that artificially overexpressing genes to promote athletic prowess may lead to unwanted and negative side effects. Some studies reported an increase in hyperactivity, aggressiveness, and other behavioral sequelae in treated mice. Overexpression of EPO in macaques has been reported to increase blood viscosity, with effects on cardiac functioning.[7] Clearly, although animal models may demonstrate the promise of gene doping, the perils of this procedure cannot be ignored because its use is contemplated in humans.

GENE DOPING IN THEORY—HUMAN MODELS

Although animal studies have been successful in demonstrating gene doping effects, the transfer of this technology to humans is met with considerable logistical and practical limitations. In mouse models, high vector doses were required to induce significant effects. It is not clear how high a vector dose would be required for human gene doping or if humans have a similar capacity to tolerate these vector doses safely and effectively.[5] Are current laboratory techniques and resources capable of handling these challenges? Gene doping targets would also need to have a sustained and regulated response to produce results similar to those in animal studies.[8] In addition to these size and distribution considerations, a potentially more serious limitation is that of control of gene expression. Successful gene doping would require tissue-specific responses. How to reliably turn gene expression on or off is critical for safety, performance, and detection purposes. Uncontrolled gene expression has the possibility of actually reducing performance,[13] making the entire gene doping procedure counterproductive.

Performance Mutations and Polymorphisms

Perhaps the first human models that demonstrate the potential for gene doping could be those with naturally occurring mutations that lead to altered gene expression. For example, Finnish cross-country skier Eero Mantyranta won 2 Olympic gold medals in 1964, far surpassing his competition. Ultimately, he was found to have a naturally occurring mutation in his EPO receptor gene that vastly increased his endurance by increasing hemoglobin levels.[7] Another case of naturally occurring performance-enhancing mutation has been documented in an extremely muscular child who was found to have loss-of-function mutations in both copies of the myostatin gene. The inactivation of this gene led to excessive muscle bulk and strength with neonatal onset.[19]

In addition to the significant effects of a single-gene mutation on athletic performance as described earlier, researchers have also begun to identify dozens of genes involved in athletic ability. Subtle variations in these genes may naturally predispose an individual to certain types of physical activities. It is fascinating to consider not only our individual genetic predispositions to "performance- and health-related fitness phenotypes"[20] but also the impact that the discovery of these genes could have on the world of gene doping. The number of candidate genes reported to be associated with endurance, muscular strength, power, body composition, training response, and other athletic traits is continuously increasing.[20,21] For example, a specific genotype in the angiotensin I–converting enzyme (ACE) gene results in reduced serum and tissue ACE activity. This genotype has been found naturally in a higher than expected rate in elite endurance athletes.[21] Nutrigenetics, or the interaction between food or supplements and genetic predisposition, is another area of interest where genetics and sport interact with positive and negative potentials.[11]

Gene doping is not the only possible method of abusing our newfound knowledge in the genetics of athletic performance. Studies have also shown that genetic variability in the ability to process testosterone can exploit weaknesses in current doping detection strategies. A specific polymorphism in a gene-involved testosterone metabolism (UGT2B17) can result in decreased levels of testosterone glucoronide being expressed in urine. This creates a problem in the detection of testosterone abuse in individuals carrying this natural gene change.[22] Knowledge of one's specific genetic ability or inability to process metabolites used in doping detection could be exploited to the advantage of the dishonest athlete. Genetic testing for such polymorphisms could become necessary as doping detection programs attempt to stay up to date with genetic knowledge and technology. These complicated practical and ethical issues raised by the identification of genetic polymorphisms have been considered by WADA, and the importance of staying current on these developments was addressed at their 2008 symposium.[3]

As more genes are identified and further characterized, the possibility of genetic testing for athletic aptitude is gaining attention in academic circles and the popular media.[23] It is therefore not unreasonable to suspect that the combination of genetic predisposition testing to determine suitability for a specific type of sport could be combined with gene doping in attempts to create a "super athlete." Although there is no evidence of such activities at the current time, the athletic world will not remain untouched in the era of personalized genomics.

RISKS OF GENE DOPING

The risks associated with gene therapy in a regulated, controlled setting are still being defined. Results of gene therapy trials performed in the 1990s indicated both a substantial variability in response to vectors and a nonlinear relationship between vector dose and toxicity. The death of an 18-year-old volunteer in a pilot study of gene therapy was attributed to systemic inflammatory response syndrome caused by an immune response to the adenoviral vector used.[24] Therefore, the risks associated with taking a new procedure and illegally abusing it in otherwise healthy individuals are real and concerning. The most significant risks are associated with both the unregulated delivery of the gene therapy by dopers and the effects of this doping on a cellular and functional level in the athlete.

The illicit production and administration of gene doping products would compound these risks. The safety, quality, and contents of a gene doping product would be unregulated, and the secretive nature of doping in general may hinder appropriate medical follow-up if needed.[11,21]

The risks secondary to altered gene expression include (1) an immune response to a viral vector, (2) an autoimmune response to a recombinant protein, (3) insertional mutagenesis, and (4) lack of expression control and the sequelae related to an artificial overproduction of a protein in a healthy subject.[5,6,8,13,17] The immune response to a viral vector can be mild, such as a fever or inflammation, but could also be overwhelming and fatal.[5] If a protein produced differs from that which is endogenously produced, autoimmune responses are possible. The prospect of insertional mutagenesis is concerning in that the vector could insert itself into the host genome and disrupt oncogenes, leading to tumor development. In some cases, the risk of germline integration, or permanent, heritable genetic changes, being introduced adds another serious ethical consideration to gene doping.[6,17] EPO overexpression leads to increased blood viscosity, which can increase the risk for heart failure or stroke.[5] Overexpression of a growth factor, such as IGF-1, can cause cardiac hypertrophy and stimulate growth of cancerous cells.[8] Increasing muscle mass by manipulating myostatin, IGF-1, or other factors is also likely to put extra stress on supporting bones and tendons, which could actually increase the risk of injury.[12]

DETECTION STRATEGIES

The only way to address the possibility of gene doping detection is to stay current with scientific techniques and potential avenues for abuse of gene therapy. WADA included gene doping in their list of banned methods in 2003, continues to monitor developments in this area closely, and sponsors research into detection strategies.[3] To be successful, doping detection needs to be accessible, fast, and reliable: 3 significant challenges when dealing with gene doping. For example, if a gene doping product is produced by introducing genes to make more proteins endogenously, how can it be distinguished from the naturally produced protein? Can evidence of gene doping be reliably assessed using body fluids? Studies have shown that gene therapy with IGF-1, while increasing the detectable levels in muscle cells, did not show an increase in circulating IGF-1 levels in the blood.[5,8] A muscle biopsy, although more sensitive, is not practical. Detection strategies can be categorized into direct (evidence of doping agent) and indirect (evidence of consequences of gene doping).

Direct Approach

Direct detection of gene doping would involve identification of the vector used or a recombinant protein that differs from naturally occurring protein. Vectors have been identified in blood after gene therapy, but the window of opportunity for detection seems to be short, which poses obvious limitations.[13] There is some evidence that some proteins produced by gene therapy undergo slightly different posttranslational modification, which opens a possible detection. Some genes may be regulated by promoters that need to be activated. Detection of activating substances such as rapamycin, tetracycline, and antiprogestins would indicate gene doping but may also be present for therapeutic reasons.[5] Although direct evidence of gene doping may be preferred, especially if legally challenged, the technical limitations of these processes may not make it the most likely solution for gene doping detection.

Indirect Approach

Indirect detection of gene doping would involve the identification of the consequences of this procedure on the athlete. Various fields of study are being investigated as a potential "biologic profile" to distinguish normal standards from those indicating gene doping. For example, transcriptomics, or the profiling of gene expression, measures changes in the concentration of messenger RNA for thousands of genes. Proteomics, or protein profiling, evaluates the set of proteins expressed from the genome and provides qualitative and quantitative analysis of their variants. Metabolomics, or the profiling of nonprotein low-molecular-weight metabolites, can also provide a possible measure of gene doping activities.[4] Although these are promising approaches, the development of normal standards, individual "passports," and variability parameters is expected to be costly, time consuming, and open to legal interpretation if a gene doping charge is made. As illustrated in the testosterone metabolism studies, natural genetic variation in the population can lead to extremely variable enzyme activity under normal circumstances and may provide enough reasonable doubt to discount a suspected case of gene doping.[25]

SUMMARY

The advancement of genetic technologies that have lead to the exciting treatment possibilities of gene therapy has also opened the door for their abuse as a performance-enhancing agent. Although gene doping may be a desirable cheating method because of the inherent detection challenges, its effects are still largely unknown and potentially lethal.

The physical, ethical, and societal pitfalls of performance-enhancing doping are numerous. Gene doping adds another level of concern not only in the sports world but also for society in general.[26,27] If gene therapy has potential for abuse in sports, it also has the potential for abuse for nonelite athletes looking for a competitive edge or even people who would like to bulk up their muscle mass or lose weight by altering their genes.

REFERENCES

1. Scollay R. Gene therapy. A brief overview of the past, present and future. Ann N Y Acad Sci 2001;953:26–30.

2. World Anti-Doping Agency. The 2010 prohibited list: international standard. Montreal, Canada; September 19, 2009. Available at: http://www.wada-ama.org/ Documents/World_Anti-Doping_Program/WADP-Prohibited-list/WADA_Prohibited_ List_2010_EN.pdf. Accessed January 26, 2010.

3. World Anti-Doping Agency. WADA St. Petersburg declaration. St. Petersburg, Russia; June 11, 2008. Available at: http://www.wada-ama.org/Documents/ Science_Medicine/Scientific%20Events/WADA_StPetersburg_Declaration_2008. pdf. Accessed December 29, 2009.

4. Baoutina A, Alexander IE, Rasko JEJ, et al. Developing strategies for detection of gene doping. J Gene Med 2008;10:3–20.

5. Wells DJ. Gene doping: the hype and the reality. Br J Pharmacol 2008;154: 623–31.

6. Gatzidou E, Gatzidou G, Theocharis S. Genetically transformed world records: a reality or in the sphere of fantasy? Med Sci Monit 2009;15(2):RA41–7.

7. Azzazy HME, Mansour MMH, Christenson RH. Gene doping: of mice and men. Clin Biochem 2009;42:435–41.

8. Harridge SDR, Velloso CP. IGF-1 and GH: potential use in gene doping. Growth Horm IGF Res 2009;19:378–82.

9. Minunni M, Scarano S, Mascini M. Affinity-based biosensors as promising tools for gene doping detection. Trends Biotechnol 2008;26(5):236–43.

10. Varlet-Marie E, Audran M, Ashenden M, et al. Modification of gene expression: help to detect doping with erythropoiesis-stimulating agents. Am J Hematol 2009;84(11):755–9.

11. Harridge SDR, Velloso CP. Gene doping. Essays Biochem 2008;44:125–38.

12. Evans CH, Ghivizzani SC, Robbins PD. Orthopedic gene therapy in 2008. Mol Ther 2009;17(2):231–44.

13. Wells DJ. Gene doping: possibilities and practicalities. Med Sport Sci 2009;54: 166–75.

14. Gaffney GR, Parisotto RP. Gene doping: a review of performance-enhancing genetics. Pediatr Clin North Am 2007;54:807–22.

15. Lunde IG, Ekmark M, Zaheer AR, et al. PPAR-delta expression is influenced by muscle activity and induces slow muscle properties in adult rat muscles after somatic gene transfer. J Physiol 2007;582:1277–87.

16. Barton-Davis ER, Shoturma DI, Musaro A, et al. Viral mediated expression of insulin-like growth factor I blocks the aging-related loss of skeletal muscle function. Proc Natl Acad Sci U S A 1998;95:15603–7.

17. Unal M, Unal DO. Gene doping in sports. Sports Med 2004;34(6):357–62.

18. Rodino-Klapac LR, Haidet AM, Kota J, et al. Inhibition of myostatin with emphasis on follistatin as a therapy for muscle disease. Muscle Nerve 2009; 39(3):283–96.

19. Schuelke M, Wagner KR, Stolz LE, et al. Myostatin mutation associated with gross muscle hypertrophy in a child. N Engl J Med 2004;350:2682–8.

20. Wolfarth B, Bray MS, Hadberg JM, et al. The human gene map for performance and health-related fitness phenotypes: the 2004 update. Med Sci Sports Exerc 2005;37:881–903.

21. Ahmetov II, Rogozkin VA. Genes, athlete status and training- an overview. Med Sport Sci 2009;54:43–71.

22. Schulze JJ, Lundmark J, Garle M, et al. Doping test results dependent on genotype of UGT2B17, the major enzyme for testosterone glucuronidation. J Clin Endocrinol Metab 2008;93(7):2500–6.

23. Lippi G, Longo UG, Maffulli N. Genetics and sports. Br Med Bull 2010;93:27–47.

24. Raper SE, Chirmule N, Lee FS, et al. Fatal systemic inflammatory response syndrome in a ornithine transcarbamylase deficient patient following adenoviral gene transfer. Mol Genet Metab 2003;80:148–58.

25. Legge M, Fitzgerald R, Jones L. An alternative consideration in drug testing in elite athletes. N Z Med J 2008;121(1278):73–7.

26. Murray TH. Reflections on the ethics of genetic enhancement. Genet Med 2002; 4(6):27S–32S.

27. Miah A. Rethinking enhancement in sport. Ann N Y Acad Sci 2006;1093:301–20.

Sports Doping in the Adolescent: The Faustian Conundrum of Hors De Combat

Donald E. Greydanus, MD, FAAP, FSAM, FIAP (H)[a,b,*],
Dilip R. Patel, MD, FAAP, FACSM, FAACPDM, FSAM[a]

KEYWORDS

• Sports doping in adolescents • Anabolic-androgenic steroids
• Adverse effects of anabolic steroids • Prevention of doping

"He (it) cures most successfully in whom the people have the greatest confidence."

(Galen, 180 AD)

For thousands of years, humans have sought the use of medicines, herbs, and other chemicals to improve their lives in various ways. Some scholars have interpreted the story of Adam and Eve in Genesis (chapter 3) as a story of the original humans seeking to be strong (wise) like God.[1] Extensive pharmacopoeias have been developed in China and India over the past eons.[2] The first classifier of medicinal herbs is noted by historians as the Chinese emperor Shen-Nung 2737 BC, and there is a classic recorded painting of him holding *Ephedra* (machuang) leaves.[3] An early historical record of medical treatments is the *Ebers Papyrus* (1500 BC), which lists more than 700 medicines of various origins (mineral, vegetable, and animal).[2,4]

In recorded history, competitive athletes have used various mixtures of animal and plant origins, taken from known and unknown products, in attempts to improve their athletic performance and gain the perceived benefits of victory.[5] For example, athletes during the Greek and Roman Games used wines, mushrooms, and opioids; stimulants (ie, strychnine) were popular at the beginning of the twentieth century. Galen, the famous Greek who became the physician to the gladiators of ancient Rome, observed the belief of athletes of his time (180 AD) that consuming mushrooms and herbal teas

[a] Department of Pediatrics & Human Development, Michigan State University College of Human Medicine, 1000 Oakland Drive, Kalamazoo, MI 49008-1284, USA
[b] Pediatrics Program, Kalamazoo Center for Medical Studies, Michigan State University/Kalamazoo Center for Medical Studies, 1000 Oakland Drive, Kalamazoo, MI 49008-1284, USA
* Corresponding author. Pediatrics Program, Kalamazoo Center for Medical Studies, Michigan State University/Kalamazoo Center for Medical Studies, 1000 Oakland Drive, Kalamazoo, MI 49008-1284.
E-mail address: Greydanus@kcms.msu.edu

Pediatr Clin N Am 57 (2010) 729–750
doi:10.1016/j.pcl.2010.02.008
0031-3955/10/$ – see front matter © 2010 Elsevier Inc. All rights reserved.

was beneficial to their overall performance.[3] In 1886, a cyclist died during a race in France because of a stimulant overdose.[3] Such sports doping practices have continued in advocates of sport and others to the present age, even though such practices have been banned by sports officials. For example, the death of a British athlete at the Tour de France in 1967 was attributed to the use of amphetamines complicated by a state of dehydration, and 9 riders were ruled ineligible for the Tour de France in 2006 because of suspected sports doping.[6]

Athletes of old and of today have been willing to take various chemicals even without any proof of their benefit, in hope of improving their general health or their sports performance.[7] Over thousands of years, athletes have consulted experts from the ancient days of sorcery and alchemy to modern-day biochemistry and pharmacology to find effective yet safe performance-enhancing drugs.[5] The milieu of "victory at any cost" that existed millennia ago continues to the present. In 1982, Goldman and colleagues[8,9] asked 198 world-class athletes if they would take a chemical that would guarantee them success but would lead to their death in 5 years; in this survey, 52% reported they would take this chemical and this report remained at this level in repeat surveys between 1982 and 1995. Connor and Mazanov[9] posed this Faustian bargain to members of the general public in Australia; they noted that only 2 of the 250 individuals surveyed agreed to take such a chemical. These sagacious members of the general public were not obsessed with victory at any cost.

As we enter a new millennium and century, it is sobering to realize that only a handful of the thousands of available herbal remedies of old or of modern chemistry have been shown to actually work as prescribed to better one's health.[2,4,10] Proof of improving sports performance with various chemicals (including herbs) is even more limited. Yet, today's athletes are taking various products in ever-increasing numbers because they are driven to succeed to obtain the perceived glories of winning in contemporary society.

Agents that have been used in the hope of winning the game of sports and the game of life include anabolic steroids, anabolic-like agents, designer steroids, creatine, protein and amino acid supplements, minerals, antioxidants, stimulants, blood doping, erythropoietin, β-blockers, sodium bicarbonate and others **Tables 1** and **2**.[11–21] For example, a survey of 13,914 college athletes published in 1997 noted a significant intake of creatine (13%), amino acids (8%) and dehydroepiandrosterone (DHEA) (1%).[19] Supplement use in athletes ranges between 40% and 60%.[20,21] The teenage athlete should be carefully counseled that there are few substances (if any) that consistently and safely improve the performance of a well-trained individual.

Table 1 Manufacturers' claims of ergogenic agents
Serve as an energy source
Decrease fatigue in sports events
Increase lean body mass and strength
Decrease adipose tissue
Alter weight in desirable directions
Improve aerobic capacity
Enhance motor capacity
Improve appearance
Enhance overall sports performance

Also, the use of these agents has considerable potential to cause physical and psychological damage. Misuse of drugs in this manner (or the sports doping phenomenon as it is called) should be discouraged. This discussion reviews some of these agents that are used. Our sports youth live in a modern-day Faustian dilemma often with the encouragement of coaches, trainers, parents, the media, and other members of society obsessed with success at any price.

PROTECTION FOR CONSUMERS

Some progress was made in the twentieth century to help consumers understand whether or not the medications or chemical agents they take are beneficial and safe. In 1906, the Pure Food and Drug Act required foods and drugs, which were sent between various states, to be provided with accurate labels. It was not required that medications be tested for safety until the 1938 Federal Food, Drug and Cosmetic Act (FFDCA). It was also not required that these drugs be proven effective for their intended use until the 1962 Harris-Kefauver Amendment of the FFDCA. However, the 1994 Dietary Supplement Health and Education Act (DSHEA) reversed some of these gains acquired over the previous 88 years. DSHEA allowed products classified as dietary supplements to avoid the scrutiny applied to drugs or medications. Thus, manufacturers of dietary supplements (defined as a vitamin, mineral, herb, other botanic, amino acid, metabolites of these products, related metabolites, related concentrations, or extracts or combinations) do not need to prove safety or efficacy of their products. All that is needed is to note that their products "maintain health or normal structure and function."[10]

This has opened up the commercial floodgates to various agents used by athletes in the hope that the products they use are ergogenic (see **Table 1**).[22–24] It is important for physicians and medical educators to be aware of these various products and to be willing to provide education to society and their patients about what is known and not known about these products.[25] With the legal floodgates open and the continuing drive for success in sports at any cost that permeates society in the United States and the world, Americans spent more than US$12 billion on dietary supplements in 1999.[18,26]

Research on these products remains limited and athletes rely on word of mouth from fellow sports enthusiasts, coaches, nutrition store personnel, advertisements, and other unscientific sources for information on what drugs, herbs, or other available agents will help them improve their athletic performance or their lives in general.[24] Most research has been done on adult men, who are involved in competitive athletics and not on teenage athletes. The potency and purity of nutritional agents are not known and the long-term effects of these various substances are also unknown at present. However, the use of ergogenic agents remains popular, and more than 30,000 individual commercial products are available throughout the world.[20,27,28] Unproven claims (see **Table 1**) remain while the hope of victory burns strong in athletes of all ages whether competing at the high school (or below) level or at the Olympic level of competition.[29,30]

DEFINITIONS

The term doping is derived from the Dutch word "dop" in reference to the practice of providing race horses with an opium mixture to act as a stimulant and enhance victory of the competing animal.[17] Sports doping refers to the attempt of improvement or stimulation of sports performance in *Homo sapiens* in the eternal quest for victory at any cost. The promise of having a drug that is a true sports doping chemical often

Table 2
Drugs misused by athletes as ergogenic products

α-Lipoic acid

Anabolic steroids (DHEA, androstenedione)

Antioxidants (vitamin C, vitamin E, β-carotene)

Amphetamines

Bee pollen

β-blockers (ie, propranolol)

β-Hydroxy-β-methylbutyrate

Blood

Caffeine

Calcium

Carnitine

Choline

Chrysin

Chromium

Clenbuterol

Coenzyme Q_{10}

Creatine

DSMO

Diuretics (furosemide, spironolactone, hydrochlorothiazide)

Engineered dietary supplements

Ephedrine

EPO

Folic acid

Ginkgo biloba

Ginseng

Glycerol

hGH

Inosine

IGF-I

Iron

Minerals:
  Boron
  Chromium
  Vanadium
  Iron
  Selenium
  Zinc

Niacin

Nicotine

Nonsteroidal antiinflammatory drugs (ibuprofen, mefenamic acid, naproxen, others)

Omega-3 fatty acids

Oxygen

Pantothenic acid

Phosphorus

Pyridoxine (vitamin B_6)

Plant steroids (phytosteroids; γ-oryzanol; ferulic acid [FRAC])
Protein supplements
Riboflavin
Sodium bicarbonate
Sport drinks
Thiamin (vitamin B_1)
Tribulus terrestris
Vitamin supplements
Vitamin B_{12} (cyanocobalamin)
Vitamin B_{15} (dimethylglycine)
Yohimbine (yohimbe)
Others
Various illicit drugs
Alcohol. marijuana, tobacco, methamphetamine, cocaine, GHB; GBL
Hallucinogens (lysergic acid diethylamide and phencyclidine·HCl)
Barbiturates, opiate narcotics, inhalants (volatile solvents, nitrous oxide, nitrites)

belies an eternal quest for the product having an ergogenic quality, and this term is derived from the Greek words érgon (to work) and gennan (to produce).

ANABOLIC STEROIDS

Anabolic steroids or anabolic-androgenic steroids (AAS) are a class of chemicals that are synthetic derivatives of testosterone and represent a drug class often abused by adolescent and adult athletes.[31] The roots of their use can be traced over 6 millennia ago when ancient farmers noted the quieting or passive effects that castration had on animals.[32] Testosterone was isolated in 1935 and developed to improve metabolism; it was used by athletes to gain strength as early as the 1940s. Concern over the use of anabolic steroids by athletes led to an inaugural definition of sports doping by the International Olympic Committee (IOC) in 1964, the banning of these drugs by the IOC, the start of antidoping programs by the IOC in 1967, and the first official testing for these chemicals at the 1976 Montreal Olympic Games.[5]

The term anabolic refers to the stimulation of protein synthesis, whereas androgenic implies the stimulation of male secondary sex characteristics. The terms steroids or steroid hormones refer to chemicals that are derived from cholesterol and include corticosteroids and sex hormones (ie, testosterone, estrogen, and progesterone). Anabolic steroids stimulate several receptors: androgen, estrogen, progestin, and glucocorticoid. Some examples of oral and injectable anabolic steroids are listed in **Table 3**. The US Food and Drug Administration (FDA) has classified these chemicals as Schedule II drugs since 1990. Dianabol has been discontinued because of the high level of abuse noted by athletes. Adequate training and protein intake are necessary for maximal effect on protein synthesis in muscle tissue and the individual response is variable. Anabolic steroids have become the sine qua non of the Faustian bargain awaiting our youth.

Epidemiology

It is clear that many youth try anabolic steroids including one-third who are not athletes.[31–35] Various studies over the past few decades confirm that 5% to 11% of high school boys and 0.5 to 2.5% of high school girls in the United States have tried anabolic steroids; of these, 50% used these chemicals before 16 years of age and

Table 3
Examples of anabolic steroids
Oral steroids
1. Oxandrolone (Oxandrin)
2. Oxymetholone (Anadrol)
3. Stanozolol (Winstrol)
Injectable steroids
1. Testosterone cypionate (Testim)
2. Testosterone enanthate (Depo-Testosterone)
3. Nandrolone phenpropionate (Durabolin)
4. Nandrolone decanoate (Deca-Durabolin)
Topical steroids
1. Testosterone gel (Androgel)
2. Testosterone transdermal (Androderm)

Data from Greydanus DE. Performance enhancing drugs and supplements In: DR Patel, DE Greydanus, R Baker, editors. Pediatric practice: sports medicine. New York: McGraw-Hill Medical Publishers; 2009. p. 63–77.

33% of these youth were not athletes.[31,33,36–49] Approximately 80% of male bodybuilders and 40% of female body builders use these drugs in contrast to 20% of college athletes; 38% of users try the injectable forms. The mean start age is about 14 years with a range of 8 to 17 years. One study looked at 1881 high school students in Georgia and noted that 5.3% of ninth grade boys and 1.5% of ninth grade girls claimed they use or had used anabolic steroids.[50] A 1988 study of 3403 high school seniors nationally indicated that 6.6% responded they were or had used these chemicals; 38.3% were less than 16 years of age; of these, 47.1% indicated that the main reason for using these drugs was to improve their sports performance.[36] The 2008 Monitor the Future Study noted the annual prevalence rates had dropped; for boys in the 8th, 10th, and 12th grades, it was 1.2%, 1.9%, and 2.7%, respectively versus 0.6%, 0.5%, and 0.7% for girls.[51] Several decades of research suggests a lifetime prevalence of 4% to 6% with teenage boys and 1.5% to 3% for teenage girls.[52]

These youth have limited knowledge of the dangers of these drugs.[41,53] Abuse of these chemicals may be increased in the nonathletic population versus the athletic adolescent population.[52] Adolescents who take anabolic steroids may also be involved in other high-risk behaviors, including illicit drug use such as cocaine, alcohol, cigarettes, marijuana, smokeless tobacco, and various injectable drugs.[43,47–55] Adolescents obtain these drugs from many sources, even from veterinary suppliers. Unless they have been banned (as in Olympic competition) and drug testing is in force, anabolic steroids are popular with all athletes. Although abuse of anabolic steroids by American professional athletes has decreased somewhat in recent years, the use of these and other drugs by famous athletes has long encouraged teenagers to try these substances.[56–58] Youth often believe that these chemicals are natural hormones and are endorsed by their sports heros.[54] Many teenagers are convinced that these drugs are valuable and worth any risk, even in very high doses.

Oral anabolic steroids are 17α-alkylation chemicals that slow liver inactivation and cause much of the liver side effects of these drugs. The injectable forms are from 19β-esterification processes and pose infectious disease risks, including hepatitis (B and C) and human immunodeficiency virus (HIV)/AIDS. The therapeutic doses of such drugs as used for treatment of various medical disorders are 8 to 30 mg depending on the particular drug being used. Because teenage athletes are often not afraid (nor informed) of risks, they may use prolonged and heavy (supraphysiologic) doses. They may use these drugs in various combinations in a method called stacking, that is, cycles of 6 to 12 weeks on and then off.[47,53,59] In 1 study, 18.2% used only 1 cycle, whereas 38.1% used oral and injectable anabolic steroids.[60] Increasing a drug dose in a cycle is called pyramiding, and doses may be 10 to more than 40 times the usual therapeutic doses.[59] While taking several drugs together (ie, stacking), some athletes use up to 200 mg per day. These athletes may not have any fear of side effects in their quest for ergogenic qualities or even in attempts to simply improve appearance.

Effects

Athletes use anabolic steroids in the hope of increasing lean body mass, strength, and/or aggressiveness; as noted, some only wish to improve appearance.[33,61] Athletes at particular risk for the use of anabolic steroids include those engaged in sports such as weight lifting, shot putting, discus throwing, bodybuilding, sprinting, football, and wrestling. If athletes take high doses of anabolic steroids while undergoing heavy resistance training, there may be an increase in body weight (with increased water retention) and lean muscle mass. One controlled study looked at adult men taking 600 mg of intramuscular testosterone and noted that they gained significant size and strength.[62] However, not all studies agree and the exact effects of anabolic steroids are complex and not fully defined. The effect of training is important because healthy volunteers who take these drugs without training show no increase in muscle strength or muscle size. Some experiments have noted that inexperienced weight lifters who take anabolic steroids may experience an increase in body weight but not strength. Whether or not athletes get a significant increase in athletic performance remains controversial, and individualized results are the norm.

Adverse Effects

Side effects of anabolic steroids are legion and reviewed in **Table 4**.[33,45,46,63] Addiction to anabolic steroids may occur.[38,44,48,56–67] One study of 164 steroid users identified 28% as being dependent on these drugs.[68] The maturation process may be accelerated in growing athletes with possible early closure of epiphyses and shortened ultimate adult height. An increase in tendon injuries has also been reported in teenagers on anabolic steroids. Liver complications are many and are related to the oral alkylated forms; these adverse effects include increase in liver function tests, peliosis hepatitis, cholestasis, hepatic failure, and hepatic neoplasms (benign and malignant). Risks for cardiovascular disorders occur, including hypertension, reports of cardiomyopathy, and various thrombogenic phenomena such as myocardial infarctions, cerebrovascular accidents, and sudden death.[69–73]

Masculinization of females may occur with changes such as hirsutism and clitoromegaly, both of which may be permanent; deepening of the voice is an irreversible effect of anabolic steroids in females. Amenorrhea, male-pattern baldness, and skin coarseness may also be seen in women; the skin changes may be permanent. Female athletes try to get a high enough dose to get the expected or desired results on muscle mass, but low enough to prevent unwanted side effects such as masculinization. Hair loss and severe acne may be seen in both sexes. Males may develop gynecomastia (partly irreversible) and prostatic enlargement (with possible increased risk for prostatic cancer). The reduction in testicular size is reversible, but abnormalities of germinal elements can persist for several weeks after cessation of anabolic steroids.

Use of Additional or Concomitant Doping Agents

Users of AAS may use other drugs as well.[48] For example, they may use human growth hormone (hGH), methamphenamine, or clenbuterol (see later discussion) to augment

Table 4
Anabolic steroids side effects
Fluid retention
Masculinization of females 　Hirsutism 　Clitoromegaly 　Alopecia (males also) 　Voice deepening
Other changes for females 　Amenorrhea 　Skin coarseness 　Acne (both sexes; can be severe)
Growing athletes: 　Acceleration of maturation 　Early epiphyseal closure 　Shortened ultimate adult height 　Increase in tendon injuries
Psychological changes See increase in: 　Aggressiveness 　Irritability 　Depression
Gastric ulcers
Liver complications 　Increase in liver function tests 　Cholestasis 　Peliosis hepatitis 　Liver failure 　Benign liver neoplasm 　Malignant liver tumor (hepatocellular carcinoma)
Hyperglycemia (hyperinsulinemia)
Prostatic enlargement (possible increase risk for prostatic cancer)
Decrease in glycoproteins (follicle-stimulating hormone and luteinizing hormone) with: 　Decreased spermatozoa 　Decreased testosterone levels 　Reduction in testicular size
Increase in tendon injuries
Reduction in high density lipoprotein, increased total cholesterol
Increased platelet aggregation, potential rise in cardiovascular disorders
Wilms tumor (at least 1 case report)

the anabolic effects of AAS. Human chorionic gonadotropin (HCG) may be added to raise testosterone synthesis and counter the anabolic steroid-induced effect of testicular atrophy. Diuretics (eg, furosemide, spironolactone, hydrochlorothiazide) may be used to reduce fluid retention, produce the desired rippled look, or dilute urine to subvert a drug-screening regimen. The use of diuretics to lose weight quickly is not an unusual plan of wrestlers. The use of such medications can result in increased weakness such that a wrestler can be injured by competing against a stronger opponent. Electrolyte dysfunction and other medical side effects of diuretics may complicate the picture. Pulmonary embolism has been reported in a high school wrestler using such a regimen.[74]

Stimulants may be taken along with AAS to increase the drive for exercise and competition, whereas anti-acne medications are used to deal with the anabolic steroid-induced acne. Antiestrogens (as tamoxifen or clomiphene) may be used to prevent male feminization effects (ie, gynecomastia) of anabolic steroids. These athletes may use other drugs as well in the course of their training, such as antibiotics, corticosteroids (ie, prednisone), and analgesics (eg, morphine, propoxyphene, meperidine, oxycodone, and others). Narcotics and other illicit drugs are abused for their pleasure-granting effects as well. Corticotrophin (ACTH) is used to raise levels of internally produced corticosteroids and to produce a sense of euphoria.

Prevention

The use of anabolic steroids poses significant risks to the user/abuser and these chemicals have been banned by the (IOC), the National Collegiate Athletic Association (NCAA), the National Football League (NFL), and many other sporting associations. However, it is often difficult for the adolescent user to stop because many young people have difficulty understanding the consequences of their actions (concrete thinking) and have difficulty avoiding the win-at-all-cost attitude prevalent in the global sports milieu.[29,30,41,56,57,75,76] It is important to educate youth about these sports doping agents.[59] Parents and coaches must be taught about these chemicals and they should not encourage the use of such potentially dangerous chemicals under the guise of "Winning is Everything!" Goldberg and colleagues[77,78] have introduced the ATLAS model or the Adolescent Training and Learning to Avoid Steroids Program with some success.

Although there may be some medical indications for these drugs (ie, treatment of HIV-associated wasting or chronic renal failure), seeking to improve sports performance should not be one of the medical indications to use these drugs.[11,44,79] Guidelines for following athletes who insist on taking anabolic steroids are provided by Blue and Lombardo.[64] The effort to ban anabolic steroids has now been complicated with the appearance of designer steroids, the first of which was norbolethone that was initially detected by a laboratory in Los Angeles in 2002.[5] Other identified designer steroids include madol (desoxy-methyl testosterone) and tetrahydrogestrinone. Unfortunately, experts and amateurs in the biochemistry industry continue to produce such drugs, and the cat and mouse game between sports dopers and sports officials will continue in perpetuum.

Other Anabolic-like Agents

DHEA

DHEA is a mildly androgenic hormone naturally produced in the adrenal glands and testes. It is the precursor to testosterone (as well as dihydrotestosterone) and estrogen. Although DHEA is banned by the FDA and has no proven ergogenic effects, it is used by athletic teens and adults as an alternative to anabolic steroids.[31,48,80] The ergogenic attempt is based on a hope and hype that DHEA will increase testosterone and an anabolic insulin-like growth factor (IGF-I). Despite animal studies having shown some DHEA-induced liver toxicity, it is marketed to adults (middle-aged and older) as an over-the-counter alternative to anabolic steroids with additional unproven claims of promoting euphoria, enhancing libido, delaying cardiovascular disease, preventing cancer, and boosting one's immunity.[17] Research is limited on DHEA.[65] One study evaluated men (average age 24 years) who used 1600 mg per day for 4 weeks; serum testosterone levels were not altered.[81] Another study called the Andro Project also noted no ergogenic qualities of DHEA.[82]

DHEA is given at a dose of 50 to 100 mg per day for 6 to 12 months in oral or injectable forms, up to 1600 mg. Side effects may occur as with ingestion of sex hormones.

At doses of more than 100 mg/day, gynecomastia (irreversible) in men and hirsutism in women can occur; cancer (prostate or endometrial) may be worsened.[83] DHEA should be considered as an anabolic steroid and teenagers should be advised not to use it. The FDA has ruled it has no medical usage, and it has been banned by the National Hockey League, the IOC, the NFL, among others (**Tables 5** and **6**).

Androstenedione

Androstenedione is another androgen produced by the adrenal gland and testes; it is a precursor of estrogen and testosterone (as well as dihydrotestosterone) and is found in Scotch pine tree pollen.[84–86] Androstenedione is available in Europe as a nasal spray and is used in the United States in a pill form. It is used as a T-booster in hope of increasing testosterone; serum testosterone/estrogen ratios are normalized within 1 day of stopping this drug. High doses (as 100–300 mg per day and 60 minutes before an event) may increase lean muscle mass and strength. Studies note that 300 mg of androstenedione increases testosterone, estrone, and estradiol levels more than 100 mg.[26] It is often used in combination with different anabolic steroids in various cycling methods.[80]

Androstenedione is a banned chemical with unknown long-term safety. Side effects are the same as noted with anabolic steroids; the potency and safety of available products are unknown. It should be avoided with growing athletes and for those at risk for prostate or breast cancer. Androstenedione and other steroidal supplements may be packaged with various other chemicals, such as ephedrine, caffeine, saw palmetto, and others.[65] Although banned by the IOC, NFL and NCAA, androstendione remains a popular sports doping agent (see **Tables 5** and **6**).

Human growth hormone (hGH)

hGH has been used especially by power and speed athletes in attempts to increase lean muscle mass and strength, often in combination with anabolic steroids.[11,31] However, ergogenic effects have not been proven, even when using supraphysiologic doses.[87] Although tests are available, it is difficult to detect all users and the user runs the risk of having an impure product obtained illegally.[88,89] Recombinant DNA technology has provided recombinant hGH (rhGH) to those able to pay the high cost of this agent (more than US$3000 per month).[89] A survey of more than 200 high school male athletes noted that 5% were on hGH.[48] The question of hGH purity as a natural product was previously raised with the development of Creutzfeld-Jacobs disease. Side effects of hGH supplementation may include jaw enlargement, gigantism,

Table 5 Banned substances and methods	

Main categories of prohibited substances	Anabolic agents
	Hormones and related substances
	   (growth hormone,
	   IGF-I, insulin, EPO)
	β2 agonists
	Hormone agonists and modulators
	Diuretics and other masking agents

Main categories of prohibited methods	Enhancement of oxygen transfer Chemical and physical manipulation Gene doping

Data from Greydanus DE, Patel DR. Sports doping: use of drugs and supplements to enhance performance. Int Public Health Journal 2009;1(4):2.

Table 6
Drugs banned from various sports competitions
Anabolic steroids (see **Table 3**)

Beta blockers
  Clenbuterol
  Metoprolol
  Propranolol

Diuretics
  Furosemide
  Hydrochlorothiazide
  Spironolactone

Narcotics
  Dextropropoxyphene (Darvon)
  Morphine
  Meperidine (Demerol)

Peptide hormones
  ACTH (corticotropin)
  EPO
  HCG
  hGH

Stimulants
  Amphetamines
  Ephedrine

Others
  Local anesthetics
  Corticosteroids
  Alcohol
  Illicit drugs, including marijuana

hypertension, hyperglycemia, fluid retention, carpal tunnel syndrome, slipped capital femoral epiphysis, and pseudotumor cerebri.[18,89] Although several amino acids (arginine, ornithine, lysine, and tryptophan) are used to induce release of hGh, doses usually used do not significantly raise hGH in the body.

γ-*Hydroxybutyrate*

γ-Hydroxybutyrate (GHB, Liquid Ecstasy, G, Georgia home boy) is a central nervous system depressant that leads to euphoria and lowering of inhibition.[90,91] GHB is popular with body builders with the hype and hope of increasing growth hormone release during sleep and enhancing muscle growth. GHB can be made at home with recipes found on the Internet and with ingredients easily purchased. It is made as a clear liquid or white powder; tablets or capsules are available. It is also used as a date-rape pill to enhance sexual assault; as a colorless, odorless and tasteless liquid, it is easily slipped into party drinks to produce sedation and amnesia; effects are noted in 10 to 20 minutes and last for 4 hours. It is quickly cleared from the body and is hard to detect. Thus, it has become a popular date-rape drug. An overdose can lead to profound respiratory depression, coma, and death.

Because the United States government is cracking down on GHB use, some are taking GHB metabolites or precursors, such as γ-butyrolactone (GBL) and even the industrial solvent, 1,4-butanediol (BD). After ingestion of GBH, it becomes GHB. Some companies are substituting BD for GHB, even though BD has been declared a potentially life-threatening drug by the FDA. It is marketed as a dietary supplement in various sleep aid and muscle builder products. Although it is promoted to enhance sexual performance, BD slows breathing and can lead to unconsciousness, emesis, seizures, and death.

Clenbuterol

Clenbuterol (Clensasma; Broncoterol) is a β2 agonist bronchodilator (substituted phenylethanolamine) that is used with anabolic steroids in attempts to improve lean body mass and decrease adipose tissue.[11,44,54,92–94] It is available in Europe, Central America, and South America. Clenbuterol can be given orally with full absorption, whereas aerosol and injection forms are also available. If used therapeutically for asthma, the dose is 0.02 to 0.04 mg per day; if used ergogenically, a dose of 0.02 to 0.16 mg per day is tried. Clenbuterol can be used in a 2-day on and 2-day off cycle for several weeks and then stopped before the athletic event, because it can be detected for 2 to 4 days after the last dose.

However, it is not proven that it increases muscle mass and reduces adipose tissue, certainly not to the extent attributed to anabolic steroids. Several side effects are observed, including tachycardia, headaches, anxiety, dizziness, nausea, tremor, and insomnia. Concern is raised that it may lead to arrhythmias, myocardial infarction, cardiac muscle hypertrophy, and cerebrovascular accidents. It is banned by many sport agencies, including the IOC, United States Olympic Committee, NCAA, and others (see **Tables 5** and **6**).

To avoid sanctions for using a medication (even with a prescription) at Olympic competition levels, rules of the World Anti-Doping Code must be followed in which the International Standard for Therapeutic Use Exemptions are used.[95] Sports doping has been viewed by authorities as being an unfair and unethical advantage in sports competition. The IOC developed a medical commission in 1967 and they have produced a list of substances that are prohibited for athletes to use as well as various antidoping regulations.[96] Specific screening for prohibited drugs was initiated at the 1972 Munich Olympic Games. In 1999, the World Anti-Doping Agency (WADA) was developed and this agency organized a worldwide effort to standardize and enforce antidoping regulations.[31] WADA has published the 2009 World Anti-Doping Code listing categories of banned substances and methods used for doping; they provide a list of substances banned in competition and in specific sports (see **Table 5**).[31] Athletes must be careful even with prescription drugs that are prescribed for them or misuse of medications that are being prescribed for someone else.[97]

Others

IGF-I is a single-chain 70 amino acid polypeptide that contributes to the growth-enhancing effects of hGH.[48] Provision of injectable r-IGF-I produces similar effects to rhGH, and to the appreciation of female athletes, there is no virilization. This product's high cost (more than US$3000 per month) limits its use. Anabolic phytosteroids (plant steroids) are marketed to athletes as plant extracts that have similar effects as anabolic steroids, but without the side effects. These products include γ-oryzanol, ferulic acid, β-sitosterol, and Smilax.[18] There is no evidence for their ergogenic properties and their purity as purchased is not guaranteed. Potential adverse effects include hyperglycemia, respiratory problems, increased blood pressure, cardiomyopathy, and others.[5] Insulin itself has been used in attempts to augment transport of glucose into muscle cells with potential adverse effects such as hypoglycemia, coma, and death.

CREATINE

Creatine is an essential amino acid synthesized from arginine, glycine, and methionine, mainly in the kidneys, and to a lesser extent in the liver and pancreas. It is available in milk, meat, fish, and other foods, although meat and fish are the main food source and supply more than half of the daily requirement.[27,28,31,80,90,98] The usual diet provides 1 to 2 g of creatine per day. It is a tasteless crystalline powder that is readily dissolved in liquids and is usually marketed as creatine monohydrate or with phosphorus.[99] At all levels of competition (from high school to professional), creatine is the most popular nutritional supplement sold today as an ergogenic agent.[27,28,31,90,98,100–104] In a well-known 1997 study by the NCAA in which more than 1400 college athletes were surveyed, 32% had used creatine in the 12 months before the survey.[98] In a study of 520 British athletes, 36.1% reported use of creatine and many believed that they were able to train longer and/or maintain strength using creatine.[104] Although annual sales of creatine are more than US$200 million, there remains little research on its effects on adolescents.[12,17,103]

All but 5% of creatine is stored in skeletal muscle (especially the fast twitch, type II muscle), two-thirds as a phosphorylated form, and one-third as free creatine. This substance serves as an energy substrate for the contraction of skeletal muscle in the body. Cells with high-energy requirements use creatine in the form of phosphocreatine, which functions as a donor of phosphate to produce adenosine triphosphate from adenosine diphosphate. Cells in the skeletal muscles store enough phosphocreatine and adenosine triphosphate (ATP) for about 10 seconds of high-intensity action.[80,100] The purpose of creatine supplementation is to increase resting phosphocreatine levels in muscles and free creatine to briefly postpone fatigue, with potential ergogenic results.[99,100] Phosphocreatine maintains high energy ATP levels, acts as a proton buffer, and can lead to reduced glycolysis. When the phosphocreatine levels decrease, glycolysis increases. Maximal exercise eventually stops because of muscle fatigue, probably because of accumulation of lactate and hydrogen ions in addition to a decrease in ATP.

Is creatine an ergogenic supplement? Studies in adult athletes suggest there may be a 5% to 15% improvement in short-term (<30 seconds), repetitive/intermittent, high-intensity exercise.[18,27,28,102,105–107] Some literature tends to suggest it is probably beneficial for those in power sports (ie, football, sprinters), but not for those in endurance sports (eg, swimming). However, not all the literature agrees that there is any improved sports performance.[31,108–112] Some athletes may have a low intracellular concentration of creatine and thus may respond to it, whereas those with a higher level do not respond. Most in vivo studies show no improvement in sports performance.[80] Also, no studies report any improvement with long-term endurance activities.

The work of Harris and colleagues[113,114] has led to the current practice of many athletes using a loading dose of 20 g per day (5 g four times a day) for 5 to 7 days followed by 2 to 5 g per day for maintenance. Other loading and maintenance doses are also used. For example, research suggests an equally beneficial effect may be seen with 3 g a day versus a loading dose of 20 g a day.[115] The loading routine may maximize the amount of phosphocreatine in muscles, whereas a maintenance dose may keep muscles filled. Positive results are best with an active exercise program, although there is no need to take creatine specifically before or during exercise. Increased muscle mass may result because of fluid (water) retention and not increased protein synthesis.[114] An increase of 0.7 to 3 kg. in 1 month has been reported; weight gain can be maintained on 5 g per day of creatine during a 10-week period of detraining and maintained 4 weeks after its use is stopped.

Although creatine is generally regarded as safe, there may be side effects and risks, especially when consuming more than 20 g per day. The best-known effect is weight gain because of fluid (water) retention. Other adverse effects that are often cited but not proven include anecdotal reports of muscle cramps, strains, dehydration in hot/

humid weather, renal function deterioration, suppression of endogenous synthesis, and possible cardiac muscle hypertrophy. Other anecdotal concerns include abdominal pain, dyspnea, nausea, emesis, diarrhea, anxiety, fatigue, migraine headaches, seizures, myopathy, and atrial fibrillation.[17,80] Long-term (ie, more than 1 year) effects are unknown and no studies are reported in children or adolescents.[20] Supplementation does reduce endogenous creatine production, with unknown results on the body. Although it is not banned by any major sports groups, the American College of Sports Medicine recommends that those less than 18 years of age should not use creatine.[115]

STIMULANTS
Ephedrine

Ephedrine is a medication that can have beneficial effects in disease states (eg, asthma), but which is not acceptable to various sports medicine committees because of potential harmful effects.[18,20,116,117] It is an example of using a stimulant drug to seek improvement in one's performance in training or competition. Although not proven to be ergogenic, it has been used by various athletes in this regard. Other stimulants include amphetamine and caffeine. They are used to reduce the sense of being tired, lessen the feeling of pain, and heighten aggressiveness.[45] As noted earlier, stimulants have been used by athletes over the eons as performance-enhancing chemicals. The Incas in South America chewed coca leaves to help them run long distances.[1]

In the case of ephedrine, many believe its sympathomimetic action gives the user an unfair advantage and is thus banned (see **Tables 5** and **6**). However, β2 agonists such as terbutaline and salbuterol are accepted in the Olympics if the athlete has documented asthma and informs the Olympic Committee of their use. The purpose is to allow the athlete proper treatment of a verified disorder (ie, asthma), but not to allow him/her to gain an unfair advantage over the competitors (ie, using stimulants).

Ephedrine alkaloids are derived from ephedra herbs (also called ma huang). Athletes use dietary supplement products that contain ma huang to improve muscle tone and energy levels, although there is no proof of these claims.[10,17] Negative effects have been identified, including more than 800 adverse reports that were investigated by the FDA between 1994 and 1997 (FDA, June 2, 1997). These incidents involved otherwise healthy young to middle-aged adults who developed various complications while on these products; these included hypertension, arrhythmias, anxiety, tremors, insomnia, seizures, paranoid psychoses, cerebrovascular accidents, myocardial infarctions, and death.[118] The FDA recommended limiting consumers to 24 mg of ephedra alkaloids and wanted labels to limit these products to 7 days and alert the public to these potential problems if high doses were taken. No official government action in this regard has been taken and the FDA was requested to provide more data. Despite such adverse reports, more than US$1 billion was spent by consumers of ephedra products in 2000.[10]

Caffeine

Caffeine is a xanthine derivative that is used by many athletes.[31,119] In a study of 520 British athletes in which 36.1% reported use of creatine, caffeine use as a sports doping agent was reported by 23.8%.[104] It may improve performance in steady state endurance activities that rely on fat for fuel, because this chemical increases lipid metabolism. It increases the release of free fatty acids from adipocytes and stimulates catecholamine activity.[44,120] Studies have noted that ingestion of 2 to 3 cups of coffee (100–150 mg of caffeine per cup) increases the endurance of individuals cycling to exhaustion on bicycle ergometers. Coffee seems to reduce the perception of fatigue and allow further performance. However, an excessive amount increases sympatho-mimetic stimulation, which can interfere with overall athletic performance. Its diuretic effect can also interfere with such performance. Excessive amounts were banned from Olympic competition and is defined as more than 12 to 15 μg/mL in the urine; this usually results from ingestion of 6 to 8 cups of coffee.[18] This ban was recently lifted. Other sources of caffeine include tea, over-the-counter pills for sleepiness, and some analgesic pills that contain caffeine.

BLOOD DOPING AND EPO

Blood doping (bloodboosting or blood packing), in which athletes receive transfusions of their own blood, is an attempt to increase aerobic performance.[31,121,122] It is impos-sible to detect by laboratory tests and the frequency of use among athletes is unknown. Hemoglobin levels may reach 19 to 20 g/dL, especially during intense competition (eg, cycling competition at high altitudes), which leads to dehydration.[44]

EPO is a renal glycoprotein that stimulates red cell production.[31,121,122] Recombinant EPO (rEPO) is used to increase aerobic capacity and thus has become popular with endurance athletes (eg, runners and cyclists)[44] rEPO is difficult to detect and has a half-life of 20 hours. As noted with blood doping, several side effects are reported, including increased blood viscosity, hypertension, coronary artery occlusion, cerebro-vascular accidents, seizures, and sudden death. Dehydration from intense sports activity may trigger some of these complications. It is difficult to detect; it is as effective in increasing aerobic capacity as blood doping and its use is banned.[121,122]

MISCELLANEOUS SPORTS DOPING AGENTS

β-Blockers (ie, propranolol, clinetrol, metoprolol) have been used to reduce anxiety, lessen hand tremor, control tachycardia, and reduce hypertension. Hand control is important in sports such as archery and riflery; these athletes may also use benzodi-azepines and barbiturates for relief of anxiety and insomnia.[44] These agents, like many others, are banned from many competitive sports (see **Tables 5** and **6**). Potential side effects of β-blockers include various well-known cardiovascular, hematologic, central nervous system, and gastrointestinal symptomatology.[5]

Ergolytic illicit drugs include alcohol (also used in small amounts for hand control), marijuana, nicotine, cocaine, amphetamines, and others.[55] Nicotine may improve central nervous system attention span in some, but may also worsen hand steadiness. Insulin has been misused in sports by some because of its anabolic and anticatabolic effects. Drug testing has been developed to detect this practice.[123] Selective androgen receptor moderators are a class of drugs with the potential for use and abuse as sports doping agents and drug testing technology is being developed to detect SARMs.[124] A selective progesterone receptor modulator is an agent that works on the progesterone receptor with an agonist action on some tissues and an antago-nist action in others. Some athletes seek to use such unapproved and controversial chemicals with the eternal sports doping hope from advertised hype that improved sports performance will occur without undesirable side effects.

Sodium bicarbonate is an alkaline salt that has been used to delay fatigue during bouts of exercise that are limited by acidosis; this may be helpful in cases where the blood flow can increase to accommodate an increase in the by-products of increased muscles at work.[17,44] Nonsteroidal antiinflammatory agents have been used to relieve pain and allow athletes to increase their performance despite painful injuries; this can lead to greater, more permanent injuries.[44] Such medications have erroneously been used to quicken healing of muscle soreness after exercise. Side effects of such medications include gastrointestinal bleeding, reduced platelet aggregation, reduced renal perfusion, increased salt/water retention, and thermal regulation dysfunction with resultant heat illness. Another agent falsely used as an antiinflammatory agent by athletes is dimethyl sulfoxide (DMSO). This chemical has been available in over-the-counter preparations and is rubbed onto sore or injured areas. Its effectiveness as an antiinflammatory agent has never been proved by research and its production does not occur under standards acceptable for human use.

There are many other substances sold as ergogenic agents, such as ginkgo biloba, ginseng, yohimbine (yohimbe), coenzyme Q_{10}, and others as listed in **Table 1**.[17,125] Nutritional supplements in sports are reviewed in other articles.[11,13,17,22,26,31,83,90] In a study of 520 British athletes in which 36.1% reported use of creatine, use of ginseng as a potential sports doping agent was reported by 8.3%.[104] Although their value in bettering health and improving sports performance remains controversial, their use continues by a population not willing to wait for scientific studies to provide helpful guidance. The purity and safety of these products are not guaranteed but this does not prevent youth and other athletes from using them in high amounts. Clinicians providing sports medicine care to youth, whether through anticipatory guidance or direct sports medicine management, should educate their young patients about the never-ending hype and hyperbole of these ergogenic products.[11,17,25,126]

SUMMARY

The ancient Olympic Games took place from 776 BC to 393 AD and sports doping was quite common among athletes of ancient societies.[5] The modern Olympic Games began in 1896 in Athens, Greece, under the influence of Baron Pierre de Coubertin who emphasized the need for sports to honor competition over winning.[3] Unfortunately, the milieu of winning is everything persists and athletes will accept the Goldman challenge in their pursuit of performance-enhancing drugs. Most consumed agents do not improve performance, and risks of severe adverse effects continue to complicate the Faustian dilemma that athletes at all levels face in the early twenty-first century. It may have begun with an apple, but sports doping has now evolved into anabolic steroids, designer steroids, and other dangerous chemicals. Sports doping is also a part of the greater issue of illicit drug use that is so prevalent in youth and adults of the world.[52,56,57] Our children and youth must be educated about proper exercise and nutrition. They are curious about using potential sports doping chemicals of all types.[127] We must teach our children and adolescents that sports doping is neither a safe nor effective way to succeed in the game of life on or off the field.[128] We need to reinstate Baron Pierre de Coubertin's view of competition over victory as the raison d'être for sports participation among our children and youth. Sports doping is an important cause of hors de combat in contemporary twenty first century sports society.

"When there is noble competition, there is victory"

(Aristotle, 4th Century BC)

REFERENCES

1. Csaky TZ. Doping. J Sports Med Phys Fitness 1972;12(2):117–23.
2. Grollman AP. Alternative medicine: the importance of evidence in medicine and medical evidence. Foreword: is there wheat among the chaff? Acad Med 2001; 76:221–3.
3. De Rose EH. Doping in athletes: an update. Clin Sports Med 2008;27:107–30.

4. Porter R. The greatest benefit to mankind: a medical history of humanity. New York: WW Norton & Co; 1998.
5. Botrè F, Pavan A. Enhancement drugs and the athlete. Neurol Clin 2008;26: 149–67.
6. Lippi G, Franchini M, Guidi GC. Switch off the light on cycling, switch off the light on doping. Br J Sports Med 2007. Available at: http://dopingjournal.org/noteworthy/achive/2007_11_01<archive.html. Accessed January 26, 2010.
7. Gregory AJ, Fitch RW. Sports medicine: performance-enhancing drugs. Pediatr Clin North Am 2007;54(4):797–806.
8. Goldman B, Bush PJ, Klatz R. Death in the locker room. London: Century; 1984. 32.
9. Connor JM, Mazanov J. Would you dope? A general population test of the Goldman dilemma. Br J Sports Med 2009;43:871–2.
10. Talalay P, Talalay P. The importance of using scientific principles in the development of medicinal agents from plants. Acad Med 2001;76:175–84.
11. Greydanus DE. Use and abuse of drugs and supplements. In: Bhave S, Patel DR, Greydanus DE, editors. Sports medicine. New Delhi: Jaypee Brothers Medical Publishers; 2008. p. 122–33. Chapter 7.
12. Greydanus DE, Patel DR. Sports doping in the adolescent athlete. Asian J Paediatr Prac 2000;4(1):9–14.
13. Jenkinson DM, Harbert AJ. Supplments and sports. Am Fam Physician 2008; 78(9):1039–46.
14. Catlin DH, Fitch KD, Ljungqvist A. Medicine and science in the fight against doping in sport. J Intern Med 2008;264(2):99–114.
15. Smith DC, McCambridge TM. Performance-enhancing substances in teens. Contemp Pediatr 2009;26(20):36–45.
16. Castillo EM, Comstock RD. Prevalence of use of performance-enhancing substances among United States adolescents. Pediatr Clin North Am 2007; 54(4):663–75.
17. Greydanus DE. Performance enhancing drugs and supplements. In: Patel DR, Greydanus DE, Baker R, editors. Pediatric practice: sports medicine. New York: McGraw-Hill Medical Publishers; 2009. p. 63–77. Chapter 7.
18. Wagner JC. Enhancement of athletic performance with drugs. Sports Med 1991; 12:150–65.
19. National Collegiate Athletic Association. NCAA study of substance use and abuse habits of college student-athletes. Indianapolis (IN): NCAA Committee on Medical Safeguards and Medical Aspects of Sports; September, 1997.
20. Petroczi A, Naughton DP. Supplement use in sport. J Occup Med Toxicol 2007; 2:4.
21. Petroczi A, Naughton DP. The age-gender-status profile of high performing athletes taking nutritional supplements: lessons for the future. J Int Soc Sports Nutr 2008;5:2.
22. Armsey TD, Green GA. Nutrition supplements. Science vs. hype. Phys Sportsmed 1997;25:77–92.
23. Catlin DH, Murray TH. Performance enhancing drugs, fair competition and Olympic sport. JAMA 1996;276:231.
24. Clarkson PM, Thompson HS. Drugs and sport: research findings and limitations. Sports Med 1997;24:366.
25. Sampson W. The need for educational reform in teaching about alternative therapies. Acad Med 2001;76:248–50.
26. Chorley JN. Dietary supplements as ergogenic agents. (American Academy of Pediatrics). Adolesc Health Update 2000;13:1–7.

27. Volek JS, Kraemer WJ. Creatine supplementation: its effect on human muscular performance and body composition. J Strength Cond Res 1996;10:200–10.
28. Williams MH, Branch JD. Creatine supplementation and exercise performance: an update. J Am Coll Nutr 1998;17:216–34.
29. Patel DR, Greydanus DE, Pratt HD. Youth sports: more than sprains and strains. Contemp Pediatr 2001;18:45.
30. Pratt HD, Patel DR, Greydanus DE. Sports and the neurodevelopment of the child and adolescent. In: DeLee JC, Drez DD, Miller MD, editors. Orthopaedics sports medicine. Philadelphia: WB Saunders; 2003. p. 624–42. Chapter 17.
31. Greydanus DE, Patel DR. Sports doping: use of drugs and supplements to enhance performance. Int J Public Health J 2009;1(4):1–7.
32. Dotson JL, Brown RT. The history of the development of anabolic-androgenic steroids. Pediatr Clin North Am 2007;54(4):761–9.
33. Kerr JM, Congeni A. Anabolic-androgenic steroids: use and abuse in pediatric patients. Pediatr Clin North Am 2007;54(4):771–85.
34. Graham MR, Davies B, Grace FM, et al. Anabolic steroid use: patterns of use and detection of doping. Sports Med 2008;38(6):505–25.
35. Sjöqvist F, Garle M, Rane A. Use of doping agents, particularly anabolic steroids, in sports and society. Lancet 2008;371(9627):1872–82.
36. Buckley WE, Yesalis CE III, Friedl KE, et al. Estimated prevalence of anabolic steroid use among male high school seniors. JAMA 1988;260:3441–6.
37. Faigenbaum AD, Zaichkowsky LD, Gardner DE, et al. Anabolic steroid use by male and female middle school students. Pediatrics 1998;101:E6.
38. Foley JD, Schydlower M. Anabolic steroid and ergogenic drugs use by adolescents. Adolesc Med State Art Rev 1993;4(2):341–52.
39. Johnson MD, Jay MS, Shoup B, et al. Anabolic steroid use by male adolescents. Pediatrics 1989;83:921–4.
40. Kindlundh AM, Isacson DG, Berglund L, et al. Doping among high school students in Uppsala, Sweden: a presentation of the attitudes distribution, side effects, and extent of use. Scand J Soc Med 1998;26:71.
41. Komoroski EM, Rickert VI. Adolescent body image and attitudes to anabolic steroid use. Am J Dis Child 1992;146:823–8.
42. Massad SJ, Shier NW, Koceja DM, et al. High school athletes and nutritional supplements: a study of knowledge and use. Int J Sport Nutr 1995;5:232.
43. Middleman AB, Faulkner AH, Woods ER, et al. High-risk behaviors among high school students in Massachusetts who use anabolic steroids. Pediatrics 1995; 96:268–72.
44. Patel DR, Greydanus DE. The adolescent athlete. In: Hofmann AD, Greydanus DE, editors. Adolescent medicine. 3rd edition. Stamford (CT): Appleton & Lange; 1997. p. 607–38. Chapter 28.
45. Pope HC Jr, Katz DL. Psychiatric and medical effects of anabolic-androgenic steroid use. Arch Gen Psychiatry 1994;51:375–82.
46. Tanner SM, Miller DW, Aongi C. Anabolic steroid use by adolescents: prevalence, motives, and knowledge of risks. Clin J Sport Med 1995;5:109–15.
47. Rogal AD, Yesalis CE III. Anabolic-androgenic steroids and the adolescent. Pediatr Ann 1992;21:175–88.
48. Sturmi JE, Diorio DJ. Anabolic agents. Clin Sports Med 1998;17:261–82.
49. Yesalis CE, Kennedy NJ, Kopstein AN, et al. Anabolic-androgenic steroid use in the United States. JAMA 1993;270:1217–21.
50. DuRant RH, Rickert VI, Ashworth CS, et al. Use of multiple drugs among adolescents who use anabolic steroids. N Engl J Med 1993;328:922–6.

51. Johnston LD, O'Malley PM, Bachman JG, et al. Monitoring the future national results on adolescent drug use. Overview of key findings. NIH publication no. 09-7401. Bethesda (MD): National Institute on Drug Abuse; 2009.
52. Harmer PA. Anabolic-androgenic steroid use among young male and female athletes: is the game to blame? Br J Sports Med 2010;44:26–31.
53. DuRant RH, Escobodo LG, Heath GW. Anabolic steroid use, strength training and multiple drug use among adolescents in the United States. Pediatrics 1995;96:23–6.
54. Heischober BS, Hofmann AD. Substance abuse. In: Hofmann AD, Greydanus DE, editors. Adolescent medicine. 3rd edition. Stamford (CT): Appleton & Lange; 1997. p. 703–39.
55. Schydlower M, Rogers PD. Adolescent substance abuse and addictions. Adolesc Med State Art Rev 1993;4:227–477.
56. Greydanus DE, Patel DR. Substance abuse in adolescents: current concepts. Curr Probl Pediatr Adolesc Health Care 2005;35(3):78–98.
57. Greydanus DE, Patel DR. Substance abuse in adolescents: current concepts. Disease-a-Month 2005;51(7):392–431.
58. Josefson D. Concern raised about performance enhancing drugs in the United States. BMJ 1998;317:702.
59. American Academy of Pediatrics. Adolescents and anabolic steroids: a subject review. Committee on sports medicine and fitness. Pediatrics 1997;99:1–7.
60. Brower KJ. Anabolic steroids. Psychiatr Clin North Am 1993;16:97–102.
61. Casavant MJ, Blake K, Griffith J, et al. Consequences of use of anabolic androgenic steroids. Pediatr Clin North Am 2007;54(4):677–90.
62. Bhasin S, Storer TW, Berman N, et al. The effects of supraphysiologic doses of testosterone on muscle size and strength in normal men. N Engl J Med 1996; 335:1–7.
63. Kanayama G, Hudson JI, Pope HG Jr. Long-term psychiatric and medical consequences of anabolic-androgenic steroid abuse: a looming public health concern? Drug Alcohol Depend 2008;98(1–2):1–12.
64. Blue JG, Lombardo JA. Steroids and steroid-like compounds. Clin Sports Med 1999;18:667–89.
65. Kashkin KB, Kleber HD. Hooked on hormones? An anabolic steroid addiction hypothesis. JAMA 1989;262:3166–70.
66. Yesalis CE III, Streit AL, Vicary JR, et al. Anabolic sterid use: indications of habituation among adolescents. J Drug Educ 1989;19:103–16.
67. Duclos M. Use, abuse, and biomedical detection of anabolic steroids and glucocorticoids in sports. Ann Endocrinol (Paris) 2007;68(4):308–14.
68. Malone DA, Dimeff RJ, Lombardo JA, et al. Psychiatric effects and psychoactive substance use in anabolic-androgenic steroid users. Clin J Sport Med 1995;5: 25–31.
69. Cohen JC. Hypercholesterolemia in male power lifters using anabolic-androgenic steroids. Phys Sportsmed 1988;16:49–59.
70. Dickerman RD, Schaller F, Prather I, et al. Sudden cardiac death in a 20-year old bodybuilder using anabolic steroids. Cardiology 1995;86:172–3.
71. Ferenchick GS. Are androgenic steroids thrombogenic? N Engl J Med 1990; 322:476.
72. Fisher M, Applyby M, Rittoo D, et al. Myocardial infarction with extensive intracoronary thrombus induced by anabolic steroids. Br J Clin Pract 1996;50: 222–3.

73. Kennedy MC, Lawrence C. Anabolic steroid abuse and cardiac death. Med J Aust 1993;158:346–8.

74. Luckstead EF, Greydanus DE. Use and abuse of drugs. In: Medical care of the athlete. Los Angeles: Practice Management Information Corp; 1993. p. 195–205. Chapter 8.

75. Greydanus DE, Pratt HD. Psychosocial considerations for the adolescent athlete: lessons learned from the United States experience. Asian J Paediatr Prac 2000;3:19–29.

76. Patel DR, Pratt HD, Greydanus DE. Adolescent growth, development and psychosocial aspects of sports participation: an overview. Adolesc Med State Art Rev 1998;9:425–40.

77. Goldberg L, MacKinnon D, Elliot D, et al. The Adolescent Training and Learning to Avoid Steroids Program: preventing drug use and promoting health behaviors. Arch Pediatr Adolesc Med 2000;154:332–8.

78. Goldberg L, Elliot D, Clark GN, et al. The Adolescent Training and Learning to Avoid Steroids (ATLAS) Program: effects of a multidimensional anabolic steroid prevention intervention. JAMA 1996;276:1555–62.

79. Dobs AS. Is there a role for androgenic anabolic steroids in medical practice? JAMA 1999;281:1326–7.

80. Creatine and androstenedione—two "dietary supplements". Med Lett Drugs Ther 1998;40:105–6.

81. Nestler JE, Barlascini CO, Clore JN, et al. Dehydroepiandrosterone reduces serum low density lipoprotein levels and body fat, but does not alter insulin sensitivity in normal men. J Clin Endocrinol Metab 1988;66:57–61.

82. Broeder CE, Quindry J, Brittingham K, et al. The Andro Project. Arch Intern Med 2000;160:3093–104.

83. Johnson WA, Landry GL. Nutritional supplements: fact vs fiction. Adolesc Med State Art Rev 1998;9:501–13.

84. Di Luigi L. Supplements and the endocrine system in athletes. Clin Sports Med 2008;27:131–51.

85. Smurawa TM, Congeni JA. Tesosterone precursors: use and abuse in pediatric athletes. Pediatr Clin North Am 2007;54(4):787–96.

86. Johnson M. Anabolic steroid use in adolescent athletes. Pediatr Clin North Am 1990;37:111.

87. Buzzini S. Abuse of growth hormone among young athletes. Pediatr Clin North Am 2007;54:823–43.

88. Erotokritou-Mulligan I, Bassett EE, Kniess A, et al. Validation of the growth hormone (GH)-dependent marker method of detecting GH abuse in sport through the use of independent data sets. Growth Horm IGF Res 2007;17(5):416–23.

89. Kamboj M, Patel DR. Abuse of growth hormone by athletes. Intern Public Health J 2009;3:10–8.

90. Lattavo A, Kopperud A, Rogers PD. Creatine and other supplements. Pediatr Clin North Am 2007;54(4):735–60.

91. Denham BE. Association between narcotic use and anabolic-androgenic steroid use among American adolescents. Subst Use Misuse 2009;44(14):2043–61.

92. Parr MK, Koehler K, Geyer H, et al. Clenbuterol marketed as dietary supplement. Biomed Chromatogr 2008;22(3):298–300.

93. Beckett AH. Clenbuterol and sport. Lancet 1992;340:1165.

94. Roberts CA. The impact of long-term clenbuterol on athletic performance in horses. Vet J 2009;182(3):377.

95. Hilderbrand RL. The world anti-doping program and the primary care physician. Pediatr Clin North Am 2007;54(4):701–11.
96. Barroso O, Mazzoni I, Rabin O. Hormone abuse in sports: the antidoping perspective. Asian J Androl 2008;10(3):391–402.
97. Alaranta A, Alaranta H, Helenius I. Use of prescription drugs in athletes. Sports med 2008;38(6):449–63.
98. The National Collegiate Athletic Association. NCAA study of substance use and abuse habits of college student-athletes. Available at: http://www.ncaa.org/sports_sciences/education/199709abuse.pdft. Assessed February 15, 2010.
99. Stricker PR. Other ergogenic agents. Clin Sports Med 1998;17:283–97.
100. Clark JF. Creatine and phosphocreatine: a review of their use in exercise and sport. Journal of Athletic Training 1997;32:45–51.
101. Engelhardt M, Neumann G, Berbalk A, et al. Creatine supplementation in endurance sports. Med Sci Sports Exerc 1998;30:1123–9.
102. Greenhaff P. Creatine and its application as an ergogenic aid. Int J Sport Nutr 1995;5:S100–10.
103. Grindstaff PD. Effects of creatine supplementation on repetitive sprint performance and body composition in competitive swimmers. Int J Sport Nutr 1997;7:330–46.
104. Petroczi A, Naughton DP, Mazanov J, et al. Performance enhancement with supplements: incongruence between rationale and practice. J Int Soc Sports Nutr 2007;4(1):19.
105. Brannon TA, Adams GR, Conniff C, et al. Effects of creatine loading and training on running performance and biochemical properties of rat skeletal muscle. Med Sci Sports Exerc 1997;29:489–95.
106. Greenhaff PL, Casey A, Short AH, et al. Influence of oral creatine supplementation on muscle torque during repeated bouts of maximal voluntary exercise for men. Clin Sci 1993;84:565–71.
107. Williams M. Nutritional ergogenics and sports performance. The President's Council on Physical Fitness and Sports Research Digest 1998;3:1–8.
108. Burke LM, Pyne DB, Telford RD. Effect of oral creatine supplementation on single effort sprint performance in elite runners. Int J Sport Nutr 1996;6:222–33.
109. Cooke WH, Grandjean PW, Barnes WS. Effect of oral creatine supplementation on power output and fatigue during bicycle ergometry. J Appl Physiol 1995;78:670–3.
110. Mujika I, Chatard JC, Lacoste L, et al. Creatine supplementation does not improve sprint performance in competitive swimmers. Med Sci Sports Exerc 1996;28:1435–41.
111. Graef JL, Smith AE, Kendall KL, et al. The effects of four weeks of creatine supplementation and high-intensity interval training on cardiorespiratory fitness: a randomized controlled trial. J Int Soc Sports Nutr 6:18. Available at: http://www.jissn.com/content/6/1/18. Accessed January 20, 2010.
112. Cristani A, Romagnoli E, Boldrini E. Sport's medicalization. Recenti Prog Med 2007;98(9):433–6.
113. Harris R, Sderlund K, Hultman E. Elevation of creatine in resting and exercise muscles of normal subjects by creatine supplementation. Clin Sci 1992;83:367–74.
114. Hultman E, Sderlund K, Timmons JA, et al. Muscle creatine loading in men. J Appl Physiol 1996;81:232–7.
115. Terjung RL, Clarkson P, Eichner ER, et al. American College of Sports Medicine roundtable. Physiological and health effects of oral creatine supplementation. Med Sci Sports Exerc 2000;32:706–17.

116. Keisler B, Hosey R. Ergogenic aids: an update on ephedra. Curr Sports Med Rep 2005;4:231–5.
117. Bent S, Tiedt TN, Odden MC, et al. The relative safety of ephedra compared to other herbal products. Ann Intern Med 2003;138:468–71.
118. FDA proposes safety measures for ephedrine dietary supplements. US Department of Health and Human Services News, June 2, 1997.
119. Burke LM. Caffeine and sports performance. Appl Physiol Nutr Metabol 2008; 33(6):1319–34.
120. Tarnopolsky M. Protein, caffeine and sports: guidelines for active people. Phys Sportsmed 1993;21:137–49.
121. Pommering TL. Erythropoietin and other blood-boosting methods. Pediatr Clin North Am 2007;54(4):691–9.
122. American College of Sports Medicine. Position stand on the use of blood doping as an ergogenic aid. Med Sci Sports Exerc 1996;28:1.
123. Thevis M, Thomas A, Schanzer W. Mass spectrometric determination of insulins and their degradation products in sports drug testing. Mass Spectrom Rev 2007. Available at: http://dopingjournal.org/noteworthy/achive/2007_11_01<archive.html. Accessed January 26, 2010.
124. Thevis M, Kohler M, Maurer J, et al. Screening for 2-quinolinone-derived selective androgen receptor agonists in doping control analysis. Rapid Commun Mass Spectrom 2007;21(21):3477–86.
125. Powers SK, Hamilton K. Antioxidants and exercise. Clin Sports Med 1999;18: 525–36.
126. Patel DR, Luckstead EF. Sport participation, risk taking and health risk behaviors. Adolesc Med State Art Rev 2000;11:78.
127. Petróczi A, Naughton DP. Popular drugs in sports: descriptive analysis of the enquiries made via the Drug Information Database (DID). Br J Sports Med 2009;43:811–7.
128. Martinsen M, Bratland-Sanda S, Eriksson AK, et al. Dieting to win to be thin? A study of dieting and disordered eating among adolescent elite athletes and non-athlete controls. Br J Sports Med 2010;44:70–6.

Analgesics and Anti-inflammatory Medications in Sports: Use and Abuse

Cynthia L. Feucht, PharmD, BCPS[a,b,*],
Dilip R. Patel, MD, FAAP, FACSM, FAACPDM, FSAM[b,c]

KEYWORDS

- Musculoskeletal injury • Nonsteroidal anti-inflammatory drugs
- Acetaminophen • Topical analgesics • Sports

Musculoskeletal injuries account for most sports-related injuries.[1] Overuse musculoskeletal injuries account for more than half of all sport-related injuries in adolescents and young adults. Overuse injuries can result in chronic or intermittent symptoms depending on the athlete's level of activity. Acute muscle injuries (strains, contusions, and lacerations) can lead to significant structural or functional damage to the muscle.[1–11] Delayed-onset muscle soreness (DOMS) (exercise-induced muscle damage [EIMD]), typically associated with new or unaccustomed exercise, often results from intense eccentric muscle activity and manifests with pain, discomfort, and decreased performance 24 to 48 hours after exercise.[1,4]

Nonpharmacological approaches are often considered as first-line treatment for musculoskeletal injuries and may include relative rest, ice, compression, and elevation.[3] Moderate to severe injuries to the athlete may result in several weeks of an inability to train or compete. Even after resuming the physical activity or sport, the athlete may continue to experience difficulties with muscle weakness and decreased flexibility.[1] As a result, treatment is often sought to alleviate pain, restore function, and allow the athlete to resume activities more quickly. Treatment options include analgesics such as nonsteroidal anti-inflammatory drugs (NSAIDs), acetaminophen, and topical over-the-counter (OTC) preparations. These classes of drugs are reviewed in this article, including their mechanisms of action, side effects, and efficacy in treating pain and inflammation associated with acute and overuse musculoskeletal injuries.

[a] Department of Pharmacy Practice, Ferris State University, Kalamazoo, MI, USA
[b] MSU/KCMS, 1000 Oakland Drive, Kalamazoo, MI 49008, USA
[c] Department of Pediatrics and Human Development, Michigan State University College of Human Medicine, East Lansing, MI, USA
* Corresponding author. MSU/KCMS, 1000 Oakland Drive, Kalamazoo, MI 49008.
E-mail address: cynthia.feucht@gmail.com

Pediatr Clin N Am 57 (2010) 751–774
doi:10.1016/j.pcl.2010.02.004
0031-3955/10/$ – see front matter © 2010 Elsevier Inc. All rights reserved.

MECHANISM OF ACTION

Arachidonic acid is released from cellular membranes as a result of tissue injury. Arachidonic acid is broken down by cyclooxygenase (COX) to produce prostaglandins and thromboxane A_2 and by lipoxygenase (LOX) enzymes to produce leukotrienes. Prostaglandins are localized hormones that, once released within the intracellular space, can produce fever, inflammation, and pain.[12] Thromboxanes are released in response to tissue injury and are responsible for producing platelet aggregation and clot formation, and for regulation of vascular tone.[12] Pain relief and decreased inflammation occur from the blockade of COX enzymes, thereby inhibiting prostaglandin E_2 and prostacyclin (PGI_2) formation (**Fig. 1**).[12,13]

Two forms of COX enzymes are cyclooxygenase-1 (COX-1) and cyclooxygenase-2 (COX-2). COX-1 is expressed in most normal tissues and cells, and is the predominant form within gastric epithelial cells.[12,14] Prostaglandin production within the gastrointestinal tract protects the gastrointestinal mucosa from gastric acidity. COX-2 is expressed when tissue damage occurs, and its release is induced by cytokines and inflammatory mediators during inflammation.[12,14]

NSAIDs are a heterogeneous class of medications that are chemically unrelated but known to have similar therapeutic effects, including antipyretic, analgesic, and anti-inflammatory activity. Their primary therapeutic effect is due to inhibition of prostaglandin synthesis by inhibiting COX-2 activity, and a correlation exists between COX-2 inhibition and anti-inflammatory activity.[15] Bradykinin and cytokines (ie, tumor necrosis factor-α [TNF-α] and interleukin-1 [IL-1]) are thought to be responsible for inducing pain with inflammation and releasing prostaglandins that enhance pain sensitivity.[16] Other mediators, such as neuropeptides (ie, substance P) are also involved in inducing pain. The gastrointestinal adverse effects of NSAIDs are predominantly, but not exclusively, due to inhibition of COX-1 enzyme (**Fig. 2**). NSAIDs are considered

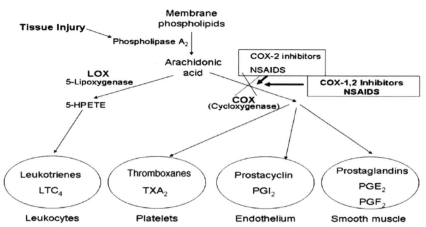

Fig. 1. When a cell membrane is injured, the arachidonic acid pathway is activated to initiate the local inflammatory response through the production of prostaglandins, thromboxanes, and leukotrienes. Their activation, however, requires the enzymes COX and LOX. The NSAIDs can block COX action and thereby prevent the formation of the COX-derived inflammatory mediators. 5-HPETE, 5-hydroperoxyeicosatetraenoic acid; LTC_4, leukotriene C4; PGE_2, prostaglandin E2; PGF_2, prostaglandin F2; PGI_2, prostacyclin; TXA_2, thromboxane. (*From* Maroon J, Bost J, Borden M, et al. Natural anti-inflammatory agents for pain relief in athletes. Neurosurg Focus 2006;21(4):E11; with permission.)

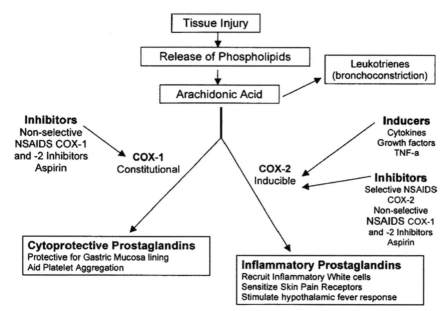

Fig. 2. The COX enzyme can exist in 2 forms: COX-1, constitutional or existing in small amounts at all times; or COX-2, inducible or only present during the inflammatory response. By selectively blocking only the COX-2–produced inflammatory prostaglandins, COX-2–inhibiting medications were believed to be superior to nonselective COX-1 and -2 inhibitors, and they were thought to have fewer gastric side effects. (*From* Maroon J, Bost J, Borden M, et al. Natural anti-inflammatory agents for pain relief in athletes. Neurosurg Focus 2006;21(4):E11; with permission.)

competitive, reversible inhibitors of COX enzymes (unlike aspirin, which is considered an irreversible inhibitor of COX enzymes) and do not affect the LOX pathway.[17]

SALICYLATED NSAIDS

Derivatives of salicylic acid include aspirin (acetylsalicylic acid), diflunisal (difluorophenyl derivative), salsalate, magnesium salicylate, and choline magnesium salicylate (**Tables 1** and **2**). Aspirin continues to be the most widely used drug and is the standard to which other NSAIDs are compared.[18] Due to its widespread availability, aspirin's potential for toxicity often goes underrecognized, and it continues to be a cause of fatal poisonings in children.[14]

Salicylates are rapidly absorbed from the gastrointestinal tract, are widely distributed throughout the body, and are highly protein bound (especially albumin).[16] Due to their high protein binding, salicylates may compete for binding with other compounds, including thyroxine, penicillin, phenytoin, bilirubin, uric acid, and other NSAIDs such as naproxen.[14] Salicylates are metabolized in the liver and excreted by the kidneys, with free salicylate excretion dependent on urinary pH and salicylate dose.[16]

Gastrointestinal adverse effects are common with salicylates and may include dyspepsia, nausea, vomiting and, more seriously, gastric ulceration, gastrointestinal hemorrhage, and erosive gastritis.[14,16] Aspirin irreversibly inhibits platelet aggregation and leads to a prolongation in the bleeding time. Gastrointestinal and platelet effects

Table 1
Salicylated NSAIDs

Drug	Onset of Action and Duration of Effect (hours)	Comments
Diflunisal	Onset: ~1 Duration: Analgesic: 8–12 Anti-inflammatory: ≤12	~4–5 times more potent analgesic and anti-inflammatory effects than aspirin; fewer platelet/GI side effects compared with aspirin; not metabolized to salicylic acid
Salsalate	Onset: N/A Duration: N/A	Fewer platelet and GI side effects than aspirin
Choline magnesium trisalicylate	Onset: ~2 Duration: N/A	Less effect on platelet aggregation and fewer GI side effects than aspirin; avoid or use with caution in renal insufficiency due to magnesium content
Magnesium salicylate	Onset: N/A Duration: 4–6	Available OTC; less effect on platelet aggregation and fewer GI side effects than aspirin; avoid or use with caution in renal insufficiency due to magnesium content

Abbreviations: GI, gastrointestinal; N/A, no data available; OTC, over-the-counter.
Data from Refs.[13,14,40]

are less likely to occur with nonacetylated salicylates (ie, salsalate, magnesium salicylate, and so forth) because they cannot acetylate COX.[16] Owing to aspirin's effect on platelet aggregation, it should be avoided in patients with hepatic impairment, hypoprothrombinemia, vitamin K deficiency, hemophilia, and within 1 week of a surgical procedure.[14]

Salicylates have been shown to have a dose-dependent effect on uric acid excretion, and in elevated doses can result in pulmonary edema, hepatotoxicity, and hyperglycemia.[14] Hypersensitivity to salicylates can result in hives, flushing, bronchoconstriction, angioedema, low blood pressure, and shock.[14] Hypersensitivity is thought to be due to COX inhibition, and cross-sensitivity occurs with other agents in the class as well as with nonsalicylated NSAIDs.[14] Patients with asthma, nasal polyps, and sensitivity to tartrazine dyes are at an increased risk for salicylate sensitivity.[19] In general, salicylates are avoided during pregnancy, especially the third trimester, due to an increased risk for perinatal death, anemia, antepartum and postpartum hemorrhage, prolonged gestation, and premature closure of the ductus arteriosus.[14]

Drug interactions can occur from salicylates displacing other agents from plasma-binding proteins. Dosages of NSAIDs, sulfonylureas, and methotrexate may need to be adjusted to prevent toxicity due to displacement. NSAIDs given concurrently with corticosteroids and warfarin may increase the risk for bleeding. NSAIDs should not be given concomitantly with the following herbals due to their anticoagulant or antiplatelet activity and increased risk for bleeding: danshen, dong quai, evening primrose, feverfew, garlic, ginger, ginkgo, red clover, horse chestnut, green tea,

Table 2
Common doses of salicylated NSAIDs

Generic Name	Trade Name	Adult Dose	Comments
Diflunisal		1000 mg, then 500 mg every 12 h Age ≥12 y: same as adult	Do not crush or chew tablet; maximum 1.5 g daily
Salsalate	Amigesic	1 g 3 times daily	Do not crush tablets; urinary acidification can decrease clearance and increase risk for toxicity
Choline magnesium trisalicylate	Trilisate	500 mg–1.5 g 2–3 times daily	Maintenance dose: 1–4.5 g daily; available as liquid formulation; urinary acidification can decrease clearance and increase risk for toxicity
Magnesium salicylate	Doan's Extra Strength Keygesic	Doan's (467 mg): 2 caplets every 6 h as needed Keygesic (650 mg): 1 tablet every 4 h as needed Age ≥12 y: same as adult	Available OTC; Doan's: maximum 8 caplets in 24 h Keygesic: maximum 4 tablets in 24 h

Data from Refs.[19,40]

policosanol, and willowbark.[19,20] In addition, NSAIDs decrease the effectiveness of angiotensin-converting enzyme (ACE) inhibitors because of the blockade of renal prostaglandin production.

Salicylates have fallen out of favor for use in adolescents and young adults because of their association with Reye syndrome. Reye syndrome is characterized by toxic hepatitis and has been associated with encephalopathy, prolonged prothrombin time, fatty infiltration of the liver, and intracranial hypertension in advanced stages.[21] Aspirin and other salicylates are contraindicated in children and young adults younger than 20 years who have a fever associated with a viral illness.[14]

NONSALICYLATED NSAIDS

Various classes of nonsalicylated NSAIDs (**Tables 3** and **4**) are among the most widely used drugs, with yearly sales in the United States for OTC drugs estimated at $30 billion.[13,22] Nonsalicylated NSAIDs are considered effective for mild to moderate pain, and have been used for a variety of musculoskeletal disorders including osteoarthritis, rheumatoid arthritis, and sports-related injuries. The choice of a particular nonsalicylated NSAID depends on its onset of action, tolerability, cost, and insurance coverage. An agent with a short onset of action, minimal adverse effects, low cost, and wide acceptability would make for an ideal nonsalicylated NSAID.

Table 3
Nonsalicylated NSAIDs

Drug	Onset of Action and Duration of Effect	Comments
Propionic acids		
Fenoprofen	Onset: ~72 h Duration: 4–6 h	~15% of patients will have side effects but few stop therapy
Flurbiprofen	Onset: ~1–2 h Duration: variable	Strong inhibitor of CYP 450 2C9 isoenzyme; substrate CYP 2C9 (minor)
Ibuprofen	Onset: Analgesic: 0.5–1 h Anti-inflammatory: ≤7 d Duration: 4–6 h	Strong inhibitor of CYP 450 2C9 isoenzyme; substrate CYP 2C9 and 2C19 (minor); equal efficacy to aspirin; ~10%–15% of patients stop therapy due to side effects
Ketoprofen	Onset: 0.5 h Duration: 6 h	~30% of patients develop side effects with GI as the most common
Naproxen	Onset: Analgesic: 1 h Anti-inflammatory: 2 weeks Duration: Analgesic: ≤7 h Anti-inflammatory: ≤12 h	Available as OTC product; more potent than aspirin in vitro, likely better tolerated than aspirin; may provide cardioprotection for some individuals with heart disease
Oxaprozin	Onset: ~0.5–4 h Duration: variable	Slower onset of effects compared with others; longer half-life allows for once a day dosing
Acetic acids		
Diclofenac	Onset: 1–4.5 h Duration: 12–24 h	More potent than aspirin; side effects experienced by ~20% and 2% stop therapy; ~15% of patients will experience an increase in liver function test; available as topical patch and gel as well as in combination with misoprostol
Etodolac	Onset: Analgesic: 2–4 h Anti-inflammatory: several days Duration: N/A	In vitro COX-2 selectivity; 100 mg of etodolac provides similar efficacy to aspirin 650 mg but may have fewer side effects
Sulindac	Onset: N/A Duration: N/A	Similar efficacy to aspirin; active metabolite; side effects experienced ~20% GI and ~10% CNS

Drug	Onset / Duration	Notes
Tolmetin	Onset: Analgesic: 1–2 h; Anti-inflammatory: days to weeks; Duration: variable	Similar efficacy to aspirin; side effects experienced by ~25%–40% and 5%–10% stop therapy
Indomethacin	Onset: ~0.5 h; Duration: 4–6 h	Compared with aspirin 10–40 times more potent; incidence of side effects 3%–50%; ~20% of patients stop therapy due to side effects
Ketorolac	Onset: Analgesic: ~10 min (IM); Duration: Analgesic: 6–8 h	Maximum duration of 5 d (oral and parenteral); strong analgesic activity but weak anti-inflammatory activity; may be given parenterally for acute pain
Oxicams		
Meloxicam	Onset: N/A; Duration: N/A	CYP 450 inhibitor of isoenzyme 2C9 (weak); substrate CYP 2C9 and 3A4 (minor); some COX-2 selective action at lower end of dosing range
Piroxicam	Onset: ~1 h; Duration: variable	Equal efficacy to aspirin; may be better tolerated than aspirin; ~20% of patients will experience side effects and 5% will stop therapy
Naphthylalkanone		
Nabumetone	Onset: ~72 h; Duration: variable	Prodrug; some COX-2 selectivity; has less GI toxicity than most NSAIDs
Fenamate		
Meclofenamate	Onset: <1 h; Duration: ≤6 h	Equal efficacy to aspirin; ~25% of patients will experience gastrointestinal adverse events
Mefenamic acid	Onset: N/A; Duration: ≤6 h	CYP 450 inhibitor of isoenzyme 2C9 (strong); substrate CYP 2C9 (minor)
COX-2 inhibitor		
Celecoxib	Onset: Analgesic: ~0.75 h to several months; Duration: ~4–8 h	CYP 450 inhibitor of isoenzymes 2C8 (moderate) and 2D6 (weak); substrate CYP 2C9 (major) and 3A4 (minor); does not inhibit platelet aggregation

Data from Refs. [13,14,40]

Table 4
Common doses of nonsalicylated NSAIDs

Generic Name	Trade Name	Adult Dose	Comments
Propionic acids			
Fenoprofen	Naflon	200 mg every 4–6 h as needed	Maximum: 3.2 g/d; do not crush tablets
Flurbiprofen	Ocufen	50–100 mg 2–3 times daily	Maximum: 300 mg/d; maximum single dose100 mg; do not crush tablets
Ibuprofen	Motrin Advil	200–400 mg every 4–6 h Maximum: 3.2 g/d	Available OTC; available in tablet (regular and chewable), capsule, suspension and infant drops; chewable tablets may contain phenylalanine
Ketoprofen	Oruvail	25–50 mg every 6–8 h as needed	Extended-release formulation is not recommended for acute pain; maximum (immediate release) 300 mg/d; maximum (extended release): 200 mg/d
Naproxen sodium	Aleve Anaprox Anaprox DS	500 mg initially, then 250 mg every 6–8 h as needed OTC label: 200 mg every 8–12 h as needed	Available OTC; dosage recommendations expressed as naproxen base; maximum (adult): 1250 mg/d (naproxen base); OTC formulation not indicated for age <12 y
Naproxen	Naprosyn Naprelan	500 mg initially, then 250 mg every 6–8 h as needed	Available as immediate-release, extended-release and suspension; extended release not recommended for acute pain; do not break, crush, or chew extended-release formulation; maximum (adult): 1250 mg/d
Oxaprozin	Daypro	600–1200 mg daily	Patients with low body weight should start with 600 mg daily; do not crush tablets
Acetic acids			
Diclofenac	Voltaren	50 mg 3 times daily	Available as immediate, extended-release formulation and powder for solution; do not crush or chew tablets; mix powder in 30–60 mL of water and drink immediately; maximum: 200 mg daily
Diclofenac patch	Flector patch	Apply 1 patch twice daily	Apply patch to most painful area of intact skin; wash hands after applying and after removal; may tape edges of patch if peeling occurs; do not wear while sunbathing; fold used patches before disposal

Drug	Brand	Dose	Notes
Etodolac	Lodine	200–400 mg every 6–8 h	Maximum: 1000 mg daily (immediate-release) and 1200 mg daily (extended-release); available as immediate- and extended-release formulation; do not crush tablets or break capsules
Sulindac	Clinoril	150–200 mg twice daily	Maximum: 400 mg daily
Tolmetin	Tolectin	400 mg 3 times daily	Maximum: 1800 mg daily; taking with food decreases bioavailability; do not crush tablets or break capsules
Indomethacin	Indocin	25–50 mg 2–3 times daily Age ≥15 y: same as adult	Available as immediate- and extended-release capsules and suspension; maximum (adult): 200 mg/d (immediate-release) and 150 mg/d (extended-release); do not crush, break or chew capsules
Ketorolac	Toradol	20 mg, then 10 mg every 4–6 h as needed <50 kg: 10 mg, then 10 mg every 4–6 h as needed	Not to exceed 5 d in duration (injection and oral combined); maximum: 40 mg daily; oral dosing intended to be a continuation of IM/IV therapy; not indicated for minor or chronic pain conditions
Oxicams			
Meloxicam	Mobic	7.5–15 mg once daily	Available as oral suspension
Piroxicam	Feldene	10–20 mg once daily	Maximum: 20 mg/d; do not break capsules
Naphthylalkanone			
Nabumetone	Relafen	1000 mg daily in 1–2 divided doses	Maximum: 2 g/d; do not crush tablets
Fenamate			
Meclofenamate		50–100 mg every 4–6 h as needed Age >14 y: same as adult	Maximum: 400 mg/d
Mefenamic acid	Ponstel	500 mg, then 250 mg every 4 h as needed Age >14 y: same as adult	Maximum duration: usually 1 week
COX-2 inhibitor			
Celecoxib	Celebrex	200 mg twice daily as needed	Contents of capsule may be sprinkled onto applesauce for administration; poor metabolizers of CYP 2C9 start at half the recommended dose

Data from Refs.[19,40]

As a class, nonsalicylated NSAIDs are usually well absorbed and highly bound to plasma proteins, and are excreted via either glomerular filtration or tubular secretion.[14] These agents accumulate at sites of inflammation, and most exhibit nonselectivity for COX-1 and COX-2 enzymes. The last decade has seen the emergence of COX-2 selective inhibitors designed to minimize gastrointestinal effects that occur due to COX-1 inhibition. Other older nonsalicylated NSAIDs have also been found to have COX-2 selectivity similar to the currently available celecoxib, based on whole blood assays.[14] Most studies on nonsalicylated NSAIDs are done in adults; however, some findings are of relevance to the adolescent age group.

SIDE EFFECTS OF NONSALICYLATED NSAIDS
Gastrointestinal

Gastrointestinal adverse effects are common with nonsalicylated NSAIDs and are often the leading reason for their discontinuation. The gastrointestinal toxicity is often dose dependent and associated with chronic use.[14] Dyspeptic symptoms are frequently experienced by patients and may include anorexia, epigastric pain, nausea, bloating, and heartburn. These symptoms have been associated with both selective and nonselective nonsalicylated NSAIDs.[13,23] Gastrointestinal toxicity may be related to prostaglandin inhibition, which is important for enhancing mucosal blood flow, mucus and bicarbonate production, and inhibition of acid production. Nonsalicylated NSAIDs also may contribute to gastrointestinal toxicity from local irritation to the gastric mucosa. More serious complications include gastric and duodenal ulcers, which may occur in up to 15% to 30% of regular nonsalicylated NSAID users.[24,25] Complications from ulcers include bleeding, perforation, and obstruction. Patients may present with a serious gastrointestinal event but have had no symptoms before presentation.[13] Factors that may increase the risk for gastrointestinal complications include the presence of *Helicobacter pylori*, advanced age, concomitant use of aspirin, anticoagulants, or corticosteroids, and duration of NSAID use (greatest within the first month).[13,26] Lifestyle factors such as smoking and alcohol use also contribute to an increased risk for side effects, but are not independent risk factors.[13,26] For those patients at risk, a proton pump inhibitor (PPI) has been shown to be effective at reducing the frequency and severity of upper gastrointestinal symptoms.[13,27]

COX-2 inhibitors were developed with the aim of reducing gastrointestinal complications associated with nonselective nonsalicylated NSAIDs. COX-2 inhibitors do not inhibit the COX-1 enzyme, which is responsible for prostaglandin production in the gastrointestinal mucosa, and therefore should have less risk for gastrointestinal toxicity. The benefit of COX-2 inhibitors with regard to less gastrointestinal toxicity remains controversial. In patients with gastrointestinal disease or risk factors for gastrointestinal complications, risk versus benefit should be assessed, and if nonsalicylated NSAIDs are used, the lowest dose for the shortest time period should be considered.[24,28]

Hepatotoxicity

Hepatotoxicity from NSAID use appears to be rare, with estimates between 3 and 23 cases per 10,000 patient years.[29,30] Two older agents (benoxaprofen and bromfenac) have been withdrawn in the United States due to reports of serious hepatotoxicity.[13] Rostom and colleagues,[31] in a systematic review, found the rate of hospitalization due to nonsalicylated NSAID-related hepatotoxicity to be 2.7 per 100,000 patients and the rate of death to be 1.9 per 100,000 patients.

A recent case report by Bennett and colleagues[29] details a 16-year-old who was previously healthy and found to be taking ibuprofen for 6 weeks before presentation. The first 2 weeks of ibuprofen use was scheduled dosing and the subsequent 4 weeks was sporadic use. The adolescent presented with dark-colored urine, jaundice, and pruritus. Laboratory results were significant for an elevated bilirubin and minimal elevation in liver enzymes.[29] The results of a liver biopsy revealed intrahepatic and canalicular cholestasis.[29] Histology was suggestive of drug-induced hepatotoxicity.[29] Over the following 4 months, the patient's symptoms resolved and laboratory values returned to normal.

Liver dysfunction related to nonsalicylated NSAIDs is rare in otherwise healthy adolescents, but should be considered in a patient with recent nonsalicylated NSAID use and presenting with cholestasis.[29] Thorough medication histories are important in determining the cause and effect. Despite the potential for hepatotoxicity, current data do not support routine monitoring of liver enzymes in individuals receiving nonsalicylated NSAIDs.

Renal Toxicity

Renal insufficiency is well known with nonsalicylated NSAID use and is likely the result of inhibition of renal prostaglandins. Renal insufficiency is estimated to occur in approximately 1% to 5% of patients, and is usually reversible on discontinuation of the NSAID.[13,32] Renal prostaglandins serve an important role in maintaining renal circulation, including vasodilation, renin secretion, and sodium and water excretion.[13] The disruption in balance between vasoconstriction and vasodilation within the kidneys may predispose a patient to renal failure. Those at the greatest risk for renal toxicity associated with nonsalicylated NSAIDs include patients with heart failure, cirrhosis, chronic kidney disease, and hypovolemic states.[13,14] Renal toxicity is characterized by elevated serum creatinine, sodium and water retention, hyperkalemia, proteinuria, interstitial nephritis, papillary necrosis, acute renal failure, acute glomerulitis, vasculitis, acute tubular necrosis, and papillary necrosis.[13,33,34] In patients at risk for renal toxicity, the risk versus benefit in using a nonsalicylated NSAID should be carefully considered and, if at all possible, NSAIDs, including COX-2 inhibitors, should be avoided.

There have been several case reports of renal toxicity in adolescents with nonsalicylated NSAID use. Nakahura and colleagues[35] discuss 5 adolescents (13–19 years old) who developed renal toxicity with the use of nonsalicylated NSAIDs. The first case was a 16-year-old girl who took ibuprofen intermittently over 9 months. Kidney biopsy results were consistent with interstitial nephritis and the patient was treated with corticosteroids. At 1 year she was asymptomatic with a decrease in serum creatinine; however, 2 years later her serum creatinine had risen and results of a repeat kidney biopsy revealed chronic interstitial fibrosis.[35] Case 3 in this report describes a 15-year-old girl who used ibuprofen every other day for 6 months. The patient was found to have proteinuria, and results of renal ultrasonography were reported normal. The patient discontinued the nonsalicylated NSAID and was asymptomatic after 1 month.[35] The other 3 cases describe adolescents who used naprosyn (1 week before hospitalization), ibuprofen (daily use for several weeks), and ketorolac (intermittently for 4 months), who all developed an increase in serum creatinine and were found to have urine eosinophilia indicative of nonsalicylated NSAID-associated nephrotoxicity.[35] In 2 of the cases nephrotoxicity resolved, and the other case reported resolution of symptoms at 1 month but continued elevation in serum creatinine.

These case reports illustrate that nonsalicylated NSAID nephrotoxicity can occur in healthy adolescents. Given the fact that several nonsalicylated NSAIDs are available as OTC preparations, adolescents should be aware of their potential adverse effects. It is important to use the lowest dose of the nonsalicylated NSAID for the shortest time period necessary, and to maintain adequate hydration while on nonsalicylated NSAIDs.

Cardiovascular Toxicity

Cardiovascular toxicity related to nonsalicylated NSAID use is generally not of concern in otherwise healthy adolescents. Cardiovascular toxicity came to light with the emergence of the selective COX-2 inhibitors. It has been theorized that the disruption in the balance between prostacyclin and thromboxane formation by selective COX-2 inhibitors may increase this risk. The selective COX-2 inhibitors, via their inhibition of prostacyclin formation, favor increased thromboxane formation and subsequent platelet aggregation.

Current data suggest that selective nonsalicylated NSAIDs may increase cardiovascular risk, but data are conflicting.[24,36–38] Heterogeneity of the studies including patient selection, duration of study, agents used, study design, and cardiovascular risk at baseline makes it challenging to summarize the cardiovascular risks associated with nonsalicylated NSAIDs. Rofecoxib was voluntarily withdrawn from the United States market in September 2004, and the Food and Drug Administration (FDA) requested Pfizer to voluntarily remove valdecoxib from the market in April 2005 because of cardiovascular risks.[39] In addition, in 2005 the FDA requested the makers of prescription and OTC nonsalicylated NSAIDs to include a boxed warning highlighting the increased risk for cardiovascular events as well as gastrointestinal toxicity, including the risk for life-threatening gastrointestinal bleeding.[39]

Drug Interactions

Drug interactions are similar to those already described for salicylated NSAIDs as well as the following additional drug interactions. Nonselective nonsalicylated NSAIDs may decrease the effectiveness of aspirin if given concomitantly due to blockade of the platelet COX-1 site.[14] It is recommended that the nonsalicylated NSAIDs be given at least 2 hours after the dose of aspirin to achieve irreversible platelet inhibition by aspirin.[13] Nonsalicylated NSAIDs may also decrease the effectiveness of thiazide and loop diuretics through blockade of renal prostaglandins.[40] In addition, nonsalicylated NSAIDs can reduce renal clearance of lithium, resulting in elevated lithium plasma levels, and the efficacy of nonsalicylated NSAIDs can be reduced with cholestyramine and colestipol due to blockade of absorption.[40] Drug interactions can occur with mefenamic acid, celecoxib, meloxicam, ibuprofen, and flurbiprofen due to their metabolism via cytochrome P450 isoenzymes. With a wide variety of drug interactions, each patient's medication profile should be reviewed, including prescription, OTC, and herbal products, to evaluate for drug-drug interactions before initiating an nonsalicylated NSAID.

EFFICACY OF NSAIDS IN MUSCULOSKELETAL INJURIES

NSAIDs have been purported to help in decreasing pain and inflammation, restore musculoskeletal function, decrease time to healing, and allow faster return to previous activity level. The benefit of using NSAIDs in the prevention of myositis ossificans traumatica following deep muscle contusions remains controversial. Concern has been raised that by inhibiting the inflammatory response, NSAIDs may slow phagocytic function and time for muscle regeneration and healing. Animal studies have been conflicting as to the effects of NSAIDs in the musculoskeletal model. Human studies have not always shown a consistent benefit of NSAIDs in treating musculoskeletal injuries. Studies have been limited at times by small sample sizes, lack of placebo group, subjective assessment, differing patient populations, and lack of control for confounding factors.

A recent review by Mehallo and colleagues[3] summarized data regarding use of NSAIDs for acute ligament and muscle injuries. Rat models for ligament sprains have shown that piroxicam strengthens the medial collateral ligament of the knee at 14 days versus celecoxib, which was found to weaken the medial collateral ligament at 14 days compared with placebo. Other animal studies have not found any benefit with selective and nonselective NSAIDs versus placebo.[3] Human studies have provided evidence for a more consistent benefit of NSAIDs in ligament sprains. A variety of NSAIDs have been shown to decrease pain and inflammation associated with acute ankle sprains.[3] Several studies have documented the efficacy of NSAIDs in decreasing pain, increasing functional ability, and allowing for a more rapid return to training.[3] Although NSAIDs have been shown to be effective for treating the pain associated with injured ligaments, their efficacy in improving joint stability remains unknown.[3] In 2 animal model studies, piroxicam was shown to improve contractile force and greater maximal failure force early post injury, but also slowed deposition of collagen and regeneration of muscle tissue.[3] Studies examining NSAIDs in human muscle strains are limited. One trial evaluated meclofenamate and diclofenac versus placebo along with physiotherapy in treating acute hamstring injuries, and found no differences among the groups with respect to pain, swelling, and isokinetic muscle performance.[3]

Howatson and van Someren[5] reviewed the use of NSAIDs in the treatment and prevention of DOMS. In one study, ketoprofen used prophylactically was found to decrease muscle soreness and enhance muscle function, while another study evaluated ibuprofen before and after exercise and demonstrated a decrease in muscle damage. In contrast, a study evaluated ibuprofen 45 minutes before downhill running and scheduled dosing for 3 days after the activity, and found no effect on muscle soreness or strength.[5] Additional studies with oxaprozin and ibuprofen with acetaminophen post exercise failed to provide benefit.[5] NSAIDs were found to attenuate loss of muscle strength and muscle soreness in 2 studies post exercise and in one study failed to provide evidence of benefit compared with placebo after elbow flexor eccentric muscle injury.[3] Conflicting evidence to support the use of NSAIDs in DOMS may be the result of differences in study methodology, patient selection, and study limitations. NSAIDs may provide benefit in decreasing muscle soreness and improving short-term muscle recovery.[3,41] Given the potential ability of NSAIDs to impair muscle healing, risk versus benefit should be considered and, if used, a short course of 3 to 7 days should be considered.[3]

TOPICAL NSAIDS

In addition to oral NSAIDs, topical formulations of NSAIDs have been used for treating musculoskeletal injuries. A systematic review conducted by Moore and colleagues[42] evaluated 37 placebo-controlled trials of topical NSAIDs in the treatment of acute soft tissue injury, sprains, strains, or trauma. Twenty-seven of the trials demonstrated a significant benefit of the topical NSAID over placebo.[42] The pooled relative benefit for all trials was 1.7 (95% confidence interval [CI]: 1.5–1.9).[42] For topical NSAIDs evaluated in 3 or more studies, pooling of data for the individual agents showed ketoprofen, felbinac, ibuprofen, and piroxicam to be superior to placebo.[42] Local skin reactions were reported in 3% or fewer, systemic adverse effects in fewer than 1%, and discontinuation due to adverse effects in 0.6% or fewer, with no significant difference noted between active treatment and placebo groups.[42] The authors note that due to the small sample size of most of the trials, publication bias may have influenced the results of the systematic review.

Diclofenac gel and topical patch were the first topical NSAIDs approved in 2007 in the United States by the FDA. Diclofenac gel (Voltaren gel) is currently approved for treatment of osteoarthritis and diclofenac topical patch (Flector patch) for the treatment of acute minor sprains, strains, and contusions.[19] When applied to the skin, diclofenac accumulates under the application site, leading to a tissue reservoir for localized effects.[43] With its topical application, systemic plasma concentrations are in the range of 1 to 3 ng/mL and relative systemic bioavailability compared with oral administration is approximately 1%.[43] The diclofenac patch is relatively safe, with skin reactions as the most common adverse event.[43] Thus, the risk for systemic adverse effects is minimal due to low plasma concentrations.

A randomized, double-blind, placebo-controlled trial using topical diclofenac in ankle sprains found it to provide a greater reduction in pain on rest and movement from day 2 and faster joint swelling reduction from day 3.[44] Five percent of the patients in the placebo group discontinued treatment due to lack of efficacy compared with none in the topical diclofenac group.[44] Another randomized, double-blind, placebo-controlled study compared topical diclofenac to placebo in patients with traumatic blunt soft tissue injury.[44] Tenderness at the center of the injured area was produced by pressure applied from calibrated calipers. The primary end point was the area under the curve (AUC) for tenderness over the first 3 days of treatment.[44] The patch was found to be significantly more effective than placebo for the primary end point ($P<.0001$).[44] Topical diclofenac also produced a greater pain intensity reduction at rest and with activity.[44] There were no significant differences between the groups with respect to adverse events, and topical diclofenac was well tolerated.[44] Additional single-blinded or nonrandomized trials have assessed the topical diclofenac patch in acute injuries and have found it to be superior to placebo in relieving pain.[44]

Studies support the use of topical diclofenac in alleviating pain related to acute injuries, but its ability to improve muscle recovery and allow participants to return to activity more quickly remains to be appropriately evaluated. Topical diclofenac, because of its low systemic bioavailability, may be beneficial in those patients who are at risk for gastrointestinal or cardiovascular toxicity from oral NSAIDs.

Acetaminophen

Acetaminophen (Tylenol) was initially used in 1893 but did not gain wide acceptance until 1949.[14] Acetaminophen is the active metabolite of phenacetin, which was widely used until the 1980s when it was withdrawn from the market due to its association with analgesic-abuse nephropathy and hemolytic anemia.[14] Acetaminophen, along with NSAIDs, has largely replaced aspirin as the analgesic of choice in children, adolescents, and young adults, because of aspirin's association with Reye syndrome. Acetaminophen is known to have analgesic and antipyretic activity similar to aspirin; however, acetaminophen has poor anti-inflammatory effects. At typical doses of 1000 mg, acetaminophen has been shown in whole blood assays of healthy volunteers to inhibit only approximately 50% of COX-1 and COX-2 enzymes.[14] Acetaminophen has good bioavailability and is evenly distributed throughout most body fluids.[14] Protein binding of acetaminophen is variable, and it undergoes extensive hepatic metabolism with glucuronidation and sulfation to form inactive metabolites that are excreted by the kidneys.[14] A small percentage (about 5%–15%) of acetaminophen is metabolized to N-acetyl-p-benzoquinoneimine (NAPQI), which normally reacts with glutathione sulfhydryl groups, is further metabolized, and then excreted.[45] When excessive amounts of acetaminophen are consumed, conjugation pathways become saturated and larger amounts of acetaminophen are converted to NAPQI.[14,45] With the shift to NAPQI, glutathione stores become depleted and the excessive NAPQI can lead to hepatotoxicity.[14,45]

Acetaminophen has mild to moderate analgesic properties as well as antipyretic activity. Acetaminophen has been used for a wide variety of indications, including fever and pain associated with many different conditions.[45] Contributing to acetaminophen's widespread use is its easy tolerability. Unlike NSAIDs, acetaminophen does not affect platelet function or uric acid levels, nor is it associated with significant gastrointestinal toxicity.[45] Acetaminophen is felt to be safe in patients with peptic ulcer disease and aspirin hypersensitivity, but is not a reasonable alternative to NSAIDs in patients with inflammatory conditions such as rheumatoid arthritis.[14] Side effects that have been reported, albeit infrequently, include rash, hypersensitivity reactions, blood dyscrasias, and renal toxicity.[45]

The most serious adverse event that may occur with acetaminophen is the risk for hepatotoxicity that occurs with overdose. The maximum adult dose of acetaminophen is 4000 mg per day and for those with chronic alcohol use, 2000 mg daily (**Table 5**).[14] Because of the vast number of preparations that contain acetaminophen, including prescription and OTC, accidental overdose can occur due to consumption of multiple products (ie, prescription analgesic agents and OTC cough and cold preparations). Whether accidental or intentional, acetaminophen overdose is a medical emergency.[14] Overdose can occur with single doses of 10 to 15 g, and doses of 20 to 25 g can be lethal.[14] Acetaminophen toxicity is divided into 4 stages. The first stage can occur within several hours of acute ingestion, is typically associated with nausea, vomiting, and stomach pain, and may resolve within 24 hours.[14,45] The second stage can start approximately 12 to 36 hours after acute ingestion, and is significant for right upper quadrant pain and elevated liver enzymes.[45] Stage 3 occurs 72 to 96 hours after ingestion of toxic doses, and hepatomegaly, jaundice, and coagulopathy may be

Table 5 Acetaminophen formulations and dosing	
Formulation	Regular: 80 mg, 160 mg, 325 mg Extra strength: 500 mg Extended release: 650 mg Liquid: 80 mg/0.8 mg, 160 mg/5 mL, 500 mg/15 mL Rectal suppository: 80 mg, 120 mg, 325 mg, 650 mg
Dosage (adult and adolescent)	325–650 mg every 4–6 h as needed 1000 mg 3–4 times daily Not to exceed 4 g/d
Comments	80 mg and 160 mg available in chewable, oral disintegrating, and meltaways Shake suspension well before dispensing Avoid chronic use in hepatic impairment Chewable tablets may contain phenylalanine Avoid or limit alcohol to <3 drinks per day Avoid other products with acetaminophen

Data from Ref.[19]

present.[14,45] Liver enzyme levels peak during this time period and renal failure can be present. The onset of encephalopathy or worsening coagulopathy after this time period indicates a poor prognosis.[14] Stage 4 is the recovery period for those who make it past stage 3.[45] Acetaminophen overdose is best managed when early diagnosis and treatment can occur. It has been estimated that about 10% of those who do not receive proper treatment will develop severe hepatic impairment, and 10% to 20% of those may eventually die from liver failure.[14,45]

Several studies have evaluated acetaminophen and compared it with an NSAID for treating pain. A study by Dalton and Schweinle[46] compared acetaminophen extended-release to ibuprofen in 260 patients who presented with grade I or II lateral ankle sprains. At the end of the study, acetaminophen was found to be not inferior to ibuprofen; 78% to 80% of patients had resumed normal activities, and mean time to resumption was approximately 4 days in both groups.[46] A study by Woo and colleagues[47] recruited 300 patients who presented to an emergency room with an isolated painful limb injury. Patients were randomized to a 3-day course of acetaminophen, indomethacin, diclofenac, or acetaminophen and diclofenac. Pain reduction was seen in all treatment arms, with score reductions not found to be clinically or statistically significant among the 4 groups over the course of the 3 days.[47] The combination therapy group had the greatest reduction in pain scores at each time point but also produced more side effects, including abdominal pain.[47] Although the literature is not as extensive as for NSAIDs regarding the use of acetaminophen for treating musculoskeletal injuries, there is evidence to support its use.

TOPICAL NONPRESCRIPTION ANALGESICS

Nonprescription, or OTC, analgesic agents and external counterirritants are widely used in the United States, with more than $2 billion spent on them each year.[48] Due to their easy access without a prescription, OTC topical analgesics are often first used in treating acute injuries before scheduling a visit to the physician. Topical analgesics can have one of several different properties; those with counterirritant effects are indicated for the acute treatment of minor aches and pains. Counterirritants exert their effect by producing a less intense pain than the pain the individual is experiencing.[48] The perception of another sensation distracts the person from the original pain produced by the injury. Counterirritants can fall into 1 of 4 categories based on their mechanism: (1) act as rubefacients, (2) production of a cooling sensation, (3) producing vasodilation, and (4) causing irritation without rubefaction.[48] A classification of topical analgesics with counterirritant properties is outlined in **Table 6**. The FDA has approved these agents for use in treating minor aches and pain for both adults and children 2 years or older.[48] Counterirritants from different categories are often combined in various preparations to enhance the efficacy of the product.

Methyl Salicylate

Methyl salicylate is a commonly used rubefacient that is available naturally in wintergreen oil, or it can be produced by esterification of salicylic acid with methyl alcohol.[48] Methyl salicylate is thought to exert its effect by producing a local vasodilation, and the counterirritant effect results from the local increase in skin temperature.[48] Most of the effects of methyl salicylate are locally mediated; however, systemic absorption can increase with the use of multiple applications, and use with local application of heat and occlusive dressings.[48] The most common adverse effects are skin irritation and rash, but more severe skin reactions along with systemic toxicity can occur.[48] The use of heating pads should be avoided while using topical methyl salicylate because

Table 6		
Classification of topical analgesics with counterirritant properties[48]		
Group Classification	Mechanism	Counterirritant
I	Rubefacients	Methyl salicylate Turpentine oil Ammonia water
II	Cooling sensation	Camphor Menthol
III	Vasodilation	Histamine dihydrochloride Methyl nicotinate
IV	Irritation without rubefaction	Capsaicin Capsicum oleoresin[a]

[a] Capsaicin is the major ingredient in capsicum oleoresin. (*Data from* Wright E. Musculoskeletal injuries and disorders. In: Berardi R, Ferreri S, Hume A, et al, editors. Handbook of nonprescription drugs, an interactive approach to self-care. 16th edition. Washington, DC: American Pharmacists Association; 2009. p. 95–113).

tissue and muscle necrosis along with interstitial nephritis have been reported when topical methyl salicylate and menthol were used.[49] Methyl salicylate should be avoided in children and in individuals with aspirin sensitivity and asthma, due to the risk for systemic absorption.[48] Drug interactions with warfarin have been reported with typical and high-dose topical methyl salicylate, resulting in an elevation of the prothrombin time/international normalized ratio.[50,51]

Camphor

Most camphor is synthetically produced and exerts a counterirritant effect via a cooling sensation. Camphor stimulates skin nerve endings producing mild pain, which allows for a masking of the deeper-seated pain.[48] The major toxicity associated with camphor is tonic-clonic seizures. The risk for toxicity correlates with the amount and extent of the camphor ingested.[48] In addition to seizures, high doses have also been associated with nausea, vomiting, dizziness, delirium, coma, and death.[48] Concentrations of camphor oil at 20% and as little as 5 mL can be lethal when ingested by children.[48] As a result, in 1982 the FDA ruled that camphorated oil products could no longer be produced and products containing camphor must have concentrations less than 11% to be considered safe for nonprescription use.[52] Unfortunately, pediatric cases of toxicity from acute ingestions have continued to be reported with OTC preparations containing camphor.[48,52,53]

Menthol

Menthol, prepared synthetically or derived from peppermint oil, is another counterirritant when used at concentrations greater than 1.25%.[48] Menthol exerts its cooling effect by activating the transient receptor potential, TRPM8, in sensory neurons.[54] Menthol has also been associated with an increase in local blood flow at the application site, resulting in a warm sensation.[54] Menthol has been associated with a low incidence of hypersensitivity reactions including itching, erythema, and skin lesions, and postmarketing data indicate minimal toxicity.[54]

Capsaicin

Capsaicin, which is derived from hot chili peppers, produces an analgesic effect due to its direct irritant properties. Topical application of capsaicin produces a warm sensation locally due to activation of the TRP vanilloid (TRPV1); this effect decreases with repeated administration due to tachyphylaxis.[55,56] Capsaicin depletes substance P (neurotransmitter for pain communication) from unmyelinated type C sensory neurons, which can produce an initial burning or itching sensation.[57] Blockade of further synthesis of substance P with repeated application leads to persistent desensitization.[57] The burning sensation diminishes with repeated use, but can lead to an increase in nonadherence and discontinuation of its use. Topical capsaicin has been recommended for use in osteoarthritis, and pain relief is usually seen within several weeks. Capsaicin is applied routinely 3 to 4 times daily to sustain its effect. Gloves should be used to minimize contact with mucous membranes.[48] As with other topical analgesics, capsaicin should not be applied to open wounds and should be discontinued if skin breakdown occurs.[48] Capsaicin has not been studied in acute sports-related injuries, and given that its analgesic effects may not be seen for several weeks, may make it less ideal for treatment.

Others

Other counterirritants not widely used include turpentine oil, histamine dihydrochloride, and ammonia water.[48] The efficacy of these agents is difficult to evaluate, because they are often used in combination with other counterirritant agents. Little data exist to support the use of eucalyptus oil and trolamine salicylate; however, trolamine salicylate continues to be available in a variety of topical analgesics. Trolamine salicylate is not a counterirritant and has been shown to be systemically absorbed.[48] In general, for trolamine salicylate 10% to 15%, is applied to the skin 3 to 4 times daily.[48] Contraindications, precautions, and drug interactions are similar to those of salicylates. Trolamine may be beneficial for those who are unable to tolerate other counterirritants or find them unacceptable.

Counterirritants are available in a wide variety of single and combination products as nonprescription analgesic agents (**Table 7**). Counterirritants are indicated for the treatment of mild aches and pains related to acute injury, and provide a useful option for self-treatment. General guidelines for use of topical counterirritant agents are outlined in **Box 1**.

USE AND ABUSE OF ANALGESICS

OTC medications are widely available and used in the United States. It is not uncommon for individuals to self treat for a wide variety of ailments, including acute musculoskeletal injuries. It has been estimated that 30% of adults have used one or more OTC medications within the past 2 days.[59] Children and adolescents are also consumers of OTC medications for cough and cold, headache, fever, menstrual, and joint and muscle pain. Chambers and colleagues,[59] administered a questionnaire to 651 junior high school students in Nova Scotia to evaluate the use of OTC medications, indications, and self-administration. Of those who used an OTC medication, 88% reported using it for muscle, joint, and back pain; acetaminophen was the most common medication used for each type of pain assessed.[59] Self-administration was common, with 58% to 76% reporting taking medication within the past 3 months without consulting any knowledgeable professional.[59]

With increasing self-administration and easily accessibility, factors that influence consumption of OTC medications have been evaluated. Van den Bulck and colleagues[60] evaluated the association between watching television and analgesic use in 2545 Belgian students (aged 13–16 years). Using a questionnaire, the investigators found that the use of analgesics differed among school years and between gender. A significant correlation was found between regular OTC analgesic use (at

Table 7
Topical analgesic agents

Preparation	Product	Ingredients
Menthol preparations	ActivOn Topical Analgesic Ultra Strength Joint and Muscle	Menthol 4.127%
	Icy Hot Extra Strength Medicated Patch	Menthol 5%
	Ben Gay Ultra Strength Pain Relieving Patch	Menthol 5%
	Absorbine Jr. Pain Relieving Liquid	Menthol 1.27%
	Aspercreme Heat Pain Relieving Gel	Menthol 10%
	Flexall Maximum Strength Relieving Gel	Menthol 16%
Camphor preparations	JointFlex Arthritis Pain Relieving Cream	Camphor 3.1%
Capsaicin preparations	Capzasin Arthritis Pain Relief No Mess Applicator	Capsaicin 0.15%
	Zostrix Arthritis Pain Relief Cream	Capsaicin 0.025%
	Zostrix HP Arthritis Pain Relief Cream	Capsaicin 0.075%
	WellPatch Natural Capsaicin Pain Relief Patch	Capsaicin 0.025%
Trolamine preparations	Aspercreme Analgesic Creme Rub	Trolamine 10%
	Mobisyl Maximal Strength Arthritis Pain Relief Creme	Trolamine 10%
	Sportscreme Deep Penetrating Pain Relieving Rub	Trolamine 10%
Combination preparations	Tiger Muscle Rub	Methyl salicylate 15% Menthol 5% Camphor 3%
	ActivOn Topical Analgesic Ultra Strength Backache	Histamine dihydrochloride 0.025% Menthol 4.127% Camphor 3.15%
	Salonpas Pain Patch	Camphor 1.12% Menthol 5.7% Methyl salicylate 6.3%
	Icy Hot Extra Strength Pain Relieving Chill Stick	Methyl salicylate 30% Menthol 10%
	Icy Hot Extra Strength Relieving Balm	Methyl salicylate 29% Menthol 7.6%
	Heet Pain Relieving Formula	Camphor 3.6% Methyl salicylate 18% Oleoresin capsicum 0.25%
	Freeze It Advanced Therapy Pain Relief, Roll On	Camphor 0.2% Menthol 3.5%

Data from Ref.[58]

least monthly) and viewing of television (odds ratio [OR] 1.16, 95% CI: 1.08–1.24).[60] Playing video games and Internet use was not significantly associated with analgesic use. The authors note that this study did not evaluate the extent to which adolescents were exposed to advertisements during television viewing.[60]

Self-administration of medications by children and adolescents can be influenced by multiple factors and is potentially dangerous. Huott and Storrow[61] surveyed 203 adolescents aged 13 to 18 years who presented to an emergency room or acute care clinic. The adolescents completed a 1-page survey assessing their knowledge of OTC medication toxicity. An informal survey of the investigators' colleagues and standard texts served as the reference point regarding medication toxicity.[61] Survey

> **Box 1**
> **General guidelines for the use of topical analgesics**
>
> Apply to affected areas of intact skin 3 to 4 times daily
>
> Massage or rub gently into the affected area
>
> Wash thoroughly with soap and water after application
>
> For patch application, clean and dry the affected areas and remove film before application
>
> Consider using gloves, especially for capsaicin application
>
> Capsaicin is contraindicated for those younger than 18 years
>
> Follow directions for each product carefully

results of the adolescents indicated that 63% considered aspirin, 57% acetaminophen, 24% iron, 22% camphor, and 17% to 21% methyl salicylate to be nonlethal, which was contradictory to the faculty's viewpoint.[61] The results of this study emphasize that education regarding the toxicity of OTC medications needs further emphasis.

While analgesic use is common among adolescents in general, the pattern of their use among student athletes in particular has not been clearly elucidated. Many student athletes experience muscle aches and pains as well as sports-related injuries, and may self-medicate with OTC analgesic agents including NSAIDs. Evidence indicates that many adolescents are unaware of the potential toxicity or risk for side effects associated with nonprescription analgesic medications. Warner and colleagues[62] distributed a self-administered questionnaire to 604 high school football athletes to compare users with nonusers of NSAIDs and discern differences in attitudes regarding daily use of NSAIDs. The study found that 75% had used NSAIDs in the past 3 months.[62] Of this cohort, 15% considered themselves daily users of NSAIDs.[62] After controlling for confounding variables, those who perceived that NSAIDs enhanced performance (adjusted odds ratio [AOR] 2.4; 95% CI 1.4–4.1), those who used prophylactic NSAIDs (AOR 2.5; 95% CI 1.5–4.3), and those who self-administered NSAIDs (AOR 2.2; 95% CI 1.01–4.9), were more likely to take NSAIDs on a daily basis.[62]

Often in athletes, student as well as elite, studies focus on medications of abuse rather than common prescription and nonprescription medications. Alaranta and colleagues[63] used a questionnaire to determine the frequency of prescribed medications in a group of elite athletes. In 2002, 446 athletes, supported by the National Olympic Committee, completed the survey and were matched to 1503 controls obtained from a population-based study done by the National Public Health Institute.[63] Among athletes, within the previous 7 days 34.5% were using a prescription medication compared with approximately 25% of the controls.[63] NSAIDs were among the most frequently prescribed medications (8.1%) in athletes, with an AOR of 3.63 (95% CI: 2.25–5.84) for use within the past 7 days.[63] Adverse events were reported in 20% of NSAID users.[63]

SUMMARY

The idea of "no pain, no gain" is a common misperception that should be dispelled. Muscle soreness can be expected with strenuous activity or due to an unaccustomed activity, but significant pain is the body's response that rest should occur to allow for healing.[6] Too often, athletes do not take the time off from training or competition to allow for adequate healing.[64] By using analgesics, in particular NSAIDs, pain may subside but further damage can result from continued exercise. Also, NSAIDs, via their inhibition of prostaglandins, may impede the healing process and muscle regeneration after an acute injury. While these agents are relatively safe they are not without side effects, and caution is warranted. There is only limited evidence (albeit it conflicting) in DOMS that NSAIDs can provide a benefit as prophylactic therapy.

Overall, analgesic agents, including NSAIDs, acetaminophen, and topical OTC agents, can effectively relieve pain associated with acute or chronic musculoskeletal injury. Data regarding the ability of NSAIDs to improve muscle recovery and allow a quicker return to activity remain controversial. This area of focus has not been adequately studied with acetaminophen and topical OTC analgesics. When considering an analgesic for alleviating pain, the lowest dose for the shortest time interval should be used. Risk for side effects should be considered and compared with the benefits of the medication. Long-term use for symptoms of sport-related injuries should be avoided, especially with NSAIDs, due to their side effect profile and concern for their impeding the healing process. Data do not adequately support the use of prophylactic NSAIDs prior to sporting events, and should be avoided.

ACKNOWLEDGMENTS

The authors thank Kim Douglas and Amy Esman, Kalamazoo Center for Medical Studies, for assistance in the preparation of this article.

REFERENCES

1. Almekinders L. Anti-inflammatory treatment of muscular injuries in sport, an update of recent studies. Sports Med 1999;28(6):383–8.
2. Garrett WE. Muscle strain injuries: clinical and basic aspects. Med Sci Sports Exerc 1990;22:436–43.
3. Mehallo C, Drezner J, Bytomski J. Practical management: nonsteroidal anti-inflammatory drug (NSAID) use in athletic injuries. Clin J Sport Med 2006;16: 170–4.
4. Micheli L. Common painful sports injuries: assessment and treatment. Clin J Pain 1989;5(Suppl 2):S51–60.
5. Howatson G, van Someren K. The prevention and treatment of exercise-induced muscle damage. Sports Med 2008;38(6):483–503.
6. Smith B, Collina S. Pain medications in the locker room: to dispense or not. Curr Sports Med Rep 2007;6:367–70.
7. Almekinders LC, Gilbert JA. Healing of experimental muscle strains and the effects of non-steroidal anti-inflammatory medication. Am J Sports Med 1986; 14:303–8.
8. Crisco JJ, Jokl P, Heinen GT, et al. A muscle contusion injury model: biomechanics, physiology and histology. Am J Sports Med 1994;22:702–10.
9. Tidball JG. Inflammatory cell response to acute muscle injury. Med Sci Sports Exerc 1995;27:1022–32.
10. Kuipers H. Exercise-induced muscle damage. Int J Sports Med 1994;15:132–5.
11. Jarvinen TA, Jarvinen TL, Kaariainen M, et al. Muscle injuries biology and treatment. Am J Sports Med 2005;33:745–64.
12. Maroon J, Bost J, Borden M, et al. Natural anti-inflammatory agents for pain relief in athletes. Neurosurg Focus 2006;21(4):E11.
13. Herndon C, Hutchinson R, Berdine H, et al. Management of chronic nonmalignant pain with nonsteroidal anti-inflammatory drugs. Pharmacotherapy 2008;28(6): 788–805.

14. Burke A, Smyth E, FitzGerald G. Analgesic-antipyretic and antiinflammatory agents; pharmacotherapy of gout. In: Brunton L, Lazo J, Parker K, editors. Goodman and Gilman's, the pharmacological basis of therapeutics. 11th edition. New York: McGraw-Hill; 2006. p. 671–715.

15. Vane J, Botting R. Mechanism of action of nonsteroidal anti-inflammatory drugs. Am J Med 1998;104(3A):2S–8S.

16. Furst Daniel E, Ulrich Robert W, Varkey-Altamirano C. Nonsteroidal anti-inflammatory drugs, disease-modifying antirheumatic drugs, nonopioid analgesics, drugs used in gout. In: Bertram GK, Susan BM, Anthony JT, editors. Basic & clinical pharmacology. 11th edition. Chapter 36. Available at: http://0-www.accesspharmacy.com.libcat.ferris.edu/content.aspx?aID=4519955. Accessed February 5, 2010.

17. Smyth Emer M, FitzGerald Garret A. The eicosanoids: prostaglandins, thromboxanes, leukotrienes, related compounds. In: Bertram GK, Susan BM, Anthony JT, editors. Basic & clinical pharmacology. 11th edition. Chapter 18. Available at: http://0-www.accesspharmacy.com.libcat.ferris.edu/content.aspx?aID=4518588. Accessed February 5, 2010.

18. Vane J, Botting R. The mechanism of action of aspirin. Thromb Res 2003;110: 255–8.

19. Lexi-Comp, Inc (Lexi-Drugs®). Lexi-Comp. Accessed December 21, 2009.

20. Natural medicines comprehensive database [database on the Internet]. Stockton (CA): Therapeutic Research Faculty; c1995–2009. Antiplatelet; [about 14 pages]. Available at: http://www.naturaldatabase.com/(S(wqklte55rbhkbvzskfpaim45))/nd/Search.aspx?cs=MHSLA%7ECP&s=ND&pt=9&Product=antiplatelet. Accessed December 21, 2009.

21. Kirchain W, Allen R. Drug-induced liver disease. In: DiPiro J, Talbert R, Yee G, et al, editors. Pharmacotherapy a pathophysiologic approach. 7th edition. New York: McGraw-Hill; 2008. p. 652.

22. Scheiman JM, Fendrick AM. Practical approaches to minimizing gastrointestinal and cardiovascular safety concerns with COX-2 inhibitors and NSAIDs. Arthritis Res Ther 2005;7(Suppl 4):S23–9.

23. Golstein JL, Eisen GM, Burke TA, et al. Dyspepsia tolerability from the patients' perspective: a comparison of celecoxib with diclofenac. Aliment Pharmacol Ther 2002;16:819–27.

24. Bombardier C, Laine L, Reicin A, et al. Comparison of upper gastrointestinal toxicity of rofecoxib and naproxen in patients with rheumatoid arthritis. N Engl J Med 2000;343:1520–8.

25. Laine L. Nonsteroidal anti-inflammatory drug gastropathy. Gastrointest Endosc Clin N Am 1996;6:489–504.

26. Gabriel SE, Jaakkimainen L, Bombardier C. Risk for serious gastrointestinal complications related to use of nonsteroidal anti-inflammatory drugs: a meta-analysis. Ann Intern Med 1991;115:787–96.

27. Ekstrom P, Carling L, Wetterhuis S, et al. Prevention of peptic ulcer and dyspeptic symptoms with omeprazole in patients receiving continuous nonsteroidal anti-inflammatory drug therapy: a Nordic multicentre study. Scand J Gastroenterol 1996;31:753–8.

28. Hippisley-Cox J, Coupland C, Logan R. Risk of adverse gastrointestinal outcomes in patients taking cyclo-oxygenase-2 inhibitors or conventional non-steroidal anti-inflammatory drugs: population based nested case-control analysis. BMJ 2005;331:1310–6.

29. Bennett W, Turmelle Y, Shepherd R. Ibuprofen-induced liver injury in an adolescent athlete. Clin Pediatr 2009;48(1):84–6.
30. Rubenstein JH, Laine L. Systematic review: the hepatotoxicity of non-steroidal anti-inflammatory drugs. Aliment Pharmacol Ther 2004;20:373–80.
31. Rostom A, Goldkind L, Laine L. Nonsteroidal anti-inflammatory drugs and hepatic toxicity: a systematic review of randomized controlled trials in arthritis patients. Clin Gastroenterol Hepatol 2005;3:489–98.
32. Whelton A. Nephrotoxicity of nonsteroidal anti-inflammatory drugs: physiologic foundations and clinical implications. Am J Med 1999;106(Suppl 5B):S13–24.
33. Clive DM, Stoff JS. Renal syndromes associated with nonsteroidal anti-inflammatory drugs. N Engl J Med 1984;310:563–72.
34. Henrich WL. Nephrotoxicity of nonsteroidal anti-inflammatory agents. Am J Kidney Dis 1983;2:478–84.
35. Nakahura T, Griswold W, Lemire J, et al. Nonsteroidal anti-inflammatory drug use in adolescents. J Adolesc Health 1998;23:307–10.
36. Solomon S, McMurray J, Pfeffer M, et al. Cardiovascular risk associated with celecoxib in a clinical trial for colorectal adenoma prevention. N Engl J Med 2005; 352:1071–80.
37. Bresalier RS, Sandler RS, Quan H, et al. Cardiovascular events associated with rofecoxib in a colorectal adenoma chemoprevention trial. N Engl J Med 2005; 352:1092–102.
38. McGettigan P, Henry D. Cardiovascular risk and inhibition of cyclooxygenase, a systematic review of the observational studies of selective and nonselective inhibitors of cyclooxygenase 2. JAMA 2006;296:1633–44.
39. COX-2 selective (includes Bextra, Celebrex, and Vioxx) and non-selective nonsteroidal anti-inflammatory drugs (NSAIDs). U.S. Food and Drug Administration, Drug Safety and Availability. Available at: http://www.fda.gov/Drugs/DrugSafety/ PostmarketDrugSafetyInformationforPatientsandProviders/ucm103420.htm. Updated September 24, 2009. Accessed December 28, 2009.
40. Drug Facts & Comparisons [database on the Internet]. Facts & comparisons. Indianapolis (IN). 4.0; 2009. Nonsteroidal anti-inflammatory agents; [about 21 pages]. Available at: http://0-online.factsandcomparisons.com.libcat.ferris.edu/ MonoDispaspx?id=570727&book=DFC. Accessed December 28, 2009.
41. Lanier A. Use of nonsteroidal anti-inflammatory drugs following exercise-induced muscle injury. Sports Med 2003;3:177–86.
42. Moore R, Tramer M, Carroll D, et al. Quantitative systematic review of topically applied non-steroidal anti-inflammatory drugs. BMJ 1998;316:333–8.
43. Peterson B, Rovati S. Diclofenac epolamine (Flector®) patch, evidence for topical activity. Clin Drug Investig 2009;29(1):1–9.
44. Zacher J, Altman R, Bellamy N, et al. Topical diclofenac and its role in pain and inflammation: an evidence-based review. Curr Med Res Opin 2008;24(4): 925–50.
45. Drug Facts & Comparisons [database on the Internet]. Facts & comparisons. Indianapolis (IN). 4.0; 2009. Acetaminophen; [about 5 pages]. Available at: http:// 0-online.factsandcomparisons.com.libcat.ferris.edu/MonoDisp.aspx?monoID= fandc-hcp10022&quick=acetaminophen&search=acetaminophen&disease=. Accessed December 31, 2009.
46. Dalton J, Schweinle J. Randomized controlled noninferiority trial to compare extended release acetaminophen and ibuprofen for the treatment of ankle sprains. Ann Emerg Med 2006;48:615–23.

47. Woo W, Man S, Lam P, et al. Randomized double-blind trial comparing oral paracetamol and oral nonsteroidal anti-inflammatory drugs for treating pain after musculoskeletal injury. Ann Emerg Med 2005;46:352–61.
48. Wright E. Musculoskeletal injuries and disorders. In: Berardi R, Ferreri S, Hume A, et al, editors. Handbook of nonprescription drugs, an interactive approach to self-care. 16th edition. Washington, DC: American Pharmacists Association; 2009. p. 95–113.
49. Heng MC. Local necrosis and interstitial nephritis due to topical methyl salicylate and menthol. Cutis 1987;39(5):442–4.
50. Yip A, Chow W, Tai Y, et al. Adverse effect of local methylsalicylate ointment on warfarin anticoagulation: an unrecognized potential hazard. Postgrad Med J 1990;66(775):367–9.
51. Joss J, LeBlond R. Potentiation of warfarin anticoagulation associated with topical methyl salicylate. Ann Pharmacother 2000;34(6):729–33.
52. Love J, Sammon M, Smereck J. Are one or two dangerous? Camphor exposure in toddlers. J Emerg Med 2004;27(1):49–54.
53. Gouin S, Patel H. Unusual cause of seizure. Pediatr Emerg Care 1996;12(4):298–300.
54. Patel T, Ishiuji Y, Yosipovitch G. Menthol: a refreshing look at this ancient compound. J Am Acad Dermatol 2007;57:873–8.
55. Vyklicky L, Novakova-Tousova K, Benedikt J, et al. Calcium-dependent desensitization of vanilloid receptor TRPV1: a mechanism possibly involved in analgesia induced by topical application of capsaicin. Physiol Res 2008;57(Suppl 3):S59–68.
56. Knotkova H, Pappagallo M, Szallasi A. Capsaicin (TRPV1 agonist) therapy for pain relief farewell or revival? Clin J Pain 2008;24:142–54.
57. Mason L, Moore A, Derry S, et al. Systematic review of topical capsaicin for the treatment of chronic pain. BMJ 2004;328:991.
58. Drugstore.com. Topical analgesics. Available at: http://www.drugstore.com/search/search_results.asp?N=0&Ntx=mode%2Bmatchallpartial&Ntk=All&srchtree=5&Ntt=topical+analgesics. Accessed January 10, 2010.
59. Chambers C, Reid G, McGrath P, et al. Self-administration of over-the-counter medication for pain among adolescents. Arch Pediatr Adolesc Med 1997;151:449–55.
60. Van den Bulck J, Leemans L, Laekeman G. Television and adolescent use of over-the-counter analgesic agents. Ann Pharmacother 2005;39:58–62.
61. Huott M, Storrow A. A survey of adolescents' knowledge regarding toxicity of over-the-counter medications. Acad Emerg Med 1997;4:214–8.
62. Warner D, Schnepf G, Barrett M, et al. Prevalence, attitudes, and behaviors related to the use of nonsteroidal anti-inflammatory drugs (NSAIDs) in student athletes. J Adolesc Health 2002;30:150–3.
63. Alaranta A, Alaranta H, Heliovaara M, et al. Ample use of physician-prescribed medications in Finnish elite athletes. Int J Sports Med 2006;27(11):919–25.
64. Alaranta A, Alaranta H, Helenius I. Use of prescription drugs in athletes. Sports Med 2008;38(6):449–63.

The Application of Osteopathic Treatments to Pediatric Sports Injuries

Delmas J. Bolin, MD, PhD[a,b,c],*

KEYWORDS

- Biomechanics • Osteopathic manipulation
- Pediatrics • Sports injury

There is little published evidence to support the use of osteopathic techniques in the treatment of pediatric athletes. Despite this, sports medicine practitioners commonly relate stories where a doctor with training in manual techniques "popped" something and an athlete was "cured." Considered alternative medicine by most allopathic physicians, there are a few instances where manipulation is an accepted treatment; for example, most pediatricians readily accept manipulation of the radial head for the treatment of nursemaids' elbow. Far from being an anecdotal trick, the nursemaids' elbow diagnosis and its treatment by manipulation represent an underlying biomechanical principle, that motion restrictions are often the symptom of a biomechanical deficit. When the deficit is corrected, function is restored. In an age of evidence-based medicine, the lack of solid literature-based evidence gives even the most open-minded pause, especially when application is made to a pediatric population. Those with additional training in manual techniques look for asymmetry and restriction of motion; once identified, a variety of osteopathic techniques can used to address the deficit and affect change.

Practitioners who look at patients through a biomechanical or osteopathic lens may identify motion restrictions that are amenable to osteopathic treatment. Manipulation should not be thought of as a solitary treatment; it is best used to correct motion restriction and then followed by appropriate muscle retraining via physical therapy to facilitate long-term resolution. In those cases where motion asymmetry persists

[a] Departments of Sports Medicine, Family Medicine, and Osteopathic Manipulative Medicine, The Via College of Osteopathic Medicine, Blacksburg, VA 24060, USA
[b] PCA Center for Sports Medicine, 1935 West Main Street, Salem, VA 24153, USA
[c] Radford University Athletics, Radford, VA 24142, USA
* PCA Center for Sports Medicine, 1935 West Main Street, Salem, VA 24153.
E-mail address: dbolin@vcom.vt.edu

Pediatr Clin N Am 57 (2010) 775–794
doi:10.1016/j.pcl.2010.02.002
0031-3955/10/$ – see front matter © 2010 Elsevier Inc. All rights reserved.

or recurs, a structural cause for the repeated dysfunction should be sought. In this article, a general discussion of osteopathic diagnosis and treatment rationale is followed by application to specific conditions associated with sports participation in the pediatric population where manual treatments may be of use.

USE AND COMPLICATIONS WITH MANUAL MEDICINE

A 2008 survey investigated the use of complementary and alternative medicine (CAM) in patients 18 years or younger. The Department of Health and Human Services found that more than 2 million youths (2.8%) had used chiropractic or osteopathic manipulation in the previous year. It was the second most common CAM behind the use of vitamins or other natural remedy. The most common reason cited for seeking care was back or neck pain.[1] Children whose parents used CAM were twice as likely to be treated with CAM. Most who used CAM did so as an adjuvant to conventional medical care.

Manual medicine, spinal manipulation in particular, is not without risk; the risk of adverse events varies by technique and is likely small. Generally, many patients can be expected to experience some discomfort after manipulation. Aggravation of symptoms is usually short lived (1–2 days) and is attributed to changes in soft tissue and ligaments associated with the regions that are mobilized.[2] In a literature review of complications associated with thrust manipulations performed by a therapist or physician and including adult and pediatric patients, catastrophic complications of manipulation were rare and were most commonly vertebral-basilar compromise (cervical manipulation) and cauda equina syndrome (lumbar manipulation).[3] The investigators associated rotatory manipulation of the cervical spine with vascular compromise. Similar results are reported in osteopathic literature, showing that most complications appear as anecdotal case reports, making efforts to attribute risk or prevalence problematic.[4]

In an effort to assess risk of manipulation in pediatric patients, Hayes and Bezilla[5] performed a retrospective chart review of 502 pediatric patients treated with osteopathic interventions (all treatments, including thrust techniques). The investigators defined aggravations as patient complaints or worsening of symptoms after manipulation. Complications were defined as cerebrovascular accident, dislocation, fracture, pneumothorax, sprains and strains, or death as an outcome of treatment. In their review, there were no manipulation-related complications; aggravations occurred and were documented in approximately 12% of manipulations. The average duration of aggravation symptoms was less than 48 hours (evidence level B).[5] In summary, most pediatric patients seem to have mild, short-lived, aggravation-type symptoms after osteopathic treatments. Complications, which seem rare, are likely underrepresented in the literature and usually associated with thrust-type manipulations.

METHODS AND BARRIERS TO SOUND RESEARCH

A paucity of literature regarding manual treatments in pediatric patients exists. Pubmed searches were performed using key words mobilization, manipulation, osteopathic, chiropractic, pediatric, child, and adolescent as well as the specific condition to be examined. The vast majority of articles identified were of an anecdotal nature.

There are many barriers to conducting high-quality osteopathic research. Chief among these is poor research question design. Most reasonable efforts have centered on applying manual techniques to nonspecific symptoms. Research questions, such as, "How effective is spinal manipulation for low back pain (a symptom)?" are unlikely to provide useful information. Such questions are based on a poor assumption, that specific treatments can be applied to general symptoms. The allopathic equivalent is to test the effectiveness of penicillin for sore throat. Penicillin is ineffective for sore throat and highly effective for streptococcal pharyngitis. A specific diagnosis should be paired with a specific treatment with a specific outcome to be measured.

The best research regarding the efficacy of manual treatments would be study of the use of a specific technique for a specific structural diagnosis. Such research is lacking for several reasons. First, there is no standardized allopathic nomenclature for the identification and description of biomechanical symptoms. Although osteopaths may identify a specific issue, for example, 3rd lumbar extended, rotated, and side-bent to the left (L_3 ERS$_L$), allopathic physicians are not generally trained to evaluate or recognize such segmental motion restrictions. Most osteopathic diagnoses are based on motion restriction, a dynamic problem. Even if a palpation-based structural diagnosis is made, there remains no gold standard (such as dynamic radiology) that can confirm the diagnosis or evaluate treatment success. With the exception of fluoroscopy, radiographic studies do not permit dynamic evaluations. Fluoroscopy is not routinely used in biomechanical analysis because of high radiation exposure. A third barrier is the persistence of methodologic issues that have not yet been overcome. There is no adequate sham manipulation or adequate blinding of patients or doctors to the procedures, which is necessary to avoid bias and improve the strength of a systematic study of specific manipulation techniques. Finally, there are no long-term follow-up studies to address whether or not the manipulation induced permanent change. Each is a significant barrier to performing a specific, highly powered, scientific inquiry into the usefulness of manual treatments.

BARRIER CONCEPTS IN THE EVALUATION OF PEDIATRIC PATIENTS

The rationale for using biomechanical approaches to a specific injury is to restore motion. Conceptually, each joint or body region has a range of motion through which it can pass. There are physiologic and anatomic barriers (**Fig. 1**). As motion in either direction from midline proceeds, ligamentous tension develops. In the case of injury or dysfunction, a restrictive barrier may alter active and passive range of motion. These restrictive barriers are referred to as somatic dysfunctions.

Most techniques used in biomechanical treatments begin with a positional diagnosis. The biomechanical evaluation uses primarily palpatory skills to identify areas of tenderness, tissue texture changes, asymmetry, and restriction of range of motion. Motion at the joint or the body part is assessed in the sagittal plane for flexion and extension, the coronal plane for lateral flexion (side bending), and the transverse plane for rotation. The primary objective of this evaluation is to identify regions that have a specific barrier to motion. For example, evaluating the motion at the 3rd lumbar vertebra in neutral, flexion, and extension, a specific motion restriction can be identified for that particular structure (if dysfunction is present). If the evaluator finds the 3rd lumbar transverse process deeper on the right and more easily rotated on the left, the segment can further be tested in flexion and extension and a positional diagnosis (eg, L_3 ERS$_L$) can be established.

Once identified, a particular osteopathic technique is chosen with the goal of removing the obstruction and restoring normal motion and function. With normal motion restored, patients are frequently referred to physical therapy for neuromuscular retraining, strengthening, and conditioning to maintain and reinforce restored positioning. It is never assumed that a biomechanical restriction happens in isolation; because of the close anatomic relationships, associated muscle and ligamentous injury requires time to heal regardless of the use of manual treatments.

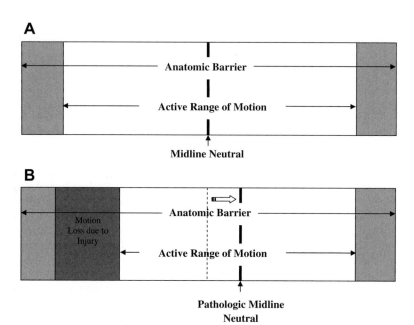

Fig. 1. Motion barrier concepts. (*A*) Normal motion. Active (physiologic) range of motion is symmetric. (*B*) Simplified loss of motion: with injury, motion is lost on 1 side, resulting in somatic dysfunction. Asymmetry results in a new midline formation. Over time, tissue contractures develop in response to motion loss and patients may compensate for lost motion at 1 site with altered motion at a second site. (*Data from* Greenman P. Principles of manual medicine. 2nd edition. Baltimore [MD]: Williams and Wilkins; 1996.)

PEDIATRIC CONSIDERATIONS AND SPECIFIC OSTEOPATHIC TECHNIQUES

Although osteopathic techniques can be applied to infants and young children,[2] this discussion is limited to the application to pediatric patients between the ages of 6 and 18. With any use of manual medicine in the pediatric population, there are key differences between pediatric and adult patients. Joint mechanics are influenced by the maturation of the ossification centers. Pediatric patients with open growth plates are vulnerable to injury; techniques used must be gentle and carefully applied. In contrast to adults, who have well-established movement patterns, children are often in the process of developing such patterns. This is relevant for post-treatment decision making. Children often use new motion patterns readily after restoration of function[2]; adults learn to compensate and must unlearn motion habits. Although complete descriptions of all manual techniques and their theoretic basis is beyond the scope of this discussion, interested readers may find more complete discussions in many sources.[2,6] Several more commonly used techniques are discussed later and listed in **Table 1**.

High- and Low-Velocity, Low-Amplitude Techniques

High-velocity, low-amplitude techniques (HVLA) and low-velocity, low-amplitude techniques (LVLA) are performed to directly engage a restrictive barrier. Using the previously described example of a spinal dysfunction (L_3 ERS$_L$), the barrier is to motion in flexion, right rotation, and right side bending. Using this technique, patients are

Table 1 Descriptions of common osteopathic manual techniques applied to pediatric sports injuries	
HVLA	Direct engagement of a motion barrier using an impulse or thrust
Muscle energy	Uses patient's muscular contraction to precisely direct away from a restrictive barrier against resistance. During relaxation phase, the motion barrier is directly engaged
Counter-strain	Passively placing a patient in a position directly opposite the barrier to indirectly treat motion deficit; typically associated with positioning to achieve maximal relief of a specific painful point
Myofascial release	Indirect technique, which uses lateral stretching, linear stretching, deep pressure, traction, and muscle stretch or compression. Aims to restore motion via tissue relaxation
Lymphatic pump	Gentle rhythmic techniques designed to improve function via improved fluid drainage from the injured area

positioned to engage the barrier at the specific vertebral level, eliminating as much motion of the segments above and below the treatment area as possible. At the barrier, the treatment consists of a quick thrust (HVLA) or a slow deliberate movement through the barrier (LVLA). A release may or may not be felt and is not essential for success of the treatment. As with any treatment, patients should be re-evaluated for improved range of motion after the procedure.

Muscle Energy

A second frequently used technique that directly engages the restriction is muscle energy. In this technique, patients are placed in a specific and controlled position and asked to contract specific muscle groups to generate motion in a particular direction against a precise counterforce.[2] Using the same positional diagnosis (as described previously), L_3 ERS_L, in this approach patients are positioned seated, lumbar spine flexed to the L_3 level, then rotated and side-bent to the right (**Fig. 2**). The treatment is performed using a patient's muscle energy (approximately 5 pounds of force) to sit upright (extension, side bending, and rotation to left) from that position while an examiner resists. This force is held for 5 seconds, then the patient briefly relaxes; during the relaxation, the slack is taken up and a new barrier in FLEXION, right rotation, and right side bending is engaged. This process is typically performed 3 times. This is a technique commonly used by physical therapists in treating motion restriction. Muscle energy poses less risk of injury to patients because they are in control of the treatment. The ability to use this treatment in the pediatric population, however, is dependent on children's ability to follow directions and to precisely control their body movements.

Strain-Counterstrain Techniques

Strain-counterstrain is a gentle indirect treatment of positional diagnosis. The basic underlying principle is that specific tender points on the body, anterior and posterior, are present and associated with specific positional diagnoses throughout the spine.[7] The concept of this treatment is that dysfunctional positioning of a body segment places ligaments and other soft tissues under strain when the body attempts to remain in neutral posture against gravity, producing discomfort in specific palpable locations. In positioning the dysfunctional segment in a position of ease, a counterstrain is applied to the area to be treated. The essence of this technique is to identify a tender point; in

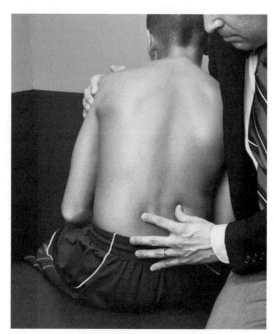

Fig. 2. Muscle energy positioning for patient with 3rd lumbar (L3) vertebrae dysfunction. The patient is positioned at the barrier to motion: flexed until motion is engaged at L3, then rotated and side-bent to the right. The technique is described in the text. Note the evaluator maintains contact with the transverse processes at L3 during the treatment. (*Courtesy of* Quinton Nottingham, PhD.)

the example described previously, the tender point would likely be identified near the transverse process of L_3. The body would be passively wrapped around this tender point until pain was subjective reduced approximately 70%. For this example (L_3 ERS_L), the patient is typically prone and the physician passively wraps around the point in extension, left rotation, and left side bending by controlling the legs. Once the position of relief is achieved, the patient is held in this position for 90 seconds. After the treatment, it is important that the patient be returned to the neutral position without activating muscles.[7] In the neutral position, the tender point and the area of dysfunction should be re-evaluated. This gentle technique can safely be used in children because it does not expose them to any external force other than positioning. Patients must be able to remain still and relaxed for the treatment period.

Myofascial Approaches

Areas of dysfunction may be identified by soft tissue palpation. These myofascial trigger points are discreet, tender, and asymmetric; have altered range of motion; and demonstrate tissue texture changes.[8] These trigger points can be treated with a variety of approaches, including ischemic inhibition, cooling spray with stretch, deep massage, injection, and myofascial release. The trigger points are thought to be related not only to positional dysfunctions but also reflective of muscle and fascial contracture as well as effects on the integrated autonomic nervous system.[9] Manual treatments of the trigger points include compression directly on the trigger point until it relaxes. This treatment is based on the concept of inducing focused regional ischemia in the tissue over the trigger point. The muscle can also be hypercontracted, that is, placed passively in a shortened position, and then manually compressed further.[8] It is thought that this treatment alters neuromuscular patterns within the muscle. A third approach is to unwind myofascial tissues at areas of constriction. This technique is based on the concept that the fascia is a continuous ligamentous stocking that can be twisted or bunched in areas of dysfunction and that unwinding loosens the tissues to allow freer motion.[6]

These 4 approaches are a sample and do not encompass several other techniques that are commonly used for manipulation. Many nonthrust techniques are used in conjunction with regular rehabilitation programs by physical therapists. Although high-velocity techniques are commonly associated with osteopathic or chiropractic adjustments, there are other approaches that can also be safely and easily applied to a variety of patient complaints.

SPECIFIC CONDITIONS
Cervical Spine

Application of manual treatments to cervical spine complaints is common. The most common complaints are headache, neck pain, and torticollis. A complete evaluation should be performed to eliminate underlying orthopedic or medical causes that constitute an absolute or relative contraindication to manual methods. In evaluating patients with headache, neck pain, or stiffness, the biomechanical principle that should be kept in mind is that patients generally position their head to keep their eyes directly in front and parallel to the ground. Historical features and structural evaluation looking for asymmetry of motion, asymmetry of deep musculature tension, and other tissue texture changes should be sought.

A practical approach to gross motion assessment is to measure cervical rotation from the manubrium to the chin on rotation to left and right. Side bending is assessed via measurement of pinna to acromion on lateral flexion. Restriction in motion may also be detected by having patients rotate left and right and returning to midline with eyes closed (while an examiner monitors the midline). This simple test may reveal patients whose sense of midline is altered to the left or right with eyes closed.[10] Compensatory increase in tone of cervical musculature may be associated with patients being off-center.

In addition to gross motion testing, segmental testing at each vertebral level can be performed.[11] It is helpful to understand the mechanics of each vertebral level, which are now well established.[12] The occipitoatlantal joint primarily flexes and extends. Side bending and rotation is coupled and always occurs in opposite directions. The atlantoaxial joint primarily rotates. Typical cervical vertebrae C3-C7 all have coupled motion with rotation and side bending to the same side. The ability to identify the precise location and direction of a segmental motion restriction is fundamental to using osteopathic technique. If there is good correlation with a patient's symptoms, signs, and physical findings, then there is a strong likelihood that improved segment mobility will decrease or even eliminate the patient's symptoms.[11] Specific instruction regarding evaluation procedures and diagnostic interpretation for the cervical spine can be found in several sources.[2,6,10,12]

Motional abnormalities of the upper 3 cervical vertebrae are significant contributors to headache, neck pain, and torticollis. Muscle energy techniques are particularly useful in this region because they avoid positioning patients in extremes of hyperextension and rotation.[11] This position places the vertebral artery and to a lesser extent the internal carotid artery in a position where injury during HVLA could occur.[13] Injury rates with cervical manipulation in children are not known; risk of catastrophic injury is estimated at between 1 in 400,000 to 1 in 2,000,000 for cervical manipulations in all patient age groups.[14,15] The use of manipulation for cervicogenic headache is associated with improvement in symptoms when motion deficits are corrected.[16] Recent systematic reviews for neck pain with or without headache suggests that manual treatments are associated with improvement in symptoms when combined with exercise programs (evidence level B).[15,17] In the treatment of children with neck pain and muscle spasm with or without headache, manipulation may be of use if a specific motion restriction is identified that correlates with symptoms.

Chest Wall Syndromes

Thoracic outlet syndrome

Thoracic outlet syndrome (TOS) is characterized by symptoms of positional parasthesia, weakness, or heaviness of the upper extremity that is associated with cervical hyperextension injury. Ninety-five percent of cases are thought to be neurogenic TOS, with compression of the brachial plexus occurring at the thoracic outlet.[17] The biomechanical basis for the condition is the compression of neurovascular structures, which supply the upper extremity by the narrowing of the thoracic outlet between the clavicle, the middle and anterior scalene muscles, the scapula, and the first rib. The condition is also associated with anomalous first ribs[18] and is common in swimmers and overhead athletes. Historical and diagnostic aspects are extensively reviewed elsewhere.[17] Traditional clinical tests, including Adson and Roo tests, lack specificity for the diagnosis.[19] Although there is no published support, osteopathic positional diagnosis of the first thoracic vertebrae and rib can be helpful when correlated with patient symptoms; the first rib is typically elevated on the affected side.

Nonoperative treatment of neurogenic TOS includes 2 months of conservative treatment with physical therapy using gentle rehabilitative exercises, nonsteroidal anti-inflammatory medications (NSAIDs), trigger point injections, manual therapy, and stretching of the neck and shoulder muscles. In the vascular surgery literature, young adolescent athletes often do not respond well to conservative therapy.[19] Surgical decompression via resection of the first rib with scalenectomy was reported in a series of 18 young (ages 13–19) patients with neurogenic TOS. All patients returned to school and competitive athletics.[20]

The osteopathic approach to patients with neurogenic TOS includes myofasical, muscle energy, and high-velocity techniques (**Fig. 3**). The indication for the use of manual techniques includes reproduction of patient symptoms and the establishment of motion restriction and positional diagnosis for the first rib or first thoracic vertebrae. The treatments usually require no more than a few minutes; patients experience rapid relief of heaviness and positional parasthesia but often experience postmanipulation soreness beginning approximately 10 minutes after the procedure, which is attributed to ligamentous stretch. After manipulation, patients are given brief courses of NSAIDs and referred for postural exercises and neuromuscular retraining at physical therapy. There are no systematic studies of the effectiveness of manual medicine for neurogenic TOS; anecdotal reports describe the successful use of manual therapies in a young athlete[18] and adult patients.[21]

The osteopathic approach (discussed previously) is presented with nothing but scant anecdotal evidence. The paucity of data for manual treatments of neurogenic TOS is in stark contrast to the well-documented evidence presented in the vascular surgery literature. Both focus attention on the thoracic outlet and both agree that the first rib and surrounding tissues can be the source of compression. Resection of the first rib is effective, if highly invasive, in curing the symptoms in young athletes.

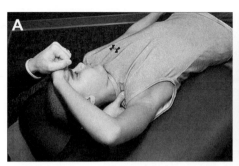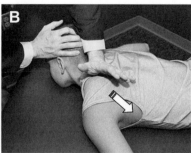

Fig. 3. Treatment of elevated first rib in pediatric patients. (*A*) Muscle energy. The patient is positioned with head rotated and side-bent away from the motion restriction. The physician's hand monitors motion at the posterior aspect of the first rib. The patient gently raises his head and fist against examiner's resistance. On relaxing, the rib is mobilized to engage the new barrier. (*B*) Impulse mobilization (HVLA). The hypothenar eminence is placed on the posterior aspect of the first rib. The patient's head is distracted with the opposite hand (no thrust is applied to the patient's head); at the barrier, a thrust downward and toward the ipsilateral breast is applied. (*Courtesy of* Quinton Nottingham, PhD.)

With advanced diagnostic imaging available, the observation that "many (neurogenic) TOS patients respond favorably to surgery, even in the absence of preoperative objective abnormalities" (quote in[17]) suggests a dynamic deficit may be underlying this condition. To add to anecdotal reports, no patient from the author's clinic has been referred for surgical rib resection with this condition since his initiation of using osteopathic treatment for clinically diagnosed TOS.22. The reconciliation of this observation with published literature awaits further high-quality investigation into the biomechanics of TOS and the effectiveness, if any, of osteopathic techniques.

Chest wall pain
Chest pain in the pediatric athletic population may arise from the ribs, costovertebral articulations, costal cartilage, and supporting structures. Appropriate evaluation and work-up is paramount in establishing musculoskeletal causes of chest pain and excluding other causes. Dysfunctions at lower ribs and thoracic vertebrae (T3-T8) typically cause vague pain between the shoulder blades often radiating around the chest wall to under the armpit or lateral and inferior to the breast. Swimmers and rowers are commonly affected.[22] These dysfunctions may arise from overuse but are not usually associated with specific injury. Examination signs include chest wall pain that is typically reproduced by palpation along involved ribs, at the rib posteriorly, and may also be present anteriorly at the costochondral junction. Palpation of the ribs during inhalation and exhalation may reveal diminished excursion of the ribs. Motion restriction on passive trunk rotation may be observed (**Fig. 4**). Successful resolution of motion restrictions and symptoms after treatment by impulse mobilization[23] or muscle energy techniques[22] has been reported.

Lower ribs may also cause symptoms: the slipping rib syndrome describes vague complaints of abdominal, flank, or low back pain with or without trauma. The symptoms are attributed to slipping of a hypermobile cartilaginous rib under adjacent ribs during muscle activity.[24] The diagnosis is aided with the hooking maneuver, in which the symptomatic floating rib is pulled under the rib above, producing a click and reproducing the pain.[25] Diagnosis is confirmed with an appropriate nerve block. The surgical literature describes several cases in which complete symptom resolution

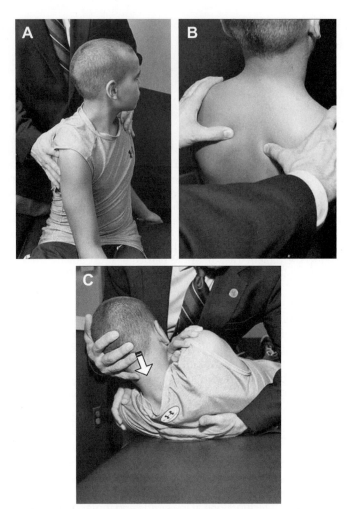

Fig. 4. Osteopathic assessment and treatment of rib and thoracic vertebrae structural issues. (*A*) Loss of passive trunk rotation—most athletic patients can rotate 90° to either side. (*B*) Palpation for relative depth and rotation of rib tubercles and transverse processes and any tissue texture change can point to areas of motion restriction. (*C*) Thrust method for the ribs and thoracic spine manipulation. After a positional diagnosis is confirmed (illustrated: T7 extended, rotated, and side-bent to right), the patient is placed with his arms folded in front. The physician monitors the level of flexion with the posterior hand until motion is engaged at the level to be treated. The patient is instructed to take a deep breath and let it out, not holding his breath, and as exhalation occurs, a quick and gentle impulse is delivered from anterior through to the posterior hand. Motion and symptoms are always re-evaluated. This method can be adapted to address lower floating rib dysfunctions. (*Courtesy of* Quinton Nottingham, PhD.)

occurred after resection of the rib tip.[26,27] Findings at surgery reveal torn ligamentous support for the ribs. In the subacute setting, it is possible to gently reposition the floating ribs using HVLA or LVLA maneuvers (see **Fig. 4**). There are anecdotal reports of symptom resolution with return to symptom-free participation even with prolonged symptoms after such treatments.[28]

SCOLIOSIS

Idiopathic scoliosis is a rotational malalignment of the vertebrae that produces a partly fixed lateral curvature of the spine.[2] Usually thoracic spine and rib cage are involved and a compensatory curve is found in the lumbar spine. Girls between the ages of 10 and 16 years are nearly 4 times more likely to develop the condition.[2] The biomechanics of scoliosis and distant claims of cures with manipulation[29] have led to efforts to define the role of manual medicine and its effectiveness. Although the cause of scoliosis is unknown, the biomechanics involved arise from the aforementioned principle that most patients compensate to achieve a position where the eyes are parallel to the horizon and face forward. Certain repetitive activities that involve asymmetric movements may predispose to soft tissue contraction; scoliosis is commonly seen in adolescent softball pitchers who bend toward their pitching arm in an effort to achieve a vertical release. Chronic backpack carrying also has altered spinal curvature over time.[30]

Long-term presence of a curvature in the spine results in fascial and muscular contractures on the concave side of the curve, which resist straightening and promote curve progression. Likewise, the muscles and fascia on the convex side of the curve are overstretched. Starling's law predicts these muscles generate different forces by virtue of their different lengths. Consequently, any attempt to alter the curve via a manipulation intuitively suggests the need for muscle retraining and tissue reorganization to achieve any long-term impact toward straightening the curve. The combination of manipulation with physical therapy has been effective in producing Cobb angle reductions of 16° to 17° with short-term[31] and longer-term[32] treatment. Exercise alone is beneficial in reducing curve progression (evidence level A).[33] This soft tissue and manipulative approach is reported in the literature with anecdotal, although well-documented, improvements in symptoms and spinal curvature for the past 20 years.[34] The addition of manipulation to physical or exercise therapy and other standard treatments may be beneficial in reducing curve progression and perhaps assisting with curvature regression (evidence level B).

LOW BACK PAIN

The sacroiliac (SI) joint and pelvis can be pain generators from the joint proper or its ligamentous attachments. Athletes involved in sports that necessitate unilateral loading of the SI joint, such as kicking or throwing, are at higher risk for SI injury and pain.[35] There are several historical features and physical examination maneuvers that are used by osteopathic practitioners to diagnose a 3-D position of the SI joint. A complete description of these is available from many sources.[2,6,10] Most patients complain of low back pain at the waistline. Historical features suggesting SI involvement include the description of pain at the sacral sulcus and radiation of the pain to the buttocks or down the posterior thigh to the level of the knee. The examination maneuvers commonly used include the standing and seated forward flexion test, palpation of the sacral sulcus and inferolateral sacral angles (ILAs), and the spring test (**Fig. 5**). In addition, the relative positions of the anterior-superior iliac spine (ASIS) and posterior-superior iliac spine (PSIS) and the relative distance of each ASIS from the umbilicus are used to determine the position of the innominate bones (ilium) in anterior or posterior rotation, inflare and outflare, or upslip or downslip.[2] These palpatory measurements are often combined with functional leg length assessment to complete the positional diagnosis. **Tables 2** and **3** summarize how dynamic and static testing is interpreted to make a positional diagnosis.

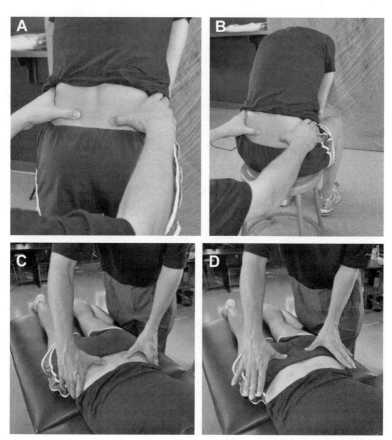

Fig. 5. Dynamic and static testing for sacral dysfunctions. (*A*) The standing forward flexion test. Examiner starts with hands on iliac crests; thumbs naturally fall at the PSIS. With thumbs resting just inferior and medial to the PSIS, have patient bend toward floor. A positive test is indicated by the thumb that moves cephalad earliest. (*B*) The seated flexion test. (*C*) Palpation of the sacral sulcus. With patient prone, the most anterior (deepest) sacral sulcus is noted. (*D*) Palpation of ILA. By palpation, determine which side of the ILA is more posterior. The spring test (not shown) is performed on the prone patient by compression of the L5-S1 junction to see if there is posterior to anterior spring. **Table 2** shows how the tests are interpreted. (*Courtesy of* Virginia College of Osteopathic Medicine.)

A brief description of the osteopathic understanding of sacral mechanics is relevant. The sacrum commonly rotates about an oblique axis left or right; less commonly, the sacrum rotates about a vertical axis left or right. Rarely, the sacrum rotates about a horizontal axis.[36] As summarized in **Table 2**, if the right sacral sulcus was thought more anterior and the left ILA more posterior, the diagnosis is a left rotation of the sacrum. The axis of rotation is determined in part by the forward flexion test results.[2]

Although this description of palpation-based diagnosis of sacral mechanics is commonly taught in osteopathic schools, there remains a discrepancy between the confidence in clinical interpretation of these tests and the literature evidence of their reliability. The palpatory skill of examiners limits interexaminer reliability of commonly used tests.[37] A study of an expert panel's "best" historical or examination techniques for the SI joint failed to identify a single "best" test or historical symptom for diagnosis

Table 2
Summary of the physical examination findings for the SI joint

FF Test Standing	FF Test Seated	Anterior Sacral Sulcus	Posterior ILA	Spring Test	Diagnosis
+L	+L	Left	Right	(−)	Right rotation on a right oblique axis
+L	+L	Right	Left	(+)	Left rotation on a right oblique axis
+L	+L	Left	Left	(−)	Left unilateral sacral flexion
+L	+L	Right	Right	(+)	Left unilateral sacral extension

The tests are as described in the text. Diagnosis is based on combined interpretation of dynamic and static testing.

Abbreviations: FF, forward flexion L, left; spring test, if posterior to anterior compression of the lumbo-sacral junction on the prone positioned patient produces no "spring" or flexible motion, the test is (+) positive by convention; (+), positive. If flexible motion is felt, the test is (−) negative.

of SI dysfunction.[38] The argument has been raised that pain is not a prerequisite for SI joint dysfunction and it is the summation of dynamic and static tests can be used to identify sacral dysfunctions in patients.[36] The dynamic and static sacral screening tests (outlined in **Tables 2** and **3**) continue to be used in the diagnosis of pediatric patients while awaiting more definitive evidence for diagnosis and treatment.

Common manual methods for addressing SI dysfunction include HVLA and muscle energy techniques. The muscle energy technique is illustrated in **Fig. 6**. A Pubmed review of this technique revealed no reports of complications; patients typically complain of soreness for 1 to 2 days after the treatment. Contraindications to the muscle energy technique include patients with suspected fracture, discitis, or herniation and inability to tolerate the treatment. Patients are typically placed on the side of the axis of dysfunction; for example, in **Fig. 6**, the treatment is of a left sacral rotation about a right oblique axis; the patient lies on his right side. The sacral sulcus is monitored by a physician, and the patient is directed to roll his torso in the direction of the sacral rotation; in **Fig. 6**, the patient has rolled his torso face-up or to his left. The muscle energy is provided by the patient gently raising his ankles toward the ceiling while the physician resists. The process is typically performed 3 times. The author has found this method helpful for addressing the abnormal findings on dynamic testing

Table 3
Osteopathic physical examination findings associated with specific pelvic (innominant) diagnosis

FF Test Standing	FF Test Seated	ASIS	PSIS	Leg Length	Diagnosis
+L	—	Left ↑	Left ↓	L < R	Left posterior innominant rotation
+L	—	Left ↑	Left ↑	L < R	Left upslipped innominant
+L	—	Left ↓	Left ↓	L > R	Left downslipped innominant
+L	—	Left ↓	Left ↑	L > R	Left anterior innominant rotation

The side of the positive forward flexion test denotes the side of dysfunction. The leg length discrepancy is a function of the position of the acetabulum relative to the innominant.

Abbreviations: FF, forward flexion; L, left; R, right; up arrow, cephalad or superior relative to the contralateral side; down arrow, caudad or inferior relative to the contralateral side.

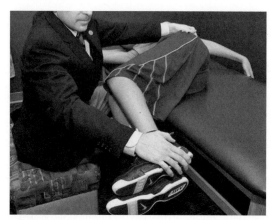

Fig. 6. Muscle energy technique for left rotation on a right oblique axis sacral torsion. Patient is positioned with knees and hips flexed until motion is felt at the sacral sulcus (physician's left hand). The patient is instructed to roll face up but leave his hips and pelvis in place. The treatment is performed by having the patient gently push his ankles toward the ceiling against isometric resistance. After 5 seconds, the patient relaxes briefly and the process is repeated after the physician repositions the legs to engage the new barrier. (*Courtesy of* Quinton Nottingham, PhD.)

(such as those listed in **Table 2**) and normalizing functional leg length discrepancy. These maneuvers are routinely followed by a course of physical therapy for gait and neuromuscular retraining. If manual treatments are used in conjunction with muscle retraining programs and a patient continues to demonstrate abnormal dynamic testing, the patient should be thoroughly re-examined for contributing orthopedic conditions. Anecdotally, the author has identified nearly 40 pediatric and adult patients who demonstrated symptoms of hip impingement and positive findings for SI joint dysfunction. Despite initial relief with manipulations and physical therapy, these patients demonstrated recurrent positive sacral screening tests as well as femoral acetabular impingement signs and ultimately were found to have underlying hip labral pathology with magnetic resonance arthrography. After arthroscopic repair and rehabilitation, the pediatric patients no longer demonstrated positive SI screening tests. This observation is intriguing and awaits further study for corroboration and clarification.

UPPER EXTREMITY

Nursemaids' elbow is probably the best-known diagnosis for which manual treatment is thought curative. The mechanism is a pull usually from above a young child's arm, which subluxes the radial head through the annular ligament. The child usually experiences pain and a loss of function of the arm. Hyperpronation with mild dorsal pressure on the radial head is considered the superior method for reduction (evidence level B).[39]

Older pediatric athletes are more likely to develop radial head symptoms in association with lateral epicondylitis. Tennis players and those athletes who perform repetitive wrist extension are at higher risk. Technical faults contribute to the development of symptoms.[40] Evaluation reveals pain with resisted extension of the wrist and at the origin of the wrist extensors. Motion testing should include pronation and supination with the elbow flexed to 90°. Motion may be limited compared with the contralateral forearm; loss of forearm motion can be associated with radial head dysfunction.[10] Treatment to correct the motion deficit can be accomplished with HVLA or muscle energy methods (illustrated in **Fig. 7**). Manipulation combined with exercise program was superior to steroid injection and exercise program for long-term resolution (after 6 weeks and at 52 weeks) and was associated with a significantly lower regression rate (evidence level A). In a study of patients 18 years of age and older[41] treatment of lateral epicondylitis with manipulation combined with an exercise program was superior to treatment with steroid injection and exercise not only in providing long-term relief (at 6 and at 52 weeks) and but also in preventing recurrence (evidence level A). The study suggests that correction of motion deficits may augment traditional treatment of lateral epicondylitis.

LOWER EXTREMITY

The rationale for manual medicine in lower-extremity injuries may be best understood when looking at the alteration of normal biomechanics that occurs with the inversion ankle sprain. In the subacute evaluation of athletes with an ankle sprain, a subtle loss of range of motion, commonly dorsiflexion, may be observed. Ankle motion loss may arise from fibular or talar malposition.

The loss of motion can be explained by the effect of the inversion mechanism on ankle mechanics. The talus and fibula are the primary contributors due to their coupled motion via the anterior talofibular ligament. The natural motion of the fibular head is to pivot in an anterolateral/posteromedial fashion with ankle motion.[42] At the lateral malleolus, there is slight cephalad motion with dorsiflexion and caudad motion with plantarflexion during gait.[43] Although small in magnitude (approximately 1.5 mm) relative to the motion of the talus, fibular motion has been confirmed radiographically.[44] Talar motion in dorsiflexion involves rotation and slight translation posteriorly into the mortise for maximal stability; in plantar flexion, the talus rotates and translates anteriorly, bringing the narrower posterior talus into the mortise.[45,46] With the inversion mechanism and weight bearing, the talus is plantar flexed and supinated and the force allows for medial rotation and anterior translation, pulling the anterior talofibibular ligament (ATF) anteriorly, and leading to ligamentous sprain. The force of the injury is transmitted to the fibula via the ATF and pulls it into an anterior position. This combination places the talus/fibula in a position that limits the ability to dorsiflex.

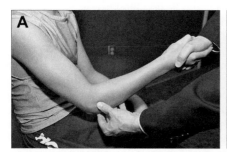 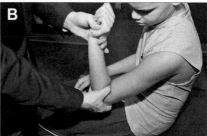

Fig. 7. Motion testing and radial head dysfunction. (*A*) With the elbow flexed to 90°, pronation and supination are tested and compared with the opposite side while monitoring the radial head. (*B*) HVLA maneuver for a subluxed radial head. The forearm is placed in pronation. With the thumb on the dorsal aspect of the radial head, the elbow is flexed to the barrier. At the barrier, a quick short thrust is performed to reposition the radial head. (*Courtesy of* Quinton Nottingham, PhD.)

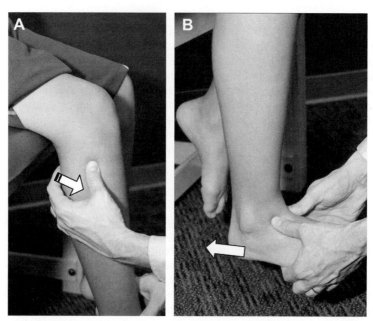

Fig. 8. Evaluation and mobilization of lower-extremity dysfunctions. (*A*) Motion of the fibular head. Mobility is assessed by gentle anterolateral/posteromedial excursion of the fibular head. Motion deficits may occur after inversion-type ankle sprains. (*B*) The swing test. The foot is held parallel to the floor and the knee gently flexed. At the motion barrier, when the ankle cannot dorsiflex further, plantar-ward pressure is felt; loss of ankle dorsiflexion after inversion injury is common. The muscle energy treatment is performed by placing the foot at the barrier; the patient gently plantarflexes 3 to 5 seconds against the physician's resistance. On relaxation, the foot is kept parallel to the floor and the knee moved into further flexion, engaging the new barrier. The process is performed 3 times. (*Courtesy of* Quinton Nottingham, PhD.)

Motion deficits at the talus and fibula are detected using the swing test and fibular motion test. Fibular head motion is assessed by grasping the fibula and pulling in the anterolateral/posteromedial plane and comparing to the unaffected side (**Fig. 8**A). Talar motion can be assessed using the swing test (see **Fig. 8**B). The swing test is performed by monitoring the motion of the talus and flexing the knee while keeping the foot parallel to the floor. At the talar barrier, the talus cannot move further into the mortise and the foot dips toward the floor; the angle of knee flexion is typically less than the unaffected side.

Treatment techniques should generally not be used in the acute injury period. In the acute period, management should consist of PRICE (*p*rotection, *r*est, *i*ce, *c*ompression, and *e*levation). After initial edema and pain is reduced, osteopathic techniques can be used to address motion restrictions attributed to specific fibular or talar dysfunctions.[47] If the talus is unable to glide or rotate into dorsiflexion (a positive swing test), muscle energy or high-velocity techniques may be appropriate. In the muscle energy technique, the ankle is moved into dorsiflexion in the same posture as the swing test. At this barrier, an athlete gently attempts plantar flexion for 3 to 5 seconds while a physician resists. As in all muscle energy techniques, physicians should not allow the foot to actually move. After a brief (1-second) relaxation period, the physician passively flexes the knee to the new barrier, maintaining the foot parallel to the floor (further into dorsiflexion). The technique is generally repeated for 2 additional cycles.

After treatment, motion is reassessed and the athlete may report that the ankle feels loose. In the author's practice, these patients are still given standard treatments and referred for therapy to restore strength and balance directed by an athletic trainer or physical therapist.

Fibular restrictions can also be treated with muscle energy techniques. For an anterior lateral maleolus, the ankle is placed into dorsiflexion and eversion to the barrier (see **Fig. 8**B). The patient gently plantar flexes and inverts the ankle against resistance for 3 to 5 seconds. After a brief relaxation period, the ankle is moved further into dorsiflexion and eversion with gentle pressure on the anterior aspect of the lateral maleolus. Gentle pressure is usually exerted on the posteromedial aspect of the fibular head proximally. After 3 cycles, motion is reassessed.

With the exception of anecdotal reports of success for manipulation in pediatric ankle sprains, most published studies for manipulation efficacy for lower-extremity injury involve young adult and adult populations. In an emergency department study of 18 patients with acute ankle sprains, the group treated with manipulation had improved immediate range of motion and decreased edema (evidence level B).[48] A sham-manipulation, single-blind study looked at load distribution via a force platform before and after manipulation in patients (ages 18 and above) with grade II ankle sprains. Manipulation leads to significant redistribution of load on the injured foot.[48] A recent review of manipulation techniques for lower-extremity conditions found modest support for the manual treatments in inversion ankle injury when combined with exercise or multimodal therapy (evidence level B).[49] Although there is sparse anecdotal support for manipulation in pediatric ankle sprains, available evidence modestly supports its use in young adults when used with standard treatments and physical therapy (evidence level B).

CUBOID SYNDROME

Cuboid subluxation or syndrome refers to pain on the lateral, dorsal, or often plantar aspect of the foot over the cuboid thought to be due to ligamentous injury and loss of joint congruity of the calcaneocuboid joint.[50] The subject has recently had a thorough literature review.[50] The disorder is commonly seen after ankle inversion injury but is also seen as a result of overuse in dance.[51] Diagnosis is usually clinical, with direct palpation of the cuboid eliciting pain. Radiography is unhelpful unless there is true fracture; ultrasound may reveal joint effusion and ligamentous injury as well as allowing for dynamic motion testing.[50] Treatment of the disorder involves restoring joint motion. There are several manipulative techniques, including HVLA and LVLA, to restore joint congruity. In a case series, 7 young athletes diagnosed and treated with mobilization and physiotherapy were able to return to activity without limitation after 1 or 2 visits.[52] Manipulation is beneficial for cuboid subluxation (evidence level B).

SUMMARY

The use of manipulation for a variety of athletic injuries remains an alternative treatment. Conditions, such as nursemaids' elbow or cuboid syndrome, that clearly resolve after appropriate restoration of function by manipulation should suggest the validity of looking more closely at underlying biomechanics to understand dysfunction and injury. As part of standard examination, motion deficits and asymmetry should be actively sought. When identified, mobilizations may be of benefit. They need not be the traditional HVLA variety; results can be achieved using muscle energy, strain-counterstrain, or soft tissue techniques to restore motion. Although manipulation may seem to offer an instant "cure," it is best used as part of a comprehensive rehabilitation approach that begins with thorough evaluation to identify contraindications and progresses to physical therapy for muscle reconditioning and retraining to offer the greatest chance for long-term resolution of symptoms.

ACKNOWLEDGMENTS

The author thanks Quinton Nottingham, PhD of Virginia Tech's Department of Business Information Technology for the photography and photo-editing of the figures in this article and Jonathon Tait, DO for his critical reading of the manuscript.

REFERENCES

1. Barnes P, Bloom B, Nahin R. Complementary and alternative medicine use among adults and children: United States, 2007. In: National Center for Complementary and Alternative Medicine NIoH, vol. 12. Hyattsville (MD): U.S. Department of Health and Human Services; 2008. p. 1–23.
2. Carreiro J. Pediatric manual medicine: an osteopathic approach. Edinburgh (UK): Churchill Livingstone Elsevier; 2009.
3. Assendelft W, Bouter L, Knipschild P. Complications of spinal manipulation: a comprehensive review of the literature. J Fam Pract 1996;42(5):475–80.
4. Vick D, McKay C, Zengerle C. The safety of manipulative treatment: review of the literature from 1925 to 1993. J Am Osteopath Assoc 1996;96:113–5.
5. Hayes N, Bezilla T. Incidence of iatrogenesis associated with osteopathic manipulative treatment of pediatric patients. J Am Osteopath Assoc 2006;106:605–8.
6. Ward R, editor. Foundations for osteopathic medicine. 2nd edition. Philadelphia: Lippincott, Williams and Wilkins; 2003.
7. Glover J, Rennie P. Strain and counterstrain techniques. In: Ward R, editor. Foundations for osteopathic medicine. 2nd edition. Philadelphia: Lippincott, Williams and Wilkins; 2003. p. 1002–16.
8. Kuchera M, McPartland J. Myofascial trigger points as somatic dysfunction. In: Ward R, editor. Foundations for osteopathic medicine. 2nd ed. Philadelphia: Lippincott, Williams and Wilkins; 2003. p. 1034–50.
9. Travell J, Simons D. Myofascial pain and dysfunction: the trigger point manual. Baltimore (MD): Williams and Wilkins; 1992.
10. Greenman P. Principles of manual medicine. 2nd edition. Baltimore (MD): Williams and Wilkins; 1996.
11. Grimshaw D. Cervicogenic headache: manual and manipulative therapies. Curr Pain Headache Rep 2001;5:369–75.
12. Bogduk N, Mercer S. Biomechanics of the cervical spine. I: normal kinematics. Clin Biomech 2000;15:633–48.
13. Di Fabio R. Manipulation of the cervical spine: risks and benefits. Phys Ther 1999;79:50–65.
14. Carey P. A report on the occurrence of cerebral vascular accidents in chiropractic practice. J Can Chiropr Assoc 1993;37:104–6.
15. Hurwitz E, Aker P, Adams A, et al. Manipulation and mobilization of the cervical spine. A systematic review of the literature. Spine 1996;21:1746–59.
16. Vernon H, McDermaid C, Hagino C. Systematic review of randomized clinical trials of complementary/alternative therapies in the treatment of tension-type and cervicogenic headache. Complement Ther Med 1999;7:142–55.
17. Nichols A. Diagnosis and management of thoracic outlet syndrome. Curr Sports Med Rep 2009;8(5):240–9.

18. Karageanes S, Jacobs A. Anomalous first rib in a high school wrestler. Clin J Sport Med 1998;8(3):240–2.
19. Sanders R, Hammond S, Rao N. Diagnosis of thoracic outlet syndrome. J Vasc Surg 2007;46:601–4.
20. Rigberg D, Gelabert H. The management of thoracic outlet syndrome in teen-aged patients. Ann Vasc Surg 2009;23:335–40.
21. Dobrusin R. An osteopathic approach to conservative management of thoracic outlet syndromes. J Am Osteopath Assoc 1989;89(8):1046–50, 1053–1047.
22. Thomas P. Thoracic back pain in rowers and butterfly swimmers: costo-vertebral subluxation. Br J Sports Med 1988;2(2):81.
23. Kelley J, Whitney S. The use of nonthrust manipulation in an adolescent for the treatment of thoracic pain and rib dysfunction: a case report. J Orthop Sports Phys Ther 2006;36(11):887–92.
24. Meuwly J, Wicky S, Schnyder P, et al. Slipping rib syndrome: a place for sonography in the diagnosis of a frequently overlooked cause of abdominal or low thoracic pain. J Ultrasound Med 2002;21(3):339–43.
25. Heinz G, Zavala D. Slipping rib syndrome. Diagnosis using the "hooking maneuver". JAMA 1977;237:794–5.
26. Porter G. Slipping rib syndrome: an infrequently recognized entity in children: a report of three cases and review of the literature. Pediatrics 1985;76(5):810–3.
27. Peterson L, Cavanaugh D. Two years of debilitating pain in a football spearing victim: slipping rib syndrome. Med Sci Sports Exerc 2003;35(10):1634–7.
28. Eastwood N. Slipping-rib syndrome. Lancet 1980;2(8198):809.
29. Bosler J. Scoliosis cured by manipulation of the neck. Med J Aust 1979;1(3):95.
30. Bettany-Saltikov J, Warren J, Stamp M. Carrying a rucksack on either shoulder or the back, does it matter? Load induced functional scoliosis in "normal" young subjects. Stud Health Technol Inform 2008;140:221–4.
31. Morningstar M, Woggon D, Lawrence G. Scoliosis treatment using a combination of manipulative and rehabilitative therapy: a retrospective case series. BMC Musculoskelet Disord 2004;14(5):32.
32. Chen K, Chiu E. Adolescent idiopathic scoliosis treated by spinal manipulation: a case study. J Altern Complement Med 2008;14(6):749–51.
33. Negrini S, Fusco C, Minozzi S, et al. Exercises reduce the progression rate of adolescent idiopathic scoliosis: results of a comprehensive systematic review of the literature. Disabil Rehabil 2008;30:772–85.
34. Lehnert-Schroth C. Introduction to the three-dimensional scoliosis treatment according to Schroth. Physiotherapy 1992;78(11):810–1.
35. Ross J. Is the sacroiliac joint mobile and how should it be treated? Br J Sports Med 2000;34:226.
36. Brolinson PK, Kozar AJ, Cibor G. Sacroiliac joint dysfunction in athletes. Curr Sports Med Rep 2003;2:47–56.
37. Carmichael J. Inter- and intra-tester reliability of palpation for sacroiliac joint dysfunction. J Manipulative Physiol Ther 1987;10:164–71.
38. Dreyfuss P, Michaelsen M, Pauza K, et al. The value of medical history and physical examination in diagnosing sacroiliac joint pain. Spine 1996;21:2594–602.
39. Krul M, van der Wouden JC, van Suijlekom-Smit LWA, et al. Manipulative interventions for reducing pulled elbow in young children. Cochrane Database Syst Rev 2009;(4):CD007759. Available at: http://www2.cochrane.org/reviews/en/ab007759.html. Accessed February 15, 2010.
40. Schnatz P, Steiner C. Tennis elbow: a biomechanical and therapeutic approach. J Am Osteopath Assoc 1993;93(7):782–8, 778.

41. Bisset L, Beller E, Jull G, et al. Mobilisation with movement and exercise, cortico-steroid injection, or wait and see for tennis elbow: randomised trial. BMJ 2006; 333(7575):939.
42. Ledermann M, Cordey J. Registration of fibular movements in vivo in relation to the tibia at the level of the ankle joint. Helv Chir Acta 1979;46(1–2):7–11.
43. Reimann R, Anderhuber F, Ebner I. Compensatory and stabilizing motions of the fibula. Acta Anat (Basel) 1982;112(3):233–41.
44. Kärrholm J, Hansson L, Selvik G. Mobility of the lateral malleolus. A roentgen stereophotogrammetric analysis. Acta Orthop Scand 1985;56(6):479–83.
45. Lundberg A, Goldie I, Kalin B, et al. Kinematics of the ankle/foot complex: plantarflexion and dorsiflexion. Foot Ankle 1989;9(4):194–200.
46. Lundberg A. Kinematics of the ankle and foot. In vivo roentgen stereophotogrammetry. Acta Orthop Scand Suppl 1989;233:1–24.
47. Blood S. Treatment of the sprained ankle. J Am Osteopath Assoc 1980;79(11): 680–92.
48. López-Rodríguez S, Fernández de-Las-Peñas C, Alburquerque-Sendín F, et al. Immediate effects of manipulation of the talocrural joint on stabilometry and baropodometry in patients with ankle sprain. J Manipulative Physiol Ther 2007;30(3): 186–92.
49. Brantingham JW, Globe G, Pollard H, et al. Manipulative therapy for lower extremity conditions: expansion of literature review. J Manipulative Physiol Ther 2009;32(1):53–71.
50. Adams E, Madden C. Cuboid subluxation: a case study and review of the literature. Curr Sports Med Rep 2009;8(6):300–7.
51. Marshall P, Hamilton W. Cuboid subluxation in ballet dancers. Am J Sports Med 1992;20:169–75.
52. Jennings J, Davies G. Treatment of cuboid syndrome secondary to lateral ankle sprains: a case series. J Orthop Sports Phys Ther 2005;35(7):409–15.

Sport Participation by Physically and Cognitively Challenged Young Athletes

Dilip R. Patel, MD, FAAP, FACSM, FAACPDM, FSAM*,
Donald E. Greydanus, MD, FAAP, FSAM, FIAP (H)

KEYWORDS
- Intellectual disability • Cerebral palsy • Myelomeningocele
- Spinal cord injury • Thermoregulation • Boosting

There is a wide spectrum of disabilities that affect the physical and intellectual domains of athletes (**Box 1**).[1–7] It is estimated that there are more than 3 million persons with physical and cognitive disabilities who are involved in organized sports in the United States, and many more in recreational sports.[8,9] Children and adolescents with disabilities are finding increasing opportunities to participate in various sport programs.[2,3,10–12] The health benefits of physical activity for athletes with disabilities are well recognized.[13,14]

Participation opportunities for physically and mentally challenged athletes have increased in the past several decades, with thousands of athletes participating in organized games such as the Paralympics (**Box 2**) and Special Olympics (**Box 3**).[6,15–17] The Paralympic Games include athletes with spinal cord injuries (SCIs), limb amputations, cerebral palsy, blindness, and other visual impairments. To a lesser extent, athletes with short stature, neuromuscular disorders, and learning disabilities have also participated. Athletes with intellectual disabilities participate in Special Olympics, whereas Deaf athletes participate in Deaflympics (**Box 4**).

This review focuses on some common medical issues that relate to sport participation by athletes with physical and cognitive disabilities.[12] Sports medicine research has not paralleled the increased interest and participation in various sports by athletes with disabilities. Research on pediatric athletes with disabilities is even more limited. The reader is referred to many comprehensive reviews and organizational resources (**Table 1**) for more specific detailed information on different sports, technical aspects, and rules.[12,16,18–35] An explanation of some common terms can be found in **Table 2**.

This article is updated from the authors' previous work (Patel DR, Greydanus DE. The pediatric athletes with disabilities. Pediatr Clin N Am 2002;49:803–27).
Department of Pediatrics and Human Development, Michigan State University College of Human Medicine, Kalamazoo Center for Medical Studies, 1000 Oakland Drive, Kalamazoo, MI 49008, USA
* Corresponding author.
E-mail address: patel@kcms.msu.edu

Box 1
Spectrum of disabilities

Amputations

Cerebral palsy

Myelomeningocele

Traumatic brain injury

Spinal cord injury

Visual impairment

Hearing impairment

Intellectual disability

Genetic syndromes

Neuromuscular disorders

Neurobehavioral disorders

CLASSIFICATION OF DISABILITY SPORTS ATHLETES

Classifying athletes with disabilities helps level the playing field so that athletes with similar functional abilities can compete with each other.[2,19,36] This helps ensure fairness in competition. The classification must also take into account the nature of the specific sport and any adaptive equipment used by the athlete.[12,29,36] The methods for classifying athletes with various disabilities have evolved during the twentieth century. In addition to medical doctors, athletic trainers and specially trained and certified classification specialists are responsible for classification.[12] Such a process involves medical and technical classifications. Medical classification delineates the basic disability present and does not necessarily provide information on the functional ability of the athlete for a given activity.[12]

Functional or technical classification is based on observation of the athlete while playing his or her sport.[20,36] A functional classification system (FCS) incorporates medical information with the ability of the athlete to perform specific skills of the sport. The function and strength of the muscle groups are determined on the basis of tests and assigned point values for each class. In this system, each class is identified by a letter (eg, T, track; S, swimming) followed by a number; a higher number denotes a more advanced ability by the athlete.[36] FCS has been used for shooting, swimming, table tennis, and track and field events; it also includes athletes with SCIs, cerebral palsy, amputation, and visual impairment.[36] Each disability sport organization may also use its own disability-specific classification system for sponsored events.[12,29]

Athletes with disabilities can also be classified based on their previous level of performance. Special Olympics use such divisioning or grouping based on the athlete's previous best times or other performance data. For example, athletes who have not more than 10% difference in best times or performance levels in a particular sport can be grouped together.

SPORT PREPARTICIPATION EVALUATION

Preparticipation evaluation (PPE) is an essential component of injury and illness prevention in athletes.[37,38] There are no guidelines specifically designed for the PPE of athletes who have different types of disabilities. The general approach to

| Box 2 |
Paralympics sports
Archery
Basketball
Boccia
Curling
Cycling
Equestrian
Fencing
Goalball
Judo
Powerlifting
Rowing
Rugby
Sailing
Shooting
Soccer
Swimming
Table tennis
Tennis
Track and field
Volleyball
Wheelchair dance
Wheelchair rugby
Alpine skiing
Biathlon
Cross-country skiing
Sled hockey
Source: www.paralympics.org

the PPE of athletes with disabilities should be similar to that of athletes without disability. Often the focus is so much on the disability that the examiner may overlook common medical issues apart from the primary disability (diagnostic overshadowing).

A detailed history is the mainstay of any PPE. It has been suggested that PPE for the athletes with disabilities should preferably be done by a team of medical professionals who are involved in the longitudinal care of these athletes and who know their baseline physical and cognitive levels of functioning.[6] These athletes should be examined in an office setting, and the mass or station method should be avoided. Examiners should be cognizant of disability-specific medical issues for the athlete. In addition to the history and physical examination, a careful evaluation of the prosthetics, orthotics, and assistive or adaptive devices being used should be

| Box 3 |
| Special Olympics sports |
| Track and field (athletics) |
| Badminton |
| Basketball |
| Bocce |
| Bowling |
| Cycling |
| Equestrian |
| Gymnastics |
| Roller skating |
| Sailing |
| Soccer |
| Swimming (aquatics) |
| Table tennis |
| Team handball |
| Tennis |
| Volleyball |
| Alpine skiing |
| Floor hockey |
| Nordic skiing |
| Speed skating |
| Source: www.specialolympics.org |

accomplished by the knowledgeable health care professionals to ensure adequacy and proper fit.

Participation Guidelines

Athletes with physical or cognitive disabilities participate in several sports, depending on their specific disabilities and the demands of the sport.[2,10,12,14,16,18,19,39] Use of adaptive equipment and modification of rules further enhance the sport participation experience for these athletes. Several factors should be considered in matching the athlete to the right sport. These include current health status of the athlete, level of competition and position played, psychological maturity of the athlete, adaptive and protective equipment, modification of the sport, and parents' and athlete's understanding of the inherent risks of injury. Thus, considering the disability and functional level of the athlete in conjunction with all other factors, the athlete should be matched to an appropriate sport.

Psychosocial Considerations

The contribution of sport participation to the psychosocial well-being of the athlete with disability is well recognized. Sport participation provides a positive social experience for these athletes. It is an opportunity for athletes and their families to share their experiences with others. Sports participation can positively affect psychological,

| Box 4 |
| Deaflympic sports |
| Track and field |
| Badminton |
| Basketball |
| Bowling |
| Cycling |
| Orienteering |
| Shooting |
| Soccer |
| Swimming (aquatics) |
| Table tennis |
| Team handball |
| Volleyball |
| Water polo |
| Wrestling |
| Alpine skiing |
| Ice hockey |
| Ice sledge hockey |
| Snowboarding |
| Source: www.deaflympics.org |

social, and moral developmental domains for the child and the adolescent, regardless of the presence of disability. Participation can enhance personal motivation, foster independence, improve coping abilities, allow athletes opportunity for social comparison, foster competitiveness and teamwork, and build self-confidence.[4,40]

Therapeutic Medication Use

Athletes with disabilities are likely to be on various therapeutic medications for associated medical disorders. The potential side effects of these medications and their effects on performance should be considered while working with these athletes.[21] The coaches, athletes, parents, and other staff should be familiar with the athlete's treatment regimen and potential medication side effects. To assess the potential for drug interaction or other inadvertent effects, one should also inquire about over-the-counter drugs and nutritional supplements the athlete may be taking. Thermoregulation can be adversely affected by sympathomimetics and anticholinergics; volume depletion and dehydration is a potential problem with diuretics and excessive caffeinated beverage usage. Potential considerations include cardiovascular side effects of β-blockers and sedating effects of narcotic analgesics, muscle relaxants, and some antiepileptic drugs.

Use of Ergogenic Aids

Athletes with disabilities are not immune from pressure to succeed and enhance their performance by various means. One unique example is noted later as the self-induced

Table 1	
Disability sport and other related organizations[a]	
Organization	Website
United States Paralympics	http://www.usparalympics.org
Disabled Sports USA	http://www.dsusa.org
Dwarf Athletic Association of America	http://www.daaa.org
National Disability Sports Alliance	http://www.ndsaonline.org
Special Olympics International	http://www.specialolympics.org
USA Deaf Sports Federation	http://www.usadsf.org
US Association of Blind Athletes	http://www.usaba.org
Wheelchair Sports USA	http://www.wsusa.org
International Paralympic Committee	http://www.paralympic.org
Comité Internationale des Sports des Sourds	http://www.ciss.org
International Sports Federation – Intellectual Disability	http://www.inas-fid.org
International Blind Sports Association	http://www.ibsa.es
International Stroke Mandeville Wheelchair Sports Federation	http://www.wsw.org.uk

[a] Partial list.

autonomic dysreflexia or boosting. No specific data are available on the prevalence of drug or supplement use for performance enhancement by athletes with disabilities. One should still be cognizant about such a possibility while working with these athletes, so they should also be screened for using ergogenic drugs and supplements.

MUSCULOSKELETAL INJURIES

Several investigators have analyzed muscusloskeletal injuries in predominantly physically challenged athletes, and the key observations are summarized in **Table 3**.[8,11,13,15,24,41–55] Data on injuries in athletes who have predominantly cognitive disabilities are limited. In a review of epidemiologic studies of sport injuries in athletes with disabilities, Ferrara and Peterson[15] concluded that the injury incidence and patterns are similar for athletes with and without disabilities. Their analysis included athletes with SCIs, amputee athletes, athletes with cerebral palsy, and visually impaired athletes. They note that various investigators have used different definitions of the injury as well as the population studied. Ferrara and colleagues[15] in their study defined an injury that caused an athlete to stop, limit, or modify participation for 1 day or more. Acute soft-tissue injuries were the most common injuries; these included skin abrasions, soft-tissue contusions, sprains, and strains. Acute fractures and dislocations were uncommon, and the investigators surmised that this may partly result from there being few contact sports in Paralympic Games. The site and type of injury depends on the particular sport and specific disability; for instance, lower-extremity injuries are more common in amputees and athletes with cerebral palsy, whereas upper-extremity injuries are more common among athletes with SCI. Use of prosthetics, orthoses, and adaptive equipment also influences the nature of injuries.

In a cross-disability study of 426 athletes with SCI, amputation, visual impairment, and cerebral palsy, Ferrara and colleagues[8] reported that 32% (n = 137) of the respondents reported at least 1 time-loss injury in past 6 months. Fifty-seven% of injuries reported by National Wheelchair Athletic Association (NWAA) athletes involved

Table 2	
Explanation of some common terms	
Impairment	Any loss or abnormality of psychological, physical, or anatomic structure or function
Disability	Global term used to encompass problems with body functions, body structures, activity limitations, and participation restrictions resulting from impairment (World Health Organization); impairment that limits a major life activity (Americans with Disabilities Act)
Handicap	A disadvantage for a given individual resulting from impairment or disability that limits or prevents the fulfillment of a role that is normal (depending on age, sex, and sociocultural factors) for that individual
Adapted sport	Sport that is specifically modified or designed for the athlete who has disability; the athlete may participate with others without disabilities (integrated settings) or only with others with disabilities (segregated settings)
Paralympics	Sports for athletes who have predominantly physical disabilities; organized sports governed by the International Paralympic Committee
Special Olympics	International sports training and competition program for persons with intellectual disability who are aged 8 y and older, irrespective of their abilities; governed by the International Special Olympics
Deaflympics	Organized sports for Deaf athletes, in which the athletes and officials are deaf

Data from Refs. [1–3,6,12,19,29,35]

the shoulder and arm/elbow; 53% of injuries reported by athletes from the United States Association for Blind Athletes (USABA) were to a lower extremity. The injuries reported by United States Cerebral Palsy Athletic Association (USCPAA) athletes involved knee (21%), shoulder (16%), forearm/wrist (16%), and leg/ankle (15%). In a study of pediatric athletes (n = 83) who participated in Junior National Wheelchair Games, Wilson and Washington[11] reported that most injuries were minor skin injuries; however, half of the participants reported symptoms of hyperthermia, whereas 9% of swimmers reported symptoms of hypothermia.

Table 3	
Epidemiologic characteristics of musculoskeletal injuries in physically challenged athletes	
Incidence	Similar to those without physical disabilities
Acute injuries	Soft-tissue injuries (skin abrasions, sprains, strains, contusions) most common Fractures and dislocations are uncommon
Overuse injuries	Most common injuries overall Most are soft-tissue or connective-tissue injuries
Severity	Most injuries considered minor (≤7 d time loss from sports)
Modifying factors	Sport Level of competition Type of disability Associated conditions Use of prosthesis, orthoses, other adaptive equipment Use of wheelchair

In a 3-year cross-disability study (n = 319), Ferrara and Buckley[45] reported an injury rate of 9.30 per 1000 athlete exposures (defined as 1 athlete participating in 1 practice or game in which there is the probability of sustaining an athletic injury), a rate similar to other able-bodied sports.[45] Fifty-two percent of injuries were considered minor (7 or fewer days of time lost from sport) and 19% were major (22 or more days of time lost from sport).

Nyland and colleagues[55] analyzed soft-tissue injuries sustained by athletes of Disabled Sports USA (n = 66), the USABA (n = 53), the USCPAA (n = 56), and Wheelchair Sports USA (n = 129) who participated at the 1996 Paralympic Games. Sixty-seven percent of athletes reported acute soft-tissue injuries. Their study supported the observation that injury patterns depend on the specific sport and the type of appropriate assistive or adaptive equipment used. The epidemiology of musculoskeletal injuries in children and adolescents with disabilities remains to be more clearly delineated.

SCI

Sport-related SCIs are not common in children and adolescents; however, SCIs can have significant lifelong consequences for independent living and sport participation.[2,4,19,56] Athletes who have SCIs are predisposed to injuries related to the use of wheelchairs, prostheses, and other adaptive devices, not unlike other athletes who are wheelchair bound.[6,39,52,57,58] Persons with SCIs are also at risk for specific medical problems related to loss of motor and sensory function as well as lack of control of autonomic function (dysautonomia) below the level of the lesion, including impaired thermoregulation and autonomic dysreflexia.[6,19,59–66]

Thermoregulation

Temperature regulation is impaired in athletes with SCI, especially with lesions above T8.[1,2,6,19] Hyperthermia and hypothermia have been reported to be serious problems in these athletes. Impaired sweating below the lesion level reduces the effective body surface area available for evaporative cooling. There is also venous pooling in lower limbs and decreased venous return, which also reduces heat loss by convection and radiation.[21] This condition can lead to increased body temperature and hyperthermia. Certain medications (eg, anticholinergics) taken by these athletes can also increase the risk of hyperthermia.

In cooler conditions such as swimming, there is increased risk for hypothermia. Impaired vasomotor and sudomotor neural control, decreased muscle mass below the lesion, and possible impaired central temperature regulating mechanisms all contribute to the development of hypothermia.[6,21] There is a lack of shiver response below the level of the lesion. These athletes also lack sensation below this level and thus may not be aware of wet clothes. Problems with appropriate temperature regulation can occur even within milder ambient temperature ranges. Adequate hydration must be maintained, and the athlete should be removed from sports activity at the first sign of any problem.[6]

Autonomic Dysreflexia

Autonomic dysreflexia has been known to occur in athletes with SCIs above T6.[16,19,21,63] There is a loss of inhibition of the sympathetic nervous system that leads to an acute uncontrolled sympathetic response; this is manifested by sweating above the lesion, chest tightness, headache, apprehension, acute paroxysmal hypertension, hyperthermia, cardiac dysrhythmia, and gastrointestinal disturbances.[6,21] Several stimuli below the level of the lesion can trigger such a response, including urinary tract infection, bladder distension, bowel distention, pressure sores, tight clothing, and acute fractures.[21] Awareness of the potential for autonomic dysreflexia is the key to prevention. At the first signs of this syndrome, the athlete should be removed from the sports activity, any recognized offending stimulus should be eliminated, and the athlete should preferably be transported to an emergency facility for further management. In many cases, autonomic dysreflexia is a self-limited response; any persistent hypertension or cardiac dysrhythmia needs further treatment.

Boosting

A phenomenon of self-induced autonomic dysreflexia, known as boosting, has been recognized in the past several years, especially in wheelchair athletes seeking to improve their race times.[9,67,68] These athletes will knowingly trigger autonomic dysreflexia by a self-induced noxious stimulus; the athlete may drink large amounts of fluids, strap legs tightly, or clamp their catheters to induce bladder distention.[9] Self-induced lower-leg fractures have also been reported. The exact mechanism of performance enhancement as a result of boosting is not known; however, it is hypothesized that it is partly due to increased blood flow to working muscles, and to glycogen sparing resulting from increased use of adipose tissue, which is induced by increased catecholamines.[9] Boosting has been shown to reduce race time and give the athlete an advantage. It is important to recognize that self-induced dysreflexia poses serious health risks for the athlete, and that this practice is considered an ergogenic aid that is not sanctioned by sports-governing bodies.

MYELOMENINGOCELE

Adolescents with myelomeningocele are at an increased risk for obesity (prevalence of up to 75%), so their participation in sports and other physical activities is especially encouraged.[1] In 75% of cases the lesions in myelomeningocele affect the lower lumbar and sacral levels, with loss of motor and sensory function below the lesion level. The presence of hydrocephalus can adversely affect cerebral function; increased intraventricular pressure and dilatation can damage the motor cortex and lead to development of spasticity above the level of the lesion.[1,2,10,12] Persons with myelomeningocele also have deficits in hand-eye and foot-eye coordination. They also have decreased aerobic power, decreased endurance, decreased peak anaerobic power, and mechanical inefficiency.[9,12,69-71] The level of the lesion and severity of hydrocephalus are important factors influencing the ability to participate in sports.[2,10] Persons with myelomeningocele are categorized according to the functional level of the spinal cord lesion.

Poor soft-tissue support, increased local pressure, and lack of sensation below the lesion level predispose persons with myelomeningocele to develop localized skin breakdown with resultant pressure sores and ulcers.[10] They are also at an increased risk for ligament sprains because of lack of strong musculotendinous units around the involved joints; decreased muscle strength and strength imbalance increase the risk for muscle strains in these athletes.[2,6,12,36] Persons with myelomeningocele lack optimal loading of their bones because of their lack of weight-bearing activities; this, often combined with nutritional inadequacy, may lead to osteopenia and an increased risk for fractures.[2,6,10,21] Fracture may occur after minimal trauma and may initially be mistaken for localized infection because of erythema and swelling.[2] These athletes may not feel pain because of lack of sensation, further delaying the diagnosis of a fracture.

Bowel and Bladder Control

Persons with myelomeningocele, SCIs, and other neuromotor disabilities lack volitional bladder and bowel control.[1,2,6,10,12] Different bowel and bladder routines, accidents, and odor may be a cause for embarrassment for the individual. In the context of sports participation, the athlete may be too preoccupied with the sport to adhere to a prescribed bladder or bowel regimen. Some athletes may be on a scheduled voiding regimen that requires intermittent catheterization, or they may have an indwelling catheter. There is also the problem of access to appropriate facilities in a timely fashion. A regular regimen of voiding, ensuring adequate hydration (before, during, and after the sports activity), and using appropriate sterile voiding techniques are helpful in preventing urinary retention and associated complications. In addition to a neurogenic bladder, these athletes also have problems with constipation and stool retention; this requires regularly following a bowel regimen.

Latex Allergy

Latex allergy is a significant concern in individuals with myelomeningocele, with a prevalence of 25% to 65%.[1,72] Because of the high prevalence of latex allergy, latex-free gloves should be used while working with persons who have myelomeningocele. Other articles containing natural rubber latex should also be avoided. Sources of latex in the medical setting include gloves, stethoscope tubing, blood pressure cuffs, catheters, wound drains, bandages, and bulb syringes; household sources include balloons, condoms, shoe soles, erasers, some toys, and sport equipment.[72]

Hydrocephalus and Shunt

The presence and severity of hydrocephalus and a ventriculoperitoneal (VP) shunt in persons with myelomeningocele are major factors that affect the functional level and ability of these athletes to participate in sports.[2,10] The VP shunt system is generally protected under the skin; however, it is at risk of injury if the overlying skin sustains sufficient impact to cause a laceration.[10] Such an injury requires immediate evaluation by a neurosurgeon. Athletes with cerebrospinal fluid shunts are not necessarily restricted from sport participation simply because of the presence of this shunt[10]; however, they should wear an appropriate helmet or headgear for protection. Blount and colleagues,[73] in their survey of neurosurgeons, reported that broken shunt catheters and shunt dysfunction were the most common complications observed. The incidence of sport-related shunt complications is reported to be significantly less than 1%. Blount and colleagues[73] noted that 90% of pediatric neurosurgeons who responded (n = 92, 55% of the sample) will allow unrestricted participation in noncontact sports by patients who have shunts, whereas for contact sports, 33% will restrict participation in all sports, 33% will restrict some contact sports, and 33% will allow unrestricted participation.

Associated Conditions

Several associated and secondary conditions (**Table 4**) should be considered when evaluating athletes who have myelomeningocele. Persons with Chiari type 2 malformations should be restricted from activities that have significant risk of injury to the cervical spine; this includes sports such as diving and football.[10] Persons with myelomeningocele who develop progressively worsening strength, increasing scoliosis, and bowel and bladder dysfunction should be evaluated for possible hydromyelia and tethered cord.[1,10,12] These athletes should be restricted from further sports

Table 4
Associated and secondary conditions in myelomeningocele

Neurologic	Arnold-Chiari malformation
	Hydrocephalus
	Tethered cord
	Syringomyelia
	Seizures
	Autonomic dysreflexia
Cognitive/behavioral	Intellectual disability
	Learning disability
	Nonverbal learning disability
	Attention-deficit hyperactivity disorder (ADHD)
Urological/renal	Neurogenic bladder
	Vesicoureteral reflux
	Hydronephrosis
	Frequent urinary tract infections
	Urinary incontinence
	Urinary retention
	Secondary chronic kidney disease and failure
	Nephrolithiasis
Gastrointestinal/nutritional	Neurogenic bowel
	Bowel incontinence, rectal prolapse
	Constipation
	Obesity
Skin	Pressure sores
	Ulcers
Endocrine	Growth hormone deficiency
	Precocious puberty
	Metabolic syndrome
Cardiovascular	Congenital heart disease
	Secondary hypertension
	Reduced aerobic capacity
	Deep venous thrombosis
	Lymphedema
Ophthalmologic	Strabismus
	Esotropia
	Papilledema
	Nystagmus
Allergic	Latex
	Sensitivies to certain foods such as bananas, water chestnuts, avocados, and kiwi fruit
Sexual	Sexual dysfunction in some men

From Patel DR, Greydanus DE, Calles Jr JL, et al. Developmental disabilities across the life span, Disease A Month. New York: Elsevier; 2010; with permission.

participation until after appropriate orthopedic intervention and reassessment of their functional abilities. Examples of high-risk sports for persons with myelomeningocele include football, cheerleading, scuba diving, water skiing, polo, and bobsledding.[10]

CEREBRAL PALSY

Cerebral palsy is primarily characterized by spasticity, athetosis, and ataxia. There is decreased musculotendinous flexibility, decreased strength, and considerable muscle imbalance; flexor muscles usually have more strength than the extensors.[1,10,12,74–77] Progressively decreasing flexibility and muscle strength, and increased tone, contribute to the development of joint contractures. Persons with cerebral palsy have a high-energy cost of movement (or decreased mechanical efficiency) and decreased peak anaerobic power; they may also have an increased cost of breathing (caused by decreased lung volume and a stiff thoracic cage) and decreased aerobic power.[74–83] Some individuals with cerebral palsy also have associated conditions such as perceptual motor problems, visual dysfunction, deafness, impaired hand-eye coordination, and intellectual disability (**Table 5**).[1,75] All these factors influence the risk for injury and ability to participate in sports, and have implications for developing training programs for athletes with cerebral palsy.

Athletes with cerebral palsy are at increased risk for overuse syndromes, muscle strains, chronic knee pain, patellofemoral problems, and chondromalacia

Table 5
Conditions associated with cerebral palsy

Neurologic	Seizures (30%–50%)
Pulmonary	Restrictive lung disease (secondary to scoliosis)
	Chronic lung disease of infancy
	Dysphagia (40%)
	Obstructive sleep apnea
	Excessive drooling
	Recurrent aspiration
Gastrointestinal	Oral motor dysfunction and feeding difficulties (80%–90%)
	Poor nutritional status and growth
	Gastroesophageal reflux disease (GERD; 25%–80%)
	Constipation (80%)
	Bowel incontinence
Genitourinary	Bladder incontinence
	Recurrent urinary tract infections
Skin	Decubitus ulcers
Vision (40%)	Refractive errors; myopia (75%)
	Strabismus, amblyopia, cataract, nystagmus, optic atrophy, cortical visual impairment
Hearing	Hearing impairment (5%–15%)
Dental	Malocclusions
Communication	Speech and language impairment (40%); dysarthria
Pain from multiple causes	Migraine, corneal abrasions, temporomandibular joint dysfunction, GERD, constipation, hip dislocation, muscle spasms, progressive scoliosis
Sleep	Sleep disturbances (25%)
Endocrine	Delayed or precocious puberty
Psychosocial and behavioral	ADHD, self-injurious behaviors, depression (20%)
Intellectual disability	Intellectual disability (30%–65%)
Learning disabilities	Learning disabilities
Musculoskeletal	Scoliosis, hip dislocation, patella alta, multiple joint contractures, foot deformities, lower-extremity rotational deformities

From Patel DR, Greydanus DE, Calles Jr JL, et al. Developmental disabilities across the life span, Disease A Month. New York: Elsevier; 2010; with permission.

patellae.[2,6,10,16] Progressively decreased flexibility of hamstrings and quadriceps contributes to proximal patellar migration.[2,6] Normal hip development is affected because of decreased flexibility and muscle imbalance around the hips; this eventually contributes to the development of coxa valga, acetabular dysplasia, and hip subluxation.[2] Hip flexion contractures and tight hamstrings can lead to increased lumbar lordosis, chronic back pain, and spondylolysis. Some athletes find it difficult to control rackets and bats because of impaired hand-eye coordination; athletes with perceptual problems may also have difficulties in throwing and catching.[2,6,12] Many will develop ankle and foot deformities that affect sport participation and require orthopedic management. The presence of tonic neck reflexes can adversely affect effective development of certain sport skills such as use of bats, hockey sticks, or rackets.[12]

Fifty percent of athletes with cerebral palsy participate in wheelchair sports and the other 50% are ambulatory.[6] The USCPAA classifies athletes on the basis of observed ability to function and formal testing of various abilities; athletes are categorized in 8 classes from the most severely affected to the least affected. The USCPAA competition events include archery, bocce, bowling, cross-country, cycling, equestrian sports, powerlifting (bench press), slalom, soccer (modified), swimming, shooting, table tennis, and track and field events.[12] The USCPAA sponsors special junior athletic events for athletes who are 7 to 18 years old, and categorizes these events into 4 divisions according to age; a special division also allows activity for those who are less than 6 years of age, in which the emphasis is on participation rather than competition.[12]

Athletes with cerebral palsy benefit from carefully designed conditioning programs that should include appropriate strength training and flexibility exercises.[10,12,16,27] Strength training should take into account the differential tone and spasticity in different muscle groups so that training is directed to appropriate muscle groups to optimize muscle balance. Stretching, started after a period of warm-up, should be slow and sustained to prevent activation of stretch reflex. Specific training will also help improve ataxia and coordination.

WHEELCHAIR ATHLETES

Wheelchair athletes include those with cerebral palsy, spina bifida, and SCIs. Use of wheelchairs influences the occurrence and patterns of certain injuries in these athletes. Sports with descending order of injury risk for wheelchair athletes are track, basketball, road racing, tennis, and field events.[6] Overuse injuries are the most common injuries in wheelchair athletes, and shoulders and wrists are the most frequently injured regions.[19,36,49,52] Shoulder pain is a common complaint in wheelchair athletes. Specific shoulder injuries in these athletes include rotator cuff impingement, rotator cuff tendonitis, biceps tendonitis, and tear of the long-head tendon. Soft-tissue injuries (most commonly seen in track, road racing, and basketball) include lacerations, abrasions, and blistering that affect the arm and hand.[19] Peripheral entrapment neuropathy is common in wheelchair athletes, the most common of which is carpal tunnel syndrome, which is reported in 50% to 75% of the athletes.[6,42,44,49] In athletes with SCIs and myelomeningocele, painless hip dislocations can occur.[2] Some athletes may develop progressive neuromuscular scoliosis that limits cardiorespiratory capacity.

Pressure Sores

Athletes with SCIs or myelomeningocele are especially at risk for developing pressure sores.[10,19] The wheelchair athlete's knees are at a higher level than the buttocks, a position that leads to increased pressure over the sacrum and ischial tuberosities.[6,12,36,49] Skin lesions remain asymptomatic because of lack of pain and touch sensations. With delay in recognition, pressure sores can become infected. Frequent, meticulous skin examinations are necessary for early detection of problem pressure areas. Any sores must be promptly treated to prevent complications. There must be adequate local padding to relieve pressure. The athlete should have appropriate chair size and fit, and should be educated and assisted as needed to frequently change position. Stump overgrowth and improperly fitting prosthetics also predispose the amputee athlete to pressure sores.

AMPUTEE ATHLETES

Use of assistive or adaptive devices, prostheses, and orthoses is common in athletes with limb amputations; these devises should be of proper fit and checked and adjusted regularly as the physical growth of the child or adolescent progresses.[2,26] Sports-governing bodies have rules that allow or disallow participation of athletes with prosthetic devices; high-school interscholastic athletics generally allow athletes to wear these devices in many sports, including football, wrestling, soccer, and baseball.[12] The factors considered in decisions to allow or disallow athletes to participate with prosthetic devices include the type of amputation and prosthesis as well as the potential for harm to others or unfair advantage for the athlete because of the prosthetic device.[12,25,26] Prosthesis technology has advanced greatly in the past 2 decades[58] not only allowing athletes increasing levels of sport participation but also possibly contributing to improved performance. This has raised questions about prostheses giving amputee athletes an advantage compared with able-bodied athletes in such sports as running. The effects of carbon fiber prostheses on the running technique and running time of transtibial amputees have come under scrutiny.[58]

   Prostheses can increase local skin pressure and contribute to abrasions, blisters, and skin rash. Prepatellar, infrapatellar, and pretibial bursitis in the below-knee amputee can result from socket irritation.[6,25,26] Athletes with lower-limb amputation compensate by increasing lateral flexion and extension of the lumbar spine, which can potentially lead to back pain.[6] Amputees are also prone to hyperextension injuries of the knee. Skills that require balance are adversely affected in persons with amputation of a limb because of altered station of the center of gravity, especially in lower-limb amputees.[12]

   In the skeletally immature athlete, overgrowth of the stump is a common problem.[2,16] The overlying skin and soft tissue may break down because of friction and pressure during sports. Awareness of this problem is the key to early detection because these athletes often lack pain sensation in extremities and may not be aware of the presence of skin lesions. Increased bony prominence and local erythema indicate consideration of stump overgrowth and further evaluation. A skeletally immature child and adolescent may need periodic stump revisions until skeletal growth is complete.[2]

VISUAL IMPAIRMENT

Visual impairment is a general term that refers to partial sight and total blindness. A person with partial sight is only able to read using large print or proper magnification. A person who is not able to read large print even with magnification is considered blind; a person with total blindness is unable to perceive a strong light shone directly into his or her eyes.[12,84,85] Legal blindness refers to visual acuity of 20/200 or less in the better eye even with correction, or a field of vision so narrowed that the widest diameter of the visual field subtends an angular distance no greater than 20° (20/200).[12,85,86]

Visual impairment does not necessarily cause motor disabilities per se; it is the lack of experience in physical activities that may limit or delay the development or acquisition of specific motor skills.[85] Thus, sports participation is an important experience for the visually impaired to learn and improve movements and motor skills. Because of fear of fall or collision with other objects, persons who have visual impairment often exhibit certain characteristic patterns of movements and posture. They have a shuffling, slow-paced gait with shorter strides; they often have stiffer posture, hyperlordosis, and protruding abdomen.[85,86]

The USABA promotes various sport activities for visually impaired athletes 14 years of age and older.[86] The USABA classification for sports, based on residual vision, has 4 categories, as shown in **Table 6**. Visually impaired athletes compete in a variety of sports including skiing, track and field events, wrestling, swimming, tandem cycling, powerlifting, goal ball, judo, gymnastics, running, bicycling, baseball, bowling, and golf.[85] Sport participation is facilitated by the use of guides, such as a sighted guide, a tether or guide wire, or a sound source, depending on the degree of visual impairment.[85]

DEAF ATHLETES

In the United States, Deaf individuals consider themselves to belong to a subculture of American society, and many do not consider themselves disabled.[87] Many prefer the term Deaf with an uppercase D, rather than the person-first terminology used to describe persons with other impairments.[87]

Hearing loss can range from mild (hearing threshold of 27–40 decibels [dB]) to profound (hearing threshold of >90 dB).[1,12] The age at which deafness occurs is an important factor in developing communication strategies for the Deaf. A child may be deaf since birth and thus before the development of speech (prelingual deafness) or may develop deafness later in childhood, after the phase of speech development (postlingual deafness, usually after first 3 years of life).[12] Some Deaf persons may have associated damage to the vestibular apparatus, affecting balance; otherwise, most Deaf persons do not have any motor or physical deficits. Deaf persons who have vestibular dysfunction and balance problems may have limitations in some activities such as climbing heights, jumping on a trampoline, diving into a pool, or tumbling activities that require rotation.[87]

Table 6 USABA visual classifications	
B1	No light perception in either eye, to light perception, but inability to recognize the shape of a hand at any distance or in any direction
B2	From ability to recognize the shape of hand to visual acuity of 20/600 or a visual field of less than 5° in the best eye with the best practical eye correction
B3	From visual acuity more than 20/600 to visual acuity of 20/200 or a visual field of less than 20° and more than 5° in the best eye with the best practical eye correction
B4	From visual acuity more than 20/200 to visual acuity of 20/70 and a visual field larger than 20° in the best eye with the best practical eye correction

Source: www.usaba.org.

Deaf athletes can potentially participate in all sports with athletes who are not deaf. Sometimes, as is true for those with unilateral deafness, some minimal additional visual cues may be helpful; athletes with unilateral and bilateral deafness may be at some disadvantage in team sports because they are not able to correctly locate the direction of sounds or perceive other auditory cues.[87,88]

In the United States, USA Deaf Sport Federation promotes and organizes sports events for Deaf athletes. On an organized level, Deaf athletes participate in Deaflympics, in which the athletes and the officials are deaf. To be eligible to participate in Deaflympics, the athletes must have a hearing loss of at least 55 dB per tone average (PTA) in the better ear (3-tone pure tone average at 500, 1000, and 2000 Hz, air conduction ISO 1969 Standard).[88] Use of any type of hearing device, such as hearing aids or other external amplification devices, is prohibited during warm-up or competition within a restricted zone area.[88]

INTELLECTUAL DISABILITY

According to the American Association of Intellectual and Developmental Disabilities (AAIDD), intellectual disability "is a disability characterized by significant limitations both in intellectual functioning and in adaptive behavior as expressed in conceptual, social, and practical adaptive skills."[89] An individual's age and culture should be taken into consideration in the assessment of intellectual and adaptive functioning.[89] Sensory, motor, communication, or behavioral factors should also be appropriately considered in cognitive assessment and interpretation of results of cognitive tests.[89]

According to the Diagnostic and Statistical Manual of Mental Disorders, fourth edition, text revision (DSM-IV-TR), intellectual disability (or mental retardation) is defined as an intelligence quotient (IQ) of approximately 70 or less on an individually administered standardized test of intelligence concurrent with deficits in adaptive functioning in 2 of the following areas: communication, self-care, home living, social or interpersonal skills, use of community resources, self-direction, functional academic skills, work, leisure, health, and safety. All definitions stipulate that the onset of disability must occur before the age of 18 years.[90]

Athletes who have intellectual disability generally participate on an organized level under the auspices of Special Olympics. There are an estimated 3 million Special Olympic athletes worldwide. The most popular sports for these athletes are track and field events, soccer, basketball, bowling, and aquatics.[4] Hearing and visual impairments are prevalent in persons who have intellectual disability.[91,92] Persons with mild intellectual disability can participate in most sports and perform close to peers who do not have intellectual disability. In general, persons who have intellectual disability have been shown to score lower than those who do not have intellectual disability on measures of strength, endurance, agility, balance, running speed, flexibility, and reaction time.[93–95] Persons who have intellectual disability also tend to have lower peak heart rate and lower peak oxygen uptake (Vo_2 peak) than those who do not have intellectual disability.

DOWN SYNDROME

Atlantoaxial instability (AAI) has been reported in 15% of persons with Down syndrome.[2] Persons with Down syndrome have abnormal collagen that results in increased ligamentous laxity and decreased muscle tone.[1,2,96–107] Laxity of the annular ligament of C1 and hypotonia contribute to the AAI; approximately 2% of persons with AAI may be symptomatic because of subluxation. Symptoms suggestive of atlantoaxial subluxation (AAS) include easy fatigability, abnormal gait, neck pain, limited range of motion of the cervical spine, torticollis, incoordination, spasticity, hyperreflexia, clonus, extensor plantar reflex, sensory deficits, and other upper motor neuron and posterior column signs.[1,2,96–107]

It has been a common practice to obtain lateral cervical spine radiographs in flexion, extension, and neutral positions to screen for asymptomatic AAI. Atlantodens interval (space between the posterior aspect of the anterior arch of the atlas and the odontoid process) of less than 4.5 mm or neural canal width of less than 14 mm in asymptomatic individuals are considered to be within normal limits, tend not to change over time, and therefore repeat radiographs are not indicated in the absence of any emerging signs or symptoms.[2,98–101] Magnetic resonance imaging (MRI) or computed tomography (CT) scan is more informative in the assessment of neural compromise associated with AAI or AAS. Although technically difficult, a dynamic or observed MRI scan of the cervical spine is reported to be highly sensitive in identifying neural compromise.[99]

Asymptomatic AAI is a concern for athletes because of increased risk for subluxation resulting in SCI during sport participation. Periodic neurologic assessment for emerging symptoms and signs suggestive of AAS and spinal cord impingement or compression is essential to identify athletes early and prevent irreversible injury to the spinal cord. The natural history of AAI and AAS in individuals who have Down syndrome has not been clearly elucidated. Radiographic evidence of AAI has not been shown to correlate with later development of AAS or predicting neural compromise.[2,4,51,99–101]

Athletes with Down syndrome participate in sports under the umbrella of Special Olympics. Because of increased risk for SCI from AAS during excessive flexion-extension movements, certain sports are contraindicated for persons with AAI as listed in **Box 5**.[93–105] Special Olympics require that all athletes with Down syndrome be screened by lateral neck radiographs before participating in sport programs. Some recommend periodic reassessment every 3 to 5 years, although some experts doubt the value of periodic screening if the initial screening was normal.[2] The highest risk for AAS has been reported to be between 5 and 10 years of age.[2,99,100]

In addition to AAI, persons who have Down syndrome also have a higher incidence of associated orthopedic and medical conditions (**Box 6**) that must be carefully considered and evaluated during sport PPE.[99–109] Fifty percent of individuals who have Down syndrome have congenital heart disease that is surgically treated in infancy and childhood and it is important to obtain detailed history during PPE.[102]

Box 5
Sports contraindicated for persons who have Down syndrome

Contact/collision sports

Gymnastics

Diving

Pentathlon

Butterfly stroke

High jump

Heading in soccer

Diving starts in swimming

Certain warm-up exercises that involve neck flexion-extension

---

Box 6
Specific conditions to be considered during PPE[a] of athletes with Down syndrome

AAI and subluxation

Anomalies and disorders of the odontoid

Occipitoatlantal instability

Cervical spondylolysis

Developmental dysplasia of the hip

Hip dislocation

Patellar instability

Neuromuscular scoliosis

Slipped capital femoral epiphysis

Arthropathy of Down syndrome

Congenital heart disease

Visual impairment

Hearing impairment

Intellectual disability

Diabetes mellitus

Obesity

Hypothyroidism

Epilepsy

[a]PPE, preparticipation evaluation.

Persons who have Down syndrome tend to have lower Vo_2 peak values and lower peak heart rates than those who do not have Down syndrome or have intellectual disability without Down syndrome.[107,108] The response to exercise on heart rate and peak oxygen consumption is also attenuated in persons who have Down syndrome, although, some studies suggest that exercise training may improve these values.

SUMMARY

There have been increased opportunities and sports participation by athletes with disabilities during the past decades. Research on pediatric athletes with disabilities remains limited. Appropriate classification of athletes on the basis of their functional and performance abilities is the key to fair participation. PPE of athletes who have disabilities is based on similar principles as for those without disability. Disability-specific medical and orthopedic conditions should be considered when working with these athletes. Sport participation recommendations are based on the specific disability and demands of the sport. Most athletes with disabilities can participate safely in several sports if appropriately matched; such participation should be encouraged and facilitated at all levels because of well-recognized psychological and medical benefits. Significant progress has been made in increasing sports participation opportunities for persons with disabilities; this is especially true for adults and, to a lesser extent, for children and adolescents. However, many barriers remain: inadequate facilities, exclusion of persons with disabilities, medical professional overprotection, lack of trained personnel and volunteers to work with children with disabilities, lack of public knowledge about disabilities, and lack of financial support for sport and physical education in schools.[9,12]

ACKNOWLEDGMENTS

The authors thank Kim Douglas, Kalamazoo Center for Medical Studies for help in preparing the manuscript.

REFERENCES

1. Batshaw ML, editor. Children with disabilities. 5th edition. Baltimore (MD): Paul Brookes Publishing; 2008.
2. Chang FM. The disabled athlete. In: Stanitiski CL, Delee JL, Drez D, editors. Pediatric and adolescent sports medicine. Philadelphia: WB Saunders; 1994. p. 48–75.
3. Gold JR, Gold MM. Access for all: the rise of the Paralympic Games. J R Soc Promot Health 2007;127(3):133–41.
4. Special Olympics Reach Report. Available at: www.specialsolympics.org; 2007. Accessed April 3, 2010.
5. Patel DR, Pratt HD, Greydanus DE. Pediatric neurodevelopment and sport participation: when are children ready to play sports? Pediatr Clin North Am 2002;49(3):505–31.
6. Halpern BC, Bochm R, Cardone DA. The disabled athlete. In: Garrett WE, Kirkendall DT, Squire DL, editors. Principles and practice of primary care sports medicine. Philadelphia: Lippincott Williams & Wilkins; 2001. p. 115–32.
7. Rimmer JH, Braddock D, Pitetti KH. Research on physical activity and disability: an emerging national priority. Med Sci Sports Exerc 1996;28:1366–72.
8. Ferrara MS, Buckley WE, Messner DG, et al. The injury experience and training history of the competitive skier with a disability. Am J Sports Med 1992;20: 55–60.
9. Steadward RD, Wheeler GD. The young athlete with a motor disability. In: Bar-Or O, editor. The child and adolescent athlete. London: Blackwell Science; 1996. p. 493–520.
10. Goldberg B. Sports and exercise for children with chronic health conditions. Champaign (IL): Human Kinetics; 1995.
11. Wilson PE, Washington RL. Pediatric wheelchair athletics: sports injuries and prevention. Paraplegia 1993;31:330–7.
12. Winnick JP, editor. Adapted physical education and sport. Champaign (IL): Human Kinetics; 2000.
13. American College of Sport Medicine (ACSM). ACSM's exercise management for persons with chronic diseases and disabilities. Champaign (IL): Human Kinetics; 1997.
14. Shephard RJ. Benefits of sport and physical activity for the disabled: implications for the individual and for society. Scand J Rehabil Med 1991;23:51–9.
15. Ferrara MS, Peterson CL. Injuries to athletes with disabilities: identifying injury patterns. Sports Med 2000;30:137–43.
16. McCann C. Sports for the disabled: the evolution from rehabilitation to competitive sport. Br J Sports Med 1996;30:279–80.
17. Reynolds J, Stirk A, Thomas A, et al. Paralympics: Barcelona 1992. Br J Sports Med 1994;28:14–7.

18. Adams RC, McCubbin JA. Games, sports, and exercises for the physically disabled. 4th edition. Philadelphia: Lea and Febiger; 1991.
19. Bergeron JW. Athletes with disabilities. Phys Med Rehabil Clin N Am 1999;10: 213–28.
20. Booth DW. Athletes with disabilities. In: Harries M, Williams C, Stanish W, et al, editors. Oxford textbook of sports medicine. 2nd edition. New York: Oxford University Press; 1998. p. 34–45.
21. Dec KL, Sparrow KJ, McKeag DB. The physically-challenged athlete: medical issues and assessment. Sports Med 2000;29:245–58.
22. DePauw KP, Gavron SJ. Disability and sport. Champaign (IL): Human Kinetics; 1995.
23. Dolnick E. Deafness as culture. The Atlantic 1993;272:37–53.
24. Ferrara MS, Buckley WE, McCann BC, et al. The injury experience of the competitive athlete with a disability: prevention implications. Med Sci Sports Exerc 1991;24:184–8.
25. Goldberg B, Hsu J, editors. Atlas of orthoses and assistive devices. American Academy of Orthopedic Surgeons. 3rd edition. St Louis (MO): Mosby; 1997.
26. Herring JA, Birch JG, editors. The child with a limb deficiency. Rosemont (IL): American Academy of Orthopedic Surgeons; 1998.
27. Lockette K, Keyes AM. Conditioning with physical disabilities. Champaign (IL): Human Kinetics; 1994.
28. Miller P, editor. Fitness programming and physical disability. Champaign (IL): Human Kinetics; 1995.
29. Paciorek MJ, Jones JA. Sports and recreation for the disabled. 2nd edition. Carmel (IN): Cooper Publishing Group; 1994.
30. Shephard RJ. Sports medicine and the wheelchair athlete. Sports Med 1988;5: 226–47.
31. Sheppard RJ. Physical activity for the disabled. Champaign (IL): Human Kinetics; 1988.
32. Sherrill C. Adapted physical activity, recreation and sport: cross disciplinary and lifespan. Madison (WI): WCB McGraw Hill; 1998.
33. Klenck C, Gebke K. Practical management: common medical problems in disabled athletes. Clin J Sport Med 2007;17(1):55–60.
34. Wind WM, Schwend RM, Larson J. Sports for the physically challenged child. J Am Acad Orthop Surg 2004;12:126–37.
35. Jacobs PL, Nash MS. Exercise recommendations for individuals with spinal cord injury. Sports Med 2004;34(11):727–51.
36. Lai AM, Stanish WD, Stanish HI. The young athlete with physical challenges. Clin Sports Med 2000;19:793–819.
37. American Academy of Pediatrics, American Academy of Family Physicians, American Orthopedic Society for Sports Medicine, et al. Preparticipation physical evaluation monograph. 4th edition. New York: McGraw Hill; 2010.
38. Jacob T, Hutzler Y. Sports-medical assessment for athletes with a disability. Disabil Rehabil 1998;20:116–9.
39. Curtis KA. Sports and recreational programs for the child and young adult. Proceedings of the Winter Park Seminar. Park Ridge (IL): American Academy of Orthopaedic Surgeons; 1983.
40. Patel DR, Greydanus DE, Pratt HD. Youth sports: more than sprains and strains. Contemp Pediatr 2000;18:45–76.
41. Batts KB, Glorioso JE Jr, Williams MS. The medical demands of the special athlete. Clin J Sport Med 1998;8:22–5.

42. Boninger ML, Robertson RN, Wolff M, et al. Upper limb nerve entrapment in elite wheelchair racers. Am J Phys Med Rehabil 1996;75:170–6.
43. Burnham R, May L, Nelson E, et al. Shoulder pain in wheelchair athletes: the role of muscle imbalance. Am J Sports Med 1993;21:238–42.
44. Burnham RS, Steadward RD. Upper extremity peripheral nerve entrapments among wheelchair athletes: prevalence, location, and risk factors. Arch Phys Med Rehabil 1994;75:519–24.
45. Ferrara MS, Buckley WE. Athletes with disabilities injury registry. Adapt Phys Act Q 1996;13:50–60.
46. Ferrara MS, Davis RW. Injuries to elite wheelchair athletes. Paraplegia 1990;28: 335–41.
47. Ferrara MS, Richter KJ, Kaschalk SM. Sport for the athlete with a physical disability. In: Scuderi GR, McCann PD, Bruno PJ, editors. Sports medicine: principles of primary care. St. Louis (MO): Mosby-Year Book, Inc; 1997. p. 598–608.
48. Ferrara MS, Palutsis GR, Snouse S, et al. A longitudinal study of injuries to athletes with disabilities. Int J Sports Med 2000;21:221–4.
49. Groah SL, Lanig IS. Neuromusculoskeletal syndromes in wheelchair athletes. Semin Neurol 2000;20:201–8.
50. Kegel B, Malchow D. Incidence of injury in amputees playing soccer. Palaestra 1994;10:50–4.
51. Laskowski ER, Murtaugh PA. Snow skiing injuries in physically disabled skiers. Am J Sports Med 1992;20:553–7.
52. McCormack DA, Reid DC, Steadward R, et al. Injury profiles in wheelchair athletes: results of a retrospective survey. Clin J Sport Med 1991;1:35–40.
53. Richter KJ, Hyman SC, Mushett CA, et al. Injuries in world class cerebral palsy athletes of the 1988 South Korea Paralympics. J Osteopath Sport Med 1991;7: 15–8.
54. Taylor D, Williams T. Sports injuries in athletes with disabilities: wheelchair racing. Paraplegia 1995;33:296–9.
55. Nyland J, Snouse SL, Anderson M, et al. Soft tissue injuries to USA paralympians at the 1996 summer games. Arch Phys Med Rehabil 2000;81:368–73.
56. Maki KC, Langbein WE, Reid-Lokos C. Energy cost and locomotive economy of handbike and rowcycle propulsion by persons with spinal cord injury. J Rehabil Res Dev 1995;32:170–8.
57. Wu SK, Williams T. Factors influencing sport participation among athletes with spinal cord injury. Med Sci Sports Exerc 2001;33(2):177–82.
58. Nolan L. Carbon fibre prostheses and running in amputees: a review. Foot Ankle Surg 2008;14(3):125–9.
59. Armstrong LE, Maresh CM, Riebe D, et al. Local cooling in wheelchair athletes during exercise-heat stress. Med Sci Sports Exerc 1995;27:211–6.
60. Bhambhani YN, Holland LJ, Eriksson P, et al. Physiological responses during wheelchair racing in quadriplegics and paraplegics. Paraplegia 1994;32: 253–60.
61. Braddom RL, Rocco JF. Autonomic dysreflexia: a survey of current treatment. Am J Phys Med Rehabil 1991;70:234–41.
62. Burnham R, Wheeler GD, Bhambhani Y, et al. Autonomic dysreflexia in wheelchair athletes. Clin J Sport Med 1994;4:1–10.
63. Erickson RP. Autonomic hyperreflexia: pathophysiology and medical management. Arch Phys Med Rehabil 1980;61:431–40.
64. McCann BC. Thermoregulation in spinal cord injury: the challenge of the Atlanta Paralympics. Spinal Cord 1996;34:433–6.

65. Sawka MN, Latzka WA, Pandolf KB. Temperature regulation during upper body exercise: ablebodied and spinal cord injured. Med Sci Sports Exerc 1989;21: S132–40.
66. van der Woude LHV, Bakker WH, Elkhuizen JW, et al. Anaerobic work capacity in elite wheelchair athletes. Am J Phys Med Rehabil 1997;76:355–65.
67. Burnham R, Wheeler G, Bhambhani Y, et al. Intentional induction of autonomic dysreflexia among quadriplegic athletes for performance enhancement: efficacy, safety, and mechanism of action. Clin J Sport Med 1994;4:1–10.
68. Harris P. Self-induced autonomic dysreflexia ("boosting") practiced by some tetraplegic athletes to enhance their athletic performance. Paraplegia 1994;32:289–91.
69. Cooper RA, Horvarth SM, Bedi JF, et al. Maximal exercise response of paraplegic wheelchair road racers. Paraplegia 1992;30:573–81.
70. Dallmeijer AJ, Kappe YJ, Veeger D, et al. Anaerobic power output and propulsion technique in spinal cord injured subjects during wheelchair ergometry. J Rehabil Res Dev 1994;31:120–8.
71. Davis GM. Exercise capacity of individuals with paraplegia. Med Sci Sports Exerc 1993;25:423–32.
72. Randolph C. Latex allergy in pediatrics. Curr Probl Pediatr 2001;31:135–53.
73. Blount JP, Severson M, Atkins V, et al. Sports and pediatric cerebrospinal fluid shunts: who can play? Neurosurg 2004;54:1190–8.
74. Richter KJ, Gaebler-Spira DG, Mushett CA. Sport and the person with spasticity of cerebral origin. Dev Med Child Neurol 1996;38:867–70.
75. Carroll KL, Leiser J, Paisley TS. Cerebral palsy: physical activity and sport. Curr Sport Med Rep 2006;5:319–22.
76. Unnithan VB, Clifford C, Bar-Or O. Evaluation by exercise testing of the child with cerebral palsy. Sports Med 1998;26:239–51.
77. Hortsman HM, Bleck EE. In: Orthopaedic management in cerebral palsy, 120. 2nd edition. London: Mac Keith Press; 2007. p. 98–211.
78. Damiano DL, Abel MF. Functional outcomes of strength training in spastic cerebral palsy. Arch Phys Med Rehabil 1998;79:119–25.
79. Figoni SF. Exercise responses and quadriplegia. Med Sci Sports Exerc 1993;25: 433–41.
80. MacPhail HE, Kramer JF. Effect of isokinetic strength training on functional ability and walking efficiency in adolescents with cerebral palsy. Dev Med Child Neurol 1995;37:763–75.
81. Parker DF, Carriere L, Hebestreit H, et al. Muscle performance and gross motor function of children with spastic cerebral palsy. Dev Med Child Neurol 1993;35: 17–23.
82. Parker DF, Carriere L, Hebestreit H, et al. Anaerobic endurance and peak muscle power in children with spastic cerebral palsy. Am J Dis Child 1992;146:169–73.
83. Pitetti KH. Exercise capacities and adaptations of people with chronic disabilities: current research, future directions, and widespread applicability. Med Sci Sports Exerc 1993;24:421–2.
84. Makris VI. Visual loss and performance in blind athletes. Med Sci Sports Exerc 1993;25:265–9.
85. Craft DH, Lieberman L. Visual impairments and deafness. In: Winnick JP, editor. Adapted physical education and sport. 3rd edition. Champaign (IL): Human Kinetics; 2000. p. 159–80.
86. Available at: www.usaba.org. United States Association for Blind Sports. Accessed February 12, 2010.
87. Palmer T, Weber KM. The deaf athlete. Curr Sport Med Rep 2006;5:323–6.

88. Audiogram Regulations. Frederic (MD): International Committee of Sports for the Deaf; 2009.
89. American Association of Intellectual and Developmental Disabilities. Intellectual disability: definition, classification, and systems of supports. 11th edition. Washington, DC: American Association of Intellectual and Developmental Disabilities; 2010. 5–20.
90. American Psychiatric Association. Mental retardation. Diagnostic and statistical manual of mental disorders. 4th edition. Washington, DC: American Psychiatric Association; 2000. Text Revision.
91. Woodhouse JM, Adler P, Duignan A. Vision in athletes with intellectual disabilities: the need for improved eye care. J Intellect Disabil Res 2004;48(Pt 8):736–45.
92. Hild U, Hey C, Baumann U, et al. High prevalence of hearing disorders at the Special Olympics indicate need to screen persons with intellectual disability. J Intellect Disabil Res 2008;52(Pt 6):520–8.
93. Fernhall BO, Pitetti KH, Rimmer JH, et al. Cardiorespiratory capacity of individuals with mental retardation including Down syndrome. Med Sci Sports Exer 1996;28:366–71.
94. Krebs P. Mental retardation. In: Winnick JP, editor. Adapted physical education and sport. 3rd edition. Champaign (IL): Human Kinetics; 2000. p. 111–26.
95. Zetaruk M, Mustapha S. Young athletes with physical or mental disability. In: Armstrong N, van Mechelen W, editors. Paediatric exercise science and medicine. 2nd edition. Oxford (England): Oxford University Press; 2008. p. 551–65.
96. Cantu RC, Bailes JE, Wilberger JE. Guidelines for return to contact or collision sport after a cervical spine injury. Clin Sports Med 1998;17:137–45.
97. American Academy of Pediatrics. Atlantoaxial instability in Down syndrome: subject review. Pediatrics 1995;96:151–4.
98. Torg JS, Ramsey-Emrhein JA. Management guidelines for participation in collision activities with congenital, developmental, or postinjury lesions involving the cervical spine. Clin J Sports Med 1997;7:273–91.
99. Brockmeyer D. Down syndrome and craniovertebral instability. Pediatr Neurosurg 1999;31:71–7.
100. Sanyer ON. Down syndrome and sport participation. Curr Sport Med Rep 2006; 5:315–8.
101. Birrer RB. The Special Olympics athlete: evaluation and clearance for participation. Clin Pediatr 2004;43:777–82.
102. Davidson MA. Primary care for children and adolescents with Down syndrome. Pediatr Clin North Am 2002;49:803–27.
103. Platt LS. Medical and orthopaedic conditions in Special Olympics athletes. J Athl Train 2001;36:74–80.
104. Mik G, Gholve PA, Scher DM, et al. Down syndrome: orthopedic issues. Curr Opin Pediatr 2008;20:30–6.
105. Roizen NJ, Patterson D. Down's syndrome. Lancet 2003;361:1281–9.
106. Caird MD, Wills BPD, Dormans JP. Down syndrome in children: the role of the orthopaedic surgeon. J Am Acad Orthop Surg 2006;14:610–9.
107. Winell J, Burke SW. Sports participation of children with Down syndrome. Orthop Clin N Am 2003;34:439–43.
108. Pittetti KH, Clinstein M, Campbell KD, et al. The cardiovascular capacities of adults with Down syndrome: a comparative study. Med Sci Sports Exerc 1992;24:13–9.
109. Nader-Sepahi A, Casey ATH, Hayward R, et al. Symptomatic atlantoaxial instability in Down syndrome. J Neurosurg 2005;103:231–7.

Stress Fractures: Diagnosis and Management in the Primary Care Setting

Dilip R. Patel, MD, FAAP, FACSM, FAACPDM, FSAM

KEYWORDS

- Stress reaction • Low-risk stress fractures
- High-risk stress fractures

Stress fracture represents an overuse injury of the bone, and is one stage on a continuum of stress injury of the bone.[1–7] Stress injury of bone can be either a fatigue reaction (or fracture) or insufficiency reaction (or fracture). Fatigue fracture results from cumulative microfractures because of excessive repetitive strain to a structurally normal bone.[7] Insufficiency fracture can result from normal stress to a structurally abnormal bone.[7] In otherwise healthy adolescent athletes, stress injury to the bone is typically a fatigue reaction or fracture. Individuals with disorders that affect bone structure, such as metabolic bone disease or osteoporosis, are at risk for insufficiency fracture.

Repetitive, excessive stress results in microfractures within the bone.[5–7] This often occurs within 6 to 8 weeks of rapid increase in physical activity, not allowing sufficient time for bone remodeling and adaptation to stress. Continued stress to the bone can lead to propagation of microfracture and eventual macrofracture. The pathogenesis of stress injury to the bone is multifactorial (**Table 1**).[7–42]

EPIDEMIOLOGY

Snyder and colleagues[43] extensively reviewed epidemiologic studies on stress fractures in athletes. It is difficult to generalize data from different studies because of methodological differences among them. Factors that influence the acquisition, results, and interpretation of data include differences in definition of injury exposure, study designs, definition of injury, and accuracy and method of diagnosis (clinical, radiological). Given these limitations, several conclusions are drawn.[43]

Stress fractures affect 1.0% to 2.6% of college athletes.[44–46] Of the recreational or competitive athletes who visit a sports medicine or orthopedic clinic, 0.5% to

Department of Pediatrics and Human Development, Michigan State University College of Human Medicine, Kalamazoo Center for Medical Studies, 1000 Oakland Drive, Kalamazoo, MI 49008, USA
E-mail address: patel@kcms.msu.edu

Pediatr Clin N Am 57 (2010) 819–827
doi:10.1016/j.pcl.2010.03.004   pediatric.theclinics.com

Table 1	
Factors associated with increased risk for stress injury of the bone	
Training related	High training volume, rapid increase in training volume
Footwear	Poor shock absorption, old shoes (more than 6 mo old), poor shoe-fit (especially in women)
Training surface	Uneven running surface, hard surface (equivocal evidence)
Gender	Female gender, may be secondary to other factors such as hormonal and nutritional
Race	Higher in white and Asian women than in African American women
Fitness level	Poor muscle strength and endurance
Bone mineral density	Low bone mineral density
Bone geometry	Reduced bone cross-sectional areas and bone resistance to bending
Anatomic	Equivocal evidence for rigid pes cavus, leg-length discrepancy, genu valgus, and increased Q angle
Hormonal	Hypoestrogenic states in female athletes, delayed menarche, amenorrhea, oligomenorrhea
Nutritional	Low calcium intake, low vitamin D intake (equivocal evidence), energy deficit

7.8% have stress fractures.[47,48] Data are not sufficient to estimate accurately the incidence of stress fracture by type of sport; however, most data suggest highest incidence in track and field and long-distance running.[14,49,50] The cumulative annual incidence of stress fractures in track and field athletes is reported to be 8.7% to 21.1%.[14,49] In track and field athletes, stress fractures account for 6% to 20% of all injuries. Of runners seen in an orthopedic clinic, stress fractures accounted for 15.6% of all injuries. Athletes in certain sports are more at risk for specific stress fractures (**Table 2**).[1,5]

Although a significantly higher incidence of stress fractures is reported in certain groups of female athletes, overall data provide equivocal evidence to support female

Table 2	
Stress fracture risk by sport	
Fracture Site	**Sport**
Tibia	Aerobics, basketball, ballet dancing, running, soccer, swimming
Fibula	Aerobics, running, skating
Femur	Jumping activities
Calcaneus	Basketball, other jumping activities
Metatarsal	Soccer, swimming
Patella	Baseball, basketball
Pubic ramus	Fencing, jumping, running
Pars interarticularis	Gymnastics
Ribs	Baseball
Scapula	Baseball
Humerus	Baseball, cricket
Ulna	Curling, javelin, tennis
Metacarpal	Handball, tennis

gender as an independent risk factor for stress fractures.[43] Similarly, age has not been found to be an independent risk factor for stress fractures.[43] Stress fractures are most frequently reported in lower extremities; tibia being most affected followed by meta-tarsals and fibula.[51,52] Stress fractures of upper extremities are rare. The duration from time of diagnosis to return to play varies depending on the type, site, and grade of severity of the fracture, and ranges from 7 to 17 weeks.[44,51,52]

DIAGNOSIS

Activity-related, insidious onset of pain that is localized to the affected area is the cardinal presenting symptom of stress fracture.[1] Initially, the pain is reduced or tran-siently relieved with rest, allowing the athlete to continue the activity; however, progression of stress injury results in increased intensity of pain and functional dete-rioration or limitation of activity, which prompts the athlete to seek medical atten-tion.[6,53–55] Pain from stress fracture is usually described as dull aching, and in the case of lower extremity injury is often aggravated by weight bearing. Onset, duration, progression, and modifying factors for the pain should be characterized. Additional history should ascertain information about other possible contributing factors for stress factors as listed in **Table 3**.[5,7,55] The affected area is usually tender to palpation. In the case of lower extremity fractures, the athlete may have a limp because of increased pain on weight bearing. If the fracture is in close proximity to a joint or involves a joint, pain is aggravated on joint movement.

Plain radiography is the initial study for confirming diagnosis of a stress fracture.[56] Plain radiographs have a high rate of false negative results because the findings suggestive of stress injury of the bone are generally not evident on plain radiographs for 2 to 4 weeks after the onset of pain.[5,56,57]

Notwithstanding the expense and accessibility, magnetic resonance imaging (MRI) has been shown to be most useful in the diagnosis of stress injury of the bone, and abnormal findings can be detected as early as within 1 to 2 days of injury.[56,58–65] MRI is useful in delineating the differential diagnosis of stress fracture that includes soft

Table 3 Main points in history	
Pain	Onset, duration, quality, progression, modifying factors, radiation, location, associated symptoms such as tingling, numbness, weakness
Training regimen	Recent increase in intensity, type of activity or sport, running surface
Footwear	Type of shoes, proper fit, how old, history of use of orthotics, inserts
Medical history	Known disorders that affect bone health, osteopenia, metabolic bone disease
Medications	Use of corticosteroid or other drugs that increase risk for osteopenia, use of depomedroxy progesterone
Performance	Anabolic androgenic steroids, growth hormone, other enhancing agents
Nutrition	Caloric intake, calcium intake, vitamin D intake, weight loss
Menstrual history	Onset of menarche, amenorrhea, oligomenorrhea
Stress fractures	Details of any previous stress fractures
Systemic symptoms	Fever, rash, joint pain, undue fatigue, unintended weight loss, loss of appetite

tissue injuries affecting the same area, and more ominous conditions such as bone malignancy and osteomyelitis. Arendt and Griffiths[58] have classified stress injury of the bone into 4 grades (**Table 4**). The MRI grading system has been found to correlate with or has a prognostic significance for time to healing and return to play. Studies have shown that the average duration of recovery time for grade 1 stress injury is 3.3 weeks, whereas it is 14.3 weeks for grade 4 injury.[6,58] MRI-based grading of stress injury of the bone has also been found to be useful in guiding management of stress fractures.

The application of ultrasonography in the diagnosis of musculoskeletal disorders is increasing. Ultrasonography has been shown to be useful in the diagnosis of stress fractures of more superficial bones such as distal tibia and bones of the foot.[56] The acuity of the fracture can be assessed by power Doppler ultrasonography, which provides a semiquantitative estimate of bone turnover.[56]

Computed tomography (CT) can be used in patients in whom MRI is contraindicated. CT is sensitive in detecting stress injury of the bone and in differentiating stress fractures from other lesions of the bone such as osteoid osteoma.[56] CT scan, especially single-photon emission CT (SPECT), has been found to be sensitive in detecting pars interarticularis stress fractures (spondylolysis).

Nuclear medicine scintigraphy is highly sensitive for evaluation of bone turnover and, therefore, for detecting stress reactions 3 to 5 days after onset of pain; however, findings are nonspecific for stress fractures.[56] It also necessitates injection of a radioactive tracer with potential associated risks.

MANAGEMENT

Management of stress fractures is guided by consideration of several factors. It is important to first recognize whether the fracture is at a high-risk (**Box 1**) or low-risk site (**Table 5**).[2,3] In general, when a high-risk stress fracture is suspected or identified, orthopedic or sports medicine consultation is recommended, although this decision may be tempered by personal experience of the primary care physician and the site and severity of the fracture. While awaiting further definitive evaluation and treatment, the athlete is advised to rest from athletic activity. In case of lower extremity fractures, he or she is placed on non–weight-bearing status. Fractures at high-risk sites are at high risk for progression to compete fracture, delayed union, nonunion, and avascular necrosis.[3,6,54]

Table 4		
Arendt and Griffiths grading of stress injury of bone based on MRI findings		
Grade of Stress Injury	**MRI Findings**	**Duration of Rest Needed for Healing, wk**
Grade 1	Positive STIR image	3
Grade 2	Positive STIR plus positive T2-weighted images	3–6
Grade 3	Positive T1- and T2-weighted images; no definite cortical break	12–16
Grade 4	Positive T1- and T2-weighted images; fracture line visible	16

Abbreviation: STIR, Short Tau Inversion Recovery or short T1 inversion recovery.

Data from Arendt EA, Griffiths HJ. The use of MR imaging in the assessment and clinical management of stress reactions of bone in high-performance athletes. Clin Sports Med 1997;16(2):292–306, Table 2, p. 293.

Box 1
Stress fractures at high-risk sites

Femoral neck

Anterior cortex of tibia

Medial malleolus

Tarsal navicular

Base of second metatarsal

Talus

Patella

Sesmoids of great toe

Fifth metatarsal

Most athletes with fractures at low-risk sites can be managed in the primary care setting. In addition to the site of the fracture, timing of the fracture in relation to the sports season, and MRI grading when available are considered in the acute management and return to play decisions.[6,53,54] Athletes with fractures at low-risk sites toward the end of a sports season or during the off-season are recommended to rest from activity that causes pain.[6] For lower extremity fractures, some athletes may need a period of non–weight bearing.[4] The athlete is allowed alternative activities such as swimming or cycling. Athletes in the middle of a sports season may desire to continue to play and finish the season.[5,6,54] These athletes who present with pain that is not limiting their ability to function may be allowed to continue to participate in the sport within the limits of pain tolerance and acuity.[6,53–55] If the intensity of pain increases with continued activity or functional limitation occurs, sports participation is discontinued and the athlete is recommended to rest.

The time to heal and return to play for stress fractures ranges from 6 to 10 weeks depending on multiple factors including the site of injury, grade of injury severity, or other associated risk factors.[6,53–55] Evidence to support use of ultrasound, electrical and electromagnetic fields, and bisphosphonates to enhance stress fracture healing is limited and equivocal.[54,66] Some studies suggest that use of nonsteroidal anti-inflammatory drugs may delay fracture healing.[66] In the management of athletes with stress fractures, the possible risk factors that contribute to pathogenesis should be carefully reviewed and modified where possible to reduce future risk. Ensure adequate nutrition, caloric intake, and calcium and vitamin D intake. Adolescents need 1300 mg per day of calcium and 400 IU of vitamin D daily.

In addition to stress fractures, the differential diagnosis of leg pain includes exertional compartment syndrome, medial tibial stress syndrome, osteomyelitis, and

---

Table 5
Stress fractures at low-risk sites

Upper extremity	Clavicle, scapula, humerus, olecranon, ulna, radius, scaphoid, metacarpals
Lower extremity	Femoral shaft, tibial shaft, fibula, calcaneus, metatarsal shaft
Thorax	Ribs
Spine	Pars interarticularis, sacrum
Pelvis	Pubic rami

bone malignancy. Any adolescent with bone pain should be evaluated carefully to establish the cause of the pain. In addition to imaging, initial laboratory studies may include comprehensive metabolic panel, compete blood count, and erythrocyte sedimentation rate.

The athlete can resume unrestricted sports participation once she or he is pain free and has normal findings on examination.[6,53–55] Routine follow-up imaging studies are not indicated in most cases.

SUMMARY

Stress fractures in adolescent athletes are common injuries seen in practice. Stress fractures most frequently affect lower extremities and are most common in long-distance runners and track and field athletes. Diagnosis is based mainly on clinical evaluation. MRI is the study of choice for further delineating the stress injury of the bone. Most stress fractures that involve low-risk sites can be managed conservatively in the primary care setting and heal in 6 to 10 weeks.

REFERENCES

1. Matheson GO, Clement DB, McKenzie DC, et al. Stress fracture in athletes. Am J Sports Med 1987;15:46–58.
2. Boden BP, Osbahr DC, Jimenez C. Low-risk stress fractures. Am J Sports Med 2001;29(1):100–11.
3. Boden BP, Osbahr DC. High-risk stress fractures: evaluation and treatment. Am Acad Orthop Surg 2000;8(6):344–53.
4. Harmon K. Lower extremity stress fractures. Clin J Sport Med 2003;13(6):358–64.
5. Bolin D, Kemper A, Brolinson G. Current concepts in the evaluation and management of stress fractures. Curr Rep Sport Med 2005;4:295–300.
6. Diehl JJ, Best TM, Kaeding CC. Classification and return-to-play considerations for stress fractures. Clin Sports Med 2006;25:17–28.
7. Pepper M, Akuthota V, McCarty EC. The pathophysiology of stress fractures. Clin Sports Med 2006;26:1–16.
8. Frey C. Footwear and stress fractures. Clin Sports Med 1997;16(2):249–57.
9. Gardner LI Jr, Dziados JE, Jones BH, et al. Prevention of lower extremity stress fractures: a controlled trial of a shock absorbent insole. Am J Public Health 1988;78(12):1563–7.
10. Finestone A, Giladi M, Elad H, et al. Prevention of stress fractures using custom biomechanical shoe orthosis. Clin Orthop 1999;360:182–90.
11. Gillespie WJ, Grant I. Interventions for preventing and treating stress fractures and stress reactions of bone of the lower limbs in young adults. Cochrane Database Syst Rev 2000;2:CD000450.
12. Ekenman I, Milgrom C, Finestone A, et al. The role of biomechanical shoe orthosis in tibial stress fracture prevention. Am J Sports Med 2002;30(6):866–70.
13. Milgrom C, Finestone A, Segev S, et al. Are overground or treadmill runners more likely to sustain tibial stress fracture? Br J Sports Med 2003;37(2):160–3.
14. Bennell KL, Malcolm SA, Thomas SA, et al. The incidence and distribution of stress fractures in competitive track and field athletes: a twelve-month prospective study. Am J Sports Med 1996;24(2):211–7.
15. Hickey GJ, Fricker PA, McDonald WA. Injuries to elite rowers over a 10-yr period. Med Sci Sports Exerc 1997;29(12):1567–72.
16. Zernicke RF, McNitt G, Fray J, et al. Stress fracture risk assessment among elite collegiate women runners. J Biomech 1994;27:854.

17. Brudvig TJ, Gudger TD, Obermeyer L. Stress fractures in 295 trainees: a one-year study of incidence as related to age, sex, and race. Mil Med 1983;148(8):666–7.
18. Milgrom C, Finestone A, Shlamkovitch N, et al. Youth is a risk factor for stress fracture: a study of 783 infantry recruits. J Bone Joint Surg Br 1994;76(1):20–2.
19. Winfield AC, Moore J, Bracker M, et al. Risk factors associated with stress reactions in female Marines. Mil Med 1997;162(10):698–702.
20. Vaitkevicius H, Witt R, Maasdam M, et al. Ethnic differences in titratable acid excretion and bone mineralization. Med Sci Sports Exerc 2002;34(2):295–302.
21. Swissa A, Milgrom C, Giladi M, et al. The effect of pretraining sports activity on the incidence of stress fractures among military recruits: a prospective study. Clin Orthop 1989;245:256–60.
22. Bennell KL, Malcolm SA, Thomas SA, et al. Risk factors for stress fractures in track and field athletes: a twelve-month prospective study. Am J Sports Med 1996;24(6):810–8.
23. Giladi M, Milgrom C, Stein M, et al. External rotation of the hip: a predictor of risk for stress fractures. Clin Orthop 1987;216:131–4.
24. Myburg KH, Hutchins J, Fataar AB, et al. Low bone density is an etiologic factor for stress fractures in athletes. Ann Intern Med 1990;113(10):754–9.
25. Marx RG, Saint-Phard D, Callahan LR, et al. Stress fracture sites related to underlying bone health in athletic females. Clin J Sport Med 2001;11(2):73–6.
26. Cobb KL, Bachrach LK, Greendale G, et al. Disordered eating, menstrual irregularity, and bone mineral density in female runners. Med Sci Sports Exerc 2003;35(5):711–9.
27. Beck TJ, Ruff CB, Mourtada FA, et al. Dual-energy X-ray absorptiometry derived structural geometry for stress fracture prediction in male US Marine Corps recruits. J Bone Miner Res 1996;11(5):645–53.
28. Milgrom C, Giladi M, Simkin A, et al. An analysis of the biomechanical mechanism of tibial stress fractures among Israeli infantry recruits: a prospective study. Clin Orthop 1988;231:216–21.
29. Giladi M, Milgrom C, Stein M. The low arch, a protective factor in stress fractures: a prospective study of 295 military recruits. Orthop Rev 1985;14:709–12.
30. Simkin A, Leichter I, Giladi M, et al. Combined effect of foot arch structure and an orthotic device on stress fractures. Foot Ankle 1989;10(1):25–9.
31. Friberg O. Leg length asymmetry in stress fractures: a clinical and radiological study. J Sports Med Phys Fitness 1982;22(4):485–8.
32. Warren MP, Brooks-Gunn J, Hamilton LH, et al. Scoliosis and fractures in young ballet dancers: relation to delayed menarche and secondary amenorrhea. N Engl J Med 1986;314(21):1348–53.
33. Loucks AB, Horvath SM. Athletic amenorrhea: a review. Med Sci Sports Exerc 1985;17(1):56–72.
34. Drinkwater BL, Nilson K, Chestnut CH, et al. Bone mineral content of amenorrheic and eumenorrheic athletes. N Engl J Med 1984;311(15):277–81.
35. Bennell KL, Malcolm SA, Thomas SA, et al. Risk factors for stress fractures in female track-and-field athletes: a retrospective analysis. Clin J Sport Med 1995;5(4):229–35.
36. Hergenroeder AC. Bone mineralization, hypothalamic amenorrhea, and sex steroid therapy in female adolescents and young adults. J Pediatr 1995;126(5 Pt 1):683–9.
37. Berenson AB, Radecki CM, Grady JJ, et al. A prospective controlled study of the effects of hormonal contraception on bone mineral density. Obstet Gynecol 2001; 98(4):576–82.

38. Specker BL. Evidence for an interaction between calcium intake and physical activity on changes in bone mineral density. J Bone Miner Res 1996;11(10):1539–44.
39. Bennell K, Matheson G, Meeuwisee W, et al. Risk factors for stress fractures. Sports Med 1999;28(2):91–122.
40. Eisman JA. Vitamin D receptor gene alleles and osteoporosis: an affirmative view. J Bone Miner Res 1995;10(9):1289–93.
41. Rigotti NA, Nussbaum SR, Herzog DB, et al. Osteoporosis in women with anorexia nervosa. N Engl J Med 1984;311(25):1601–6.
42. Frusztajer NT, Dhuper S, Warren MP, et al. Nutrition and the incidence of stress fractures in ballet dancers. Am J Clin Nutr 1990;51(5):779–83.
43. Snyder RA, Koester MC, Dunn WR. Epidemiology of stress fractures. Clin Sports Med 2006;25:37–52.
44. Johnson AW, Weiss CB Jr, Wheeler DL. Stress fractures of the femoral shaft in athletes—more common than expected: a new clinical test. Am J Sports Med 1994;22(2):248–56.
45. Lloyd T, Triantafyllou SJ, Baker ER, et al. Women athletes with menstrual irregularity have increased musculoskeletal injuries. Med Sci Sports Exerc 1986;18(4):374–9.
46. Hame SL, LaFemina JM, McAllister DR, et al. Fractures in the collegiate athlete. Am J Sports Med 2004;32(2):446–51.
47. Clement DB, Taunton JE, Smart GW, et al. A survey of overuse running injuries. Phys Sportsmed 1981;9(5):47–58.
48. Witman P, Melvin M, Nicholas JA. Common problems seen in a metropolitan sports injury clinic. Phys Sports Med 1981;9(3):105–8.
49. Nattiv A, Puffer JC, Casper J, et al. Stress fracture risk factors, incidence, and distribution: a 3 year prospective study in collegiate runners. Med Sci Sports Exerc 2000;32(Suppl 5):S347.
50. James SL, Bates BT, Osternig LR. Injuries to runners. Am J Sports Med 1978;6(2): 40–50.
51. Arendt E, Agel J, Heikes C, et al. Stress injuries to bone in college athletes: a retrospective review of experience of a single institution. Am J Sports Med 2003;31(6): 959–68.
52. Taunton JE, Clement DB, Webber D. Lower extremity stress fractures in athletes. Phys Sports Med 1981;9(1):77–86.
53. Brukner P, Bradshaw C, Bennell K. Managing common stress fractures: let risk level guide treatment. Phys Sports Med 1998;26(8):39–47.
54. Raasch WG, Hergan DJ. Treatment of stress fractures: the fundamentals. Clin Sports Med 2006;25:29–36.
55. Kaeding C, Yu J, Wright R, et al. Management and return to play of stress fractures. Clin J Sport Med 2005;15(6):442–7.
56. Sofka CM. Imaging of stress fractures. Clin Sports Med 2006;25:53–62.
57. Daffner RH, Pavlov H. Stress fractures: current concepts. AJR Am J Roentgenal 1992;159:245–52.
58. Arendt EA, Griffiths HJ. The use of MR imaging in the assessment and clinical management of stress reactions of bone in high-performance athletes. Clin Sports Med 1997;16(2):292–306 Table 2, p. 293.
59. Shin AY, Morin WD, Gorman JD, et al. The superiority of magnetic resonance imaging in differentiating the cause of hip pain in endurance athletes. Am J Sports Med 1996;24:168–76.
60. Slocum KA, Gorman JD, Puckett ML, et al. Resolution of abnormal MR signal intensity in patients with stress fractures of the femoral neck. AJR Am J Roentgenol 1997; 168:1295–9.

61. Bergman AG, Fredericson M, Ho C, et al. Asymptomatic tibial stress reactions: MRI detection and clinical follow-up in distance runners. AJR Am J Roentgenal 2004;183:635–8.
62. Lazzarini KM, Troiano RN, Smith RC. Can running cause the appearance of marrow edema on MR images of the foot and ankle? Radiology 1997;202:540–2.
63. Fredericson M, Jennings F, Beaulieu C, et al. Stress fractures in athletes. Top Magn Reson Imaging 2006;17(5):309–25.
64. Kiuru MJ, Niva M, Reponen A, et al. Bone stress injuries in asymptomatic elite recruits: a clinical and magnetic resonance imaging study. Am J Sports Med 2005;33(2):272–6.
65. Provencher MT, Baldwin AJ, Gorman JD, et al. Atypical tensile-sided femoral neck stress fractures: the value of magnetic resonance imaging. Am J Sports Med 2004;32(6):1528–34.
66. Koester MC, Spindler KP. Pharmacologic agents in fracture healing. Clin Sports Med 2006;25:63–73.

Managing the Adolescent Athlete with Type 1 Diabetes Mellitus

Martin B. Draznin, MD

KEYWORDS

- Diabetes • Hypoglycemia • Hyperglycemia
- Adolescent • Athlete • Management

Providing safe and successful diabetes management assistance and advice to an adolescent athlete is a challenging task. It should also be a very rewarding task. To make accurate and useful recommendations one must master required elements: key knowledge about the athlete, the sport, the team and coach, the effects of exercise on diabetes and of diabetes on the ability to exercise, and the resources that can be accessed or employed to support an adolescent athlete who has type 1 diabetes. This article points to sources of information that can be successfully employed by the physician and athlete, and illustrates the use of some of them. The reader is encouraged to access tables and charts of data from work that has been done by research centers; this article is designed to help the reader make effective use of that information. The physician who undertakes the management of an adolescent with diabetes should access and use the International Society for Pediatric and Adolescent Diabetes 2009 *Clinical practice consensus guidelines* (http://www.ispad.org)[1] as a framework within which each athlete's management should be individualized based on his or her unique needs and circumstances.

PREPARTICIPATION CONSIDERATIONS

The physician must get to know the athlete; aptitudes, attitudes, intelligence, intensity, and family variables may all come into play. It is also often necessary to "get into the head" of the athlete regarding rituals, such as lucky things done or worn, to bring success. It is useful to explore the youth's ideas about performance at different levels of blood glucose, attitudes about knowing blood glucose by how it feels versus testing with a blood glucose meter, and fears about hypoglycemia. Also, explore how and

Pediatric Endocrine Subspecialty Clinics, Michigan State University Kalamazoo Center for Medical Studies, Michigan State University College of Human Medicine, 1000 Oakland Drive, Kalamazoo, MI 49008, USA
E-mail address: draznin@kcms.msu.edu

Pediatr Clin N Am 57 (2010) 829–837
doi:10.1016/j.pcl.2010.02.003
0031-3955/10/$ – see front matter © 2010 Elsevier Inc. All rights reserved.

when concentration or visualization is used to prepare for sports so that diabetes-related actions will be incorporated and reliably executed without the athlete feeling loss of ability to excel.

The next thing to know is the sport: the balance between aerobic and anaerobic exercise, how intensively the sport is played and practiced, the duration of the exercise, the risks of injury, and especially the risk for injury to self or others if distracted by hypoglycemia. These are only a few of the critical aspects of a sport. It is vital to understand the nature and intensity of the training and of the competition—and how those two aspects may affect the athlete in different ways—so that appropriate adjustments in management can be made.

One must know the teammates and the coach: their attitudes, abilities, methods, and willingness to assist in the diabetes management are critical to a successful plan for participation. This is included but not always emphasized in the scientific literature regarding athletes with diabetes. Where appropriate, and with permission of the athlete and family, direct contact with teammates and the coach may be very helpful.

Knowledge of the physiology of exercise, at least at a basic level, is needed in order to understand the changes in fuel use, blood sugar levels, or insulin effects.

Knowledge, both of the effects of diabetes complications on participation in the particular sport and of the risks of sports participation in the presence of complications is important.

Knowledge of the diabetes management resources that benefit the athlete is another key area. Necessary information includes: how insulin works, what delivery devices are used for the insulin, what monitoring devices are in use, which insulin administration protocols are being followed, what sources of carbohydrate are available to support exercise, or to treat hypoglycemia, who has access and knowledge of the use of emergency glucagon kits for severe episodes of hypoglycemia, and how to access support groups and information that the athlete can employ for improvement of the process.

Follow-up of the recommendations to assess how well they have worked during the sports season, is not an element of knowledge to be gained, but it is the only sure way to allow for necessary adjustments.

THE ATHLETE

Getting to know the athlete before the start of the season will give the best chance for making a plan that has the participation and buy-in of the adolescent. The preparticipation interview regarding diabetes management for sports is ideally part of routine diabetes care, and it certainly may be done in the primary care setting by a knowledgeable physician.

Important factors include the type of diabetes management currently employed by the athlete; types of insulin and delivery devices; and how well the management is working, eg, glycohemoglobin level, number of severe episodes of hypoglycemia, or any ill effects on growth from the diabetes. To make useful adjustments in insulin dosing or carbohydrate intake, the athlete or his or her support team must be willing and able to make the kinds of calculations needed. These include carbohydrate counting, knowing the insulin-to-carbohydrate ratio for food coverage and the insulin dose for excessively high blood glucose, and tracking the blood glucose trends before, during, and after training and competition by frequent monitoring of capillary blood glucose levels. We use the slogan "just test it."

When the athlete is a highly intelligent and curious individual, reinvention of management ideas may occur between office visits. One basketball player in our clinic discovered that the effect of the short-acting insulin analog given soon before eating did not persist long enough to adequately cover his evening meal—he had previously needed to wait 45 minutes after using regular insulin before eating to get good effect. He hit upon using 50% of each type of insulin so that he had no waiting and regained excellent control. This kind of discovery humbles and gladdens diabetes doctors!

THE FAMILY AND THE ATHLETIC STAFF

The family plays a vital, if not always front-seat role, in diabetes care of an adolescent. Involve family members in the planning because they, along with the adolescent, are the primary contacts for educating the coaching staff about the needs of the adolescent to safely participate. Discussion about the appropriate blood glucose-level strategy is a central part of the preparticipation interview. Ideas that a high blood sugar at the start of exercise will lead to a better performance are probably not correct.[2] Using out-of-range starting glucose levels to protect against hypoglycemia does not seem successful in youth seen in this clinic. It is also important that the athlete test real-time capillary blood glucose levels during the exercise, counting on how it feels to recognize hypoglycemia is not always accurate and can be dangerous.

Defining roles for the athlete, family and coaching staff should be decided early in the season: who will have the fast-acting source of carbohydrate, whether there will be a glucagon kit and who will know how and when to give it, and where the testing supplies will be kept and when they may be used. Validation of worries about hypoglycemia and developing a plan with the athlete to help avoid it will build the trust needed to keep the athlete on track with blood sugars. The fear of hypoglycemia is a major impediment to improving blood glucose control. To not recognize that, and thus miss the opportunity to help minimize risks while maintaining good control of levels, is to ask for hyperglycemia as the pre-exercise condition.

THE SPORT

Different sports have their own effects on diabetes management. Moderate aerobic exercise is associated with hypoglycemia while bursts of anaerobic exercise may actually raise blood glucose.[3] The very helpful tables of carbohydrate use and "exercise exchanges" (minutes of exercise requiring 15 g of carbohydrate based on size and type of exercise) from the work of Riddell and Bar-or[4] can be found in the *Handbook of exercise in diabetes*, and their table of exercise exchanges can be found online in the International Society for Pediatric and Adolescent Diabetes (ISPAD) Clinical Practice Consensus Guideline for 2009 entitled *Exercise in children and adolescents with diabetes*.[5] Recognize that these, like all other numeric calculations for diabetes care, are starting points, they are only approximations of the truth, which is to be found by testing levels when the individual athlete is exercising. It is only by monitoring the outcomes that they can be validated and adjustments made to fit an individual.

There is also a need to be certain that information regarding the effect of training and practice, as differentiated from the effect of competition, be kept in mind. Many sports have much longer practice times than game participation times in order to promote endurance, yet the athletes often "leave it all on the field" during a game. The role of exercise duration and the role of exercise intensity need to be assessed. One question to ask is: How much is practice biased toward aerobics and conditioning and how much is a game like repetitive sprints?

In addition, depending on the sport, some of the most intensely pleasurable experiences are related to level of skill, such as a perfectly executed golf or tennis swing, a weightless-feeling basketball during a well-executed hook shot, or the sensation of the "sweet spot" of the bat crushing the baseball with no shock to the hands. Clear-headed concentration is needed both to attain those skills and to enjoy them. "Practice does not make perfect, perfect practice makes perfect" is not just a slogan, it is the core of motor memory training and well-controlled levels of blood glucose will facilitate this process. Risk of injury during episodes of hypoglycemia is a serious matter in sports with rapid movements; sports in which collisions routinely occur; and in sports such as climbing, scuba diving, and swimming, in which diminished attention could lead to a catastrophic event. The primary safety concern is avoidance of unrecognized hypoglycemia.

Additionally, in activities where an injured or incapacitated partner might risk the health or life of the other partner, such as technical climbing, mountaineering, or scuba diving, there is also a moral imperative to minimize the risk of hypoglycemia. Gradual acclimatization to these sports should be recommended with much attention to the effect on blood glucose so that appropriate adjustments in management can be made. For example, it did not seem necessary to stop mountaineers with diabetes from climbing Mt Everest or Denali because they were capable climbers. Helping them to keep their diabetes safe was the needed intervention.[6] World-class athletes with diabetes have earned Olympic Gold Medals and been professional athletes for decades, even with the older more cumbersome diabetes management systems.[7] One vignette regarding practice and competition comes to mind from our clinic. A very competitive sprint swimmer with diabetes had miserable experiences and slowing times when swimming 500-yard races in practice. We even went so far as to test him for the overtraining phenomenon, which is a transient hypopituitary state that is the equivalent of the oligomenorrhea seen in some intensely training female endurance athletes. In spite of his complaints about the 500-yard races, his times in the 50-yard races were quite good; in fact, he obtained a high ranking in the state and he felt well when sprinting. He elected to tolerate the "misery" of endurance training as he was in no danger and he had a successful year.

TEAMMATES AND COACH

Teammates and coaches are usually managed by the athlete and family. When an athlete is valuable to a team, or when the coach is a parent of the athlete with diabetes, the clinic may be able to interact directly, with permission of the athlete and family of course. One young woman distance runner's coach was willing and able to attend diabetes clinic with her on a few occasions. After discussions with the diabetes-care team about how exercise may affect diabetes, she and the athlete together made the necessary adjustments to carbohydrate-intake schedules for successful, safe training and a successful season. It is equally important that all athletes with diabetes, even those less "valuable" to the team, be given every opportunity to participate that a teammate without diabetes would have. Remedial education by consultation with coaches may be indicated when the athlete is restricted by the prejudices or fears of others rather than by ability and effort.

EXERCISE PHYSIOLOGY

Numerous comprehensive articles and chapters related to diabetes and exercise have described the effects of exercise on fuel metabolism in persons with diabetes.[8–10]

The initiation of exercise elicits hormonal signals to release fuels. Glucose from liver glycogen; use of the glucose stored as glycogen in muscle, leading to generation of lactic acid that is then cycled through the liver to make new glucose; mobilization of fatty acids, especially in fit endurance athletes; and gluconeogenesis from amino acids all may be set in motion.

The nondiabetic individual has near instantaneous insulin modulation to keep blood glucose levels within normal range during exercise; the athlete with diabetes relies on the release of insulin from subcutaneous depots, the increased exposure of insulin to receptors on muscle cells as blood flow increases, and some element of non–insulin-induced muscle uptake. The lack of a closed-loop system can result in hyperglycemia during the initial exercise, hypoglycemia later on as the level of injected insulin can not respond to a falling level of glucose, and excess generation of ketone bodies if available insulin is insufficient to modulate use of fat for energy. In spite of the lack of automatic and easy regulation, young athletes can often manage very well.

More recently detailed attention has been paid to the effects of having diabetes to slightly lower exercise capacity.[11] However, the take-home message from observing athletes in sports activity is that, whereas there are real differences of laboratory-tested performance between athletes who do and do not have diabetes; these differences do not seem to be reflected in the everyday world outside the laboratories. In other words, athletes who have diabetes may be as capable, and feel nearly as well while exercising as if they did not have it, at least until or unless they have complications of diabetes that may limit them in other ways.

IMPLICATIONS OF DIABETES COMPLICATIONS
Hypoglycemia and Ketoacidosis

The main acute complications are hypoglycemia and ketoacidosis. Ketoacidosis may be engendered by exercise, whereas ketoacidosis that exists before exercise usually leaves sufferers feeling too ill to play. Antecedent hypoglycemia has long been known to blunt counterregulatory response to subsequent hypoglycemia. It also blunts the response to exercise.[12] This information should be shared with the athlete, so that much more attention is paid to checking blood glucose levels after there has been a significant low.

Ocular Changes

Long-term complications are not seen as early in the course of the diabetes during the current era of striving for tight metabolic control. It is still necessary to screen for them as they can have profound effects on participation in sports. Ocular changes have become less frequent during childhood and adolescence owing to improved care plans and patient success in adhering to them. It is rare to see proliferative retinopathy in youth. Nonproliferative retinopathy can be a risk factor during sudden impacts or breath-holding during extreme exertion such as weight lifting, which can lead to rapid increase of blood pressure and rupture of microaneurysms.

Neuropathy

Peripheral neuropathy is likewise uncommon in children and adolescents with diabetes. The risks would be due to clumsiness from lack of proper sensation in the feet. Autonomic neuropathy leading to loss of cardiac responsiveness, that is, low beat-to-beat variability of the heart rate while at rest and slow adaptation to change in posture or activity, may lead to syncope. This is not seen much in adolescents.

Other

Poorly controlled hypertension can be a problem, sapping performance and being exacerbated by exertion. Renal compromise would mostly be manifested early on by hypertension. Advanced renal disease is much less common with modern care of adolescents. Whereas associated autoimmune conditions are not complications of diabetes, in that they cannot be prevented by excellent diabetes care, hypothyroidism impairs performance, celiac disease could impair ability to be very active, and the uncommon occurrence of Addison's disease or of pernicious anemia in youth with diabetes would also make exercise difficult or hazardous.

DIABETES MANAGEMENT FOR THE ATHLETE

Modern diabetes management systems have made it possible to prolong healthy life in children and youth with diabetes who can and will master their use.[1,13] They are also much more flexible, allowing for safe participation in sports and exercise. It must be acknowledged that there were superb athletes who had nothing more flexible for diabetes regulation than the difficult, cumbersome, and inflexible care systems from early years and they succeeded anyway.

Insulin and Insulin Regimens

Modern insulin has identical amino acid sequence and activity compared with the human molecule. The amino acid sequences can also be deliberately altered to allow specific action profiles to enhance effectiveness. Its concentration in the vial pen or pump is high and uniform so that the discomfort of injections is minimal. There are only miniscule amounts of impurities and their action from day to day is reproducible. Even the need to suspend insoluble intermediate acting forms and to mix insulin from two vials in one syringe has nearly disappeared in pediatric diabetes practices in United States.

Many, if not most, children and adolescents with diabetes now use what are called basal-bolus insulin regimens using a long-acting analog by injection or short-acting insulin delivered by an insulin pump at continuous low levels to provide basal, or foundation, insulin to prevent ketogenesis and provide needed insulin during fasting. Injections of short acting insulin or pump bolus infusions are used to cover the carbohydrate part of meals, and to correct high levels of blood glucose. Insulin is available in vials to be injected by syringe, in prefilled pen devices used with disposable needles for quick and precise dosing, and via insulin pumps. There are possibly as many protocols to setup and adjust these systems as there are diabetes clinics!

What makes intensive management of diabetes work for patients is the ability to quickly, and with some precision, measure blood glucose levels at appropriate times with the monitoring devices needing only tiny drops of blood. Fortunately, the discomfort level has become much less with the modern devices. There are also continuous monitoring devices that record or report the level of glucose in subcutaneous tissue fluids to assist in understanding how well insulin-dosing matches the needs of the patient. It is not clear that these can be used during strenuous exercise due to mechanical considerations or loss of the signal, but, if they could, they would provide helpful data.

Carbohydrates for Hypoglycemia

Rapidly absorbed sources of carbohydrate to treat hypoglycemia include 4 g or 5 g glucose tablets. "Take 4 or 3 for routine hypoglycemia, retest in 15 minutes, and repeat until under control" is the "rule of 15" used to treat low blood glucose with less risk of an overshoot. Athletes often take these tablets by the handful to keep up. Other sources of glucose include hard candies, cake icing in tubes, glucose gels, sport drinks (although it takes 250 mL of a 6% drink to provide 15 g), and soft drinks (a few ounces is enough but the carbonation may be problematic).

Modulation of Insulin Delivery for Exercise

How could or should the insulin delivery be altered to accommodate exercise? In growing children and adolescents, especially during the adolescent growth spurt, reducing insulin should be reserved for times when increased oral intake of carbohydrates cannot maintain safe blood glucose levels. Pediatricians tend to be in favor of increasing pre-exercise food intake to prevent hypoglycemia in exercising children and adolescents with diabetes; reducing insulin is a second step. To start, insulin in the basal-bolus systems is usually divided between 50% for basal needs and 50% for carbohydrate coverage. It is then adjusted based on blood glucose readings. It may be useful to lower the basal insulin.

One may also decrease pre-exercise meal coverage with short-acting insulin, but must be aware that the increased availability of fuels in the circulation may lead to hyperglycemia and ketogenesis if the meal insulin is lowered too much. Also, vexatious is what to do when postexercise blood glucose is high. Should one fully correct the high level as if no exercise had occurred, or perhaps only a half correction is enough? With an insulin pump, one can change one or more of the basal rates, have an entirely different set of rates and ratios for exercise versus nonexercise days, or even disconnect the pump for up to two hours to avoid hypoglycemia during exercise.

A useful insulin dose-alteration scheme devised by an internist with diabetes[14] employs a lowered basal pump rate for exercise intensive days; he uses 25% but that amount can be adjusted for the individual athlete. The key difference of his system from just having a different basal rate is that insulin glargine is then given to replace the "missing" 75% of the basal dose when the pump rate is lowered. This prevents the blood glucose from rising too much during nonexercise intervals. It also leaves insulin in the circulation when the pump is disconnected for more than two hours, but it is at a lower level than the usual pump delivery would yield, which prevents hypoglycemia during exercise. This has worked well for athletes from our clinic who have used it. For many types of sports, insulin pumps should be removed to avoid damage to the pump, or because the pump is not waterproof, this scheme works well. In the athletes using an older scheme of insulin dosing with an intermediate insulin, the pre-exercise dose may need to be reduced and short-acting insulin used to control high readings or the postexercise dose of intermediate-acting insulin may need to be reduced also to prevent late-onset hypoglycemia.

Glucagon

For extremely dangerous episodes of hypoglycemia in which the athlete is unconscious or confused to the extent that oral administration of glucose tablets or anything else would risk aspiration, glucagon should be injected directly into a large muscle such as the deltoid, or quadriceps femoris. The dose of glucagon should have been calculated in advance and the family must instruct whoever will administer it if it not a family member. Usually 1 mg for body weights above 100 lb will suffice, and 0.5 mg if the athlete is smaller. When the blood glucose level is raised enough to restore a more conscious athlete, oral feedings will probably be needed as well.

RESOURCES

Where should the athlete, family, and physician obtain information about adjustments in diabetes management to allow safe exercising, practicing, and competing? The ISPAD *Clinical Practice Consensus Guideline*,[5] available at http://www.ispad.org, is highly recommended. On the Internet, http://www.childrenwithdiabetes.org is a very helpful and practical consumer-driven Web site. Also, http://www.desa.org is the Web site of an organization of committed athletes with diabetes, mostly adults. A British Web site, http://www.runsweet.com, has a number of commentaries on many different sports, again by adult athletes and based more on personal experiences than scientific studies. All of these Web sites provide thought-provoking insights that physicians would do well to access when working with today's web-savvy athlete. Physicians need to know where they get their independent information and what it is likely to best help them. Web sites such as the ones listed are very valuable, there may be some that are less so, or even dangerous.

SUMMARY

The essence of successful diabetes management depends on assessment of outcome so that necessary adjustments in the regimen can be made. No perfect process exists that can be applied to diabetes care in a "fire-and-forget" manner. Intensive diabetes management will not succeed without multiple capillary blood glucose measurements at strategic times to allow for course corrections, to avoid hyperglycemia and long-term complications on the one hand and severe hypoglycemia on the other. Similarly, the recommendations that physicians make to athletes with diabetes must be validated by the athletes' outcome testing and awareness. If the clinic and the athlete are able to communicate during the season without need for office visits, or if the plan is comprehensive enough to include recommendations for adjustments, a safe season should be the reward. Constant attention to details, agility in making adjustments to match needs, and focus on the outcome are helpful for diabetes management and are not different from the kinds of actions needed by athletes to progress in their sport. Physicians should emphasize those similarities for their patients' benefit! The energy, focus, and drive that make it possible to be a successful athlete ought to be harnessed to make diabetes management successful also.

REFERENCES

1. ISPAD Clinical practice consensus guidelines 2009 compendium. Available at: http://www.ispad.org. Accessed February 6, 2010.
2. Stettler C, Jenni S, Allemann S, et al. Exercise capacity in subjects with type 1 diabetes mellitus in eu- and hyperglycaemia. Diabetes Metab Rev 2006;22(4): 300–6.
3. Bussau VA, Jones TW, Ferreira LD, et al. The 10-s maximal sprint. A novel approach to counter an exercise-mediated fall in glycemia in individuals with type 1 diabetes. Diabetes Care 2006;29(3):601–6.
4. Riddell MC, Bar-or O. Children and adolescents. In: Ruderman N, Devlin JT, Schneider SH, et al, editors. Handbook of exercise in diabetes. Alexandria (Egypt): American Diabetes Association; 2002. p. 547–66.
5. Robertson K, Adolfsson P, Riddell M, et al. Exercise in children and adolescents with diabetes. Pediatr Diabetes 2009;10(Suppl 12):154–68 In: Hanas R, Donaghue K, Klingnsmith G, et al, editors. ISPAD Clinical practice consensus guidelines 2009 compendium. Available at: http://www.ispad.org. Accessed February 6, 2010.
6. Mountaineering stories. Available at: http://www.runsweet.com. Accessed February 6, 2010.
7. Rowing and swimming. Available at: http://www.runsweet.com. Accessed February 6, 2010.

8. Riddell MC, Iscoe KE. Physical activity, sport, and pediatric diabetes. Pediatr Diabetes 2006;7:60–70.
9. Oetliker JS, Alleman S, Ith M, et al. Fuel metabolism during exercise in euglycemia and hyperglycemia in patients with type 1 diabetes mellitus—a prospective single-blinded randomized crossover trial. Diabetologia 2008;51(8):1457–65.
10. Rosa JS, Glassetti PR. Altered molecular adaptation to exercise in children with type1 diabetes: beyond hypoglycemia. Pediatr Diabetes 2009;10:213–36.
11. Komatsu WR, Gabbay MA, Castro ML, et al. Aerobic exercise capacity in normal adolescents and those with type 1 diabetes mellitus. Pediatr Diabetes 2005;6(3): 145–9.
12. Davis ST, Galassetti P, Wasserman DH, et al. Effects of antecedent hypoglycemia on subsequent counterregulatory responses to exercise. Diabetes 2000;49: 73–81.
13. Kamboj MK, Draznin MB. Diabetes mellitus. In: Patel DR, Greydanus DE, Baker RJ, editors. Pediatric practice: sports medicine. New York (NY): McGraw-Hill; 2009. p. 157–66.
14. Edelman S. The un-tethered regimen. Available at: http://www.childrenwithdiabetes. org. Accessed February 6, 2010.

Medical and Orthopedic Conditions and Sports Participation

Eugene Diokno, MD[a],*, Dale Rowe, MD[b,c]

KEYWORDS

- Juvenile arthritis • Scoliosis • Spondylolysis
- Scheuermann disease • Slipped vertebral apophysis

Adolescents with chronic conditions are often restricted unnecessarily from sports participation or other physical activities for fear of injury or other complications. For some of the orthopedic conditions, athletes are also advised prolonged periods of rest and restrictions from sports. The benefits of sport participation, with few exceptions, far outweigh any concerns for potential injuries or complications in these adolescents. This article reviews sport participation guidelines for some of these medical and orthopedic conditions.

ARTHRITIS

With the increasing problem of the obesity epidemic, it has been shown that youths with low levels of physical activity and high body fat are at increased risk for cardiovascular disease. In contrast, it is a challenge for our patients who suffer from chronic illnesses to be encouraged to stay active and fit while keeping their condition under control.[1] One such condition is juvenile idiopathic arthritis (JIA), which is the most common chronic rheumatoid disease in childhood. Exercise is an integral part of managing this condition to preserve joint mobility and maintain muscle mass and strength.[2,3] However, data show that these patients are less active than their peers.[4] It is vital to have a multidisciplinary team approach to achieve success and adherence to a sound and practical exercise program.[5]

---

[a] Primary Care Sports Medicine Program, Arnold Palmer Sports Health Center, Union Memorial Hospital, 3333 North Calvert Street, Baltimore, MD 21218, USA
[b] Department of Orthopedic Surgery, Michigan State University College of Human Medicine, East Lansing, MI, USA
[c] Orthopedic Residency Program, Kalamazoo Center for Medical Studies, Kalamazoo, MI, USA
* Corresponding author.
E-mail address: diokno@comcast.net

Pediatr Clin N Am 57 (2010) 839–847
doi:10.1016/j.pcl.2010.03.005
0031-3955/10/$ – see front matter © 2010 Elsevier Inc. All rights reserved.

pediatric.theclinics.com

Despite having no significant effects on endurance and functional ability of patients with JIA, an aquatic-based program studied by Takken and colleagues[6] has been shown to positively influence the health-related quality of life of these patients. Takken and colleagues[7] found this to be a safe program, with no signs of worsening in the health status of patients. A land-based aerobic program that included warm-up and stretching used by Singh-Grewal and colleagues[8] in a randomized controlled trial resulted in improved physical function as measured in the Child Health Assessment Questionnaire. There was better compliance with the control group that involved the qigong regimen, which is similar to tai chi.[8] An intensive Cochrane review did not show statistically significant evidence that exercise therapy can improve functional ability, quality of life, aerobic capacity, or pain, but it did affirm that exercise does not exacerbate arthritis.[9]

Participation in sports needs to be individualized for each patient with JIA, as is the case for any chronic condition. Aerobic, flexibility, static, dynamic, and neuromuscular demands of the sport should be considered, as well as the potential for contact or collision.[2] The availability of safety equipment has to be explored, alongside the need for splints or orthosis.[2] The family and coaches have to assess the athlete's ability to self-limit participation.[2]

JIA often persists into adulthood, although fewer than 10% become severely disabled.[10] Promoting sports during childhood and adolescence hopefully will help individuals to acquire healthy practices and maintain an active lifestyle as they transition into adulthood.

EYE INJURIES

Eye injuries are rare among high-school and college athletes but have the potential for high morbidity.[11,12] Baseball and basketball in the United States and soccer in European countries are most commonly implicated to cause eye injuries.[13] Injuries range from the more benign eyelid laceration, corneal abrasion, foreign bodies, and hyphema to the more serious blow-out fracture, retinal detachment, or globe rupture. Children and adolescents are still developing their muscle coordination and reaction time, making them more vulnerable to these injuries.[14]

Injured players may return to play immediately, depending on the extent of the trauma, but, if they received a topical anesthetic in the eye, then they should not be allowed to resume play.[14] The affected eye should be pain free and have adequate recovery of vision.[14] Symptoms like foreign-body sensation, vision loss, proptosis interfering with vision, pain, loss of visual field, or a flash sensation are warnings for an ophthalmology evaluation and clearance for return to play.[15]

The American Academy of Pediatrics (AAP) and American Academy of Ophthalmology issued a joint policy statement in 2004 recommending that all youths in organized sports should wear appropriate eye protection.[16] There are sport-specific eye protectors such as a face guard attached to the helmet in baseball or a full-face shield in hockey. Protective eye wear for sports should meet the requirements of certifying bodies like the Protective Eyewear Certification Council, American Society for Testing and Materials (ASTM), Hockey Equipment Certification Council (HECC) and the National Operating Committee on Standards in Athletic Equipment (NOCSAE). Regular spectacles and contact lenses do not offer protection, so the appropriate eyewear is still strongly recommended.[15] Functionally one-eyed athletes should wear protective eyewear as well as those whose ophthalmologists recommend eye protection after surgery or trauma.[15] Sport-appropriate and properly fitting eye protectors reduce the risk of significant eye injury by at least 90%, so young athletes should develop the habit of using this protective gear early to avoid potentially blinding injuries.[4]

SOLITARY KIDNEY

Should an athlete with a solitary kidney be allowed to participate in contact sports? The answer to this question remains inconsistent, controversial, and difficult. In 1994, a survey of 438 members of the American Medical Society of Sports Medicine (AMSSM) showed that 54% would allow participation, but that this decreased to 42% when the athlete was their own child.[17] More recently, Grinsell and colleagues[18] showed only 34% of respondents from the American Society of Pediatric Nephrology (ASPN) would allow participation, and Sharp and colleagues[19] likewise found that 32% of pediatric urologists surveyed would agree to contact sports for these patients. However, studies suggest that the risk of renal injury in contact or collision sports is extremely low. Recreational activities such as cycling, skiing, sledding, snowboarding, and horseback riding have shown higher risks of renal injury.[18–21] A review of data from the National Pediatric Trauma Registry (NPTR) by Wan and colleagues[22] during a 10-year span from 1990 to 1999 concluded that abdominal and testicular injuries are rare in team and individual contact and collision sports. Another extensive NPTR study reported that much more common causes of catastrophic kidney loss were those from motor vehicle crashes, pedestrians being struck by a vehicle or other object, and falls.[23]

Several factors are considered when arriving at the decision of precluding an athlete with a solitary kidney from participating in contact or collision sports. These include the perception of injury risk (whether accurate or not), weighing the benefits of participation versus the tragic consequence of the potential loss of the remaining kidney, absence of a clear consensus, and ethical and medicolegal concerns. Restriction not based on clinical evidence can result in depriving an athlete of the physical, social, and educational rewards of their involvement in sports. Some would even argue that we let athletes with solitary brain, heart, and spinal cord play, and these have higher injury rates.[18]

The AAP recommends a "qualified yes" for athletes who have a solitary kidney, with an individual assessment.[24] As with athletes with a solitary testicle, providing protective equipment is essential. It is imperative that an open discussion on potential risks and benefits of sports participation take place among the athlete, the parents, and the clinician before making the informed decision not only about whether to play contact sports but also about participating in certain recreational activities.

SKIN CONDITIONS

Unlike most other organ systems that show benefits from increased physical activity, skin actually develops pathologic conditions directly attributed to sports participation.[25] Skin is subjected to direct repetitive trauma producing abrasions, blisters, chafing, corns, calluses, and black heel. Most of these lesions will not lead to significant interruption of athletic participation if recognized early and treated appropriately.[26]

Making return-to-play decisions for infectious dermatologic conditions is another issue altogether. Skin infections are commonly encountered in the athletic setting. Player hygiene; close physical contact in locker rooms, buses, and benches; moist environments; and sharing of towels, equipment, and even housing accommodation all contribute to the host factors of the incubation and transmission process.[27] An epidemiologic study on wrestling done by the National Collegiate Athletic Association

(NCAA) Injury Surveillance System from 1988/1989 to 2003/2004 recorded that infectious dermatoses accounted for the most missed practice time, amounting to more than 17% of the reported events.[28]

For bacterial (most commonly staphylococcal or streptococcal) infections including impetigo, folliculitis, furuncles (boils), carbuncles, abscesses, and cellulitis, the NCAA will preclude an athlete from participating if they are at risk of transmitting the infection. According to the NCAA protocol, the athlete must meet the following criteria: (1) no new lesions within the past 48 hours, (2) completion of 72 hours of antibiotic therapy, and (3) no moist, exudative, or purulent lesions at time of play.[29] The National Federation of State High School Associations (NFHS) endorses these guidelines for wrestling and football, which they consider high risk for significant contact with opponent or equipment.[30] Methicillin-resistant *Staphylococcus aureus* (MRSA), frequently called the superbug, has been the latest sports epidemic because of the emergence of antibiotic resistance. Increasing prevalence and reports of significant morbidity and mortality have brought MRSA to the attention of the sports community. The Centers for Disease Control and Prevention (CDC) reinforces the NCAA guidelines of excluding the athlete if the wound cannot be properly covered during participation, and even if it can be covered but still poses a risk to the health of the infected athlete, such as a further injury to the affected area.[31]

Herpetic infections include simplex, fever blisters, zoster, and gladiatorum. To be allowed to participate, a wrestler must: (1) be free of systemic symptoms of viral infection; (2) have no new blisters for 72 hours before the examination; (3) have no moist lesions, and any remaining lesions must be dried and have a firm adherent crust; (4) have been on antiviral therapy for at least 120 hours before meet time; and (5) not cover active lesions.[29]

Tinea lesions need oral or topical treatment for a minimum of 72 hours for skin lesions and 14 days on scalp lesions before the athlete is allowed to return to play.[29,30] Wrestlers with solitary or clustered lesions will be disqualified if the lesions are in a location that cannot be adequately covered.[29] If wrestlers have contracted scabies, they should have a negative prep at tournament time.[29] Because there are no clear rules for most other sports, it is recommended that the guidelines for wrestling be used for any contact or collision sports or other sports that involve shared equipment or facilities like a gymnasium or pool.[32] As the NCAA/CDC poster says, "If in doubt, check it out."

SCOLIOSIS

Most scoliosis is not related to instability, especially if it is classified as early- or late-onset hereditary scoliosis. Pain is an uncommon feature for these patients; however, if present it may require some restrictions to control the symptoms. Most of these patients will not require restrictions to protect from instability.[33,34] Some congenital scoliosis may present with such sharp angulations that the spinal cord is impaired or at risk. In these cases, restriction from contact and high-level sports requiring bending or aerial activities should be advised. Patients who have undergone surgical fusion for scoliosis and are fully healed can often participate in noncontact sports. Although the authors often advise their patients to avoid contact, some do participate without significant injury. No good studies have been published to offer scientific guidelines for postoperative patients. Consultation with the spinal surgeon will often be necessary.[35,36]

Patients with scoliosis are often treated with a thoracic lumbar sacral orthosis (TLSO, eg, Boston brace) or cervical TLSO (Milwaukee brace). These braces pose a risk of injury to other athletes participating in the game or practice, and can restrict movements for the patient. In many cases, the orthotics can be removed during the game or practice.[37] Consultation with the orthopedic surgeon is advised in these cases.[38]

KYPHOSIS

Scheuermann kyphosis or juvenile idiopathic round back is a hereditary deformity of the thoracic spine. In mild and moderate cases this is a structurally stable condition. In these cases, no restrictions from sports are necessary. Some patients have pain, which may require some modification of participation to control the pain. Moderate deformities (>50°) are often treated with an orthotic such as a Milwaukee or Boston brace. These orthotics can often be removed during games or practices to allow the athletes to participate in sports. These modifications of the treatment regimens also improve patients' willingness to comply with the brace treatment plans.[39–41] Some kyphotic deformities are so severe that spinal cord compromise is found. These patients should be restricted from sports until there is a full evaluation by the spine surgeon.[35]

Atypical Scheuermann kyphosis, or rower's back, is a deformity of the thoracolumbar or lumbar spine associated with a large defect in the anterior superior vertebral end plate. This condition is classically seen in athletes who are required to flex and extend the spine repeatedly, such as gymnasts, rowers, wrestlers, football players, weight lifters, tennis players, and bicycle riders.[35] These lesions are stable but often painful. The pain is frequently relieved by restriction of the sporting activity for a period of 6 months. A TLSO brace can often be used to provide relief sooner and allow athletes to return to sports within a 2- to 3-month period. However, returning to the sport often results in recurrence of the pain. Sometimes activity modifications are necessary. Rarely, surgical intervention can relieve the pain and allow participation in high-level athletes.

SPONDYLOLYSIS

Lytic lesions of the pars interarticularis of the lumbar spine are common in athletes who repeat extension of the spine. This condition is common in gymnastics, defensive linemen in football, weight lifters, and cheerleaders. These patients present with pain because of the acute nature of the fracture.[35] Restrictions from participation are necessary to treat the stress injury, along with a TLSO to splint the spine, and physical therapy. After the lesion heals or develops a painless fibrous union, usually following 4 to 6 weeks of treatment, the athlete can return to gradual training and participation as long as the pain does not return.[38,39,42]

SPONDYLOLISTHESIS

Chronic pars interarticularis fractures with fibrocartilaginous union can be silent and found incidentally on radiographs done for another reason. If the slip is less that 50%, the athlete can often be allowed to participate as long as pain remains absent or mild. Routine follow-up of the slip with radiographs is necessary during the growing years.[35] If the slip is greater than 50% or progressive, the spine may be unstable, and restrictions are advised until the patient can be fully evaluated by a spine surgeon. Some patients have undergone spinal fusions to treat spondylolisthesis. Once the fusion is solid, patients may return to full sport activities, including contact sports, without problems.[42]

DEGENERATIVE DISC DISEASE

Injury to the discs produce annular tears and loss of water content that leads to reduced height and a black disc on the T2 magnetic resonance image. They are associated with pain that can be disabling. Sports such as weight lifting and football have been shown to increase disc disease, as have improper or excessive training for any sport. Sports participation should be limited until the patient has rested for a brief period with nonsteroidal antiinflammatory drugs, then started on a strengthening and stretching program, once pain free. A physical therapist is often invaluable in obtaining patients' optimal recovery. Once the pain has been totally relieved, with demonstration of muscle strength without spasm, the athlete can return to training and sports. If the pain is chronic, evaluation by a spine surgeon will be necessary.[39]

ADOLESCENT DISC HERNIATION

Intervertebral discs can herniate portions of the nucleolus fibrosis, producing compression of lumbar spinal nerves. Patients with these conditions present with back pain and sciatica. Often, they also have reactive or sciatic scoliosis. Initial restrictions from participation in sports are necessary, along with physical therapy. Once the initial pain has subsided, often after 6 to 12 weeks of treatment, the patients may gradually return to sports. Continued sciatica and back pain may require more restrictions and an evaluation by a spine surgeon.

SLIPPED VERTEBRAL APOPHYSIS

This condition involves the fracture and displacement of the ring apophysis into the spinal canal with neurologic damage and symptoms. Because this tissue is hyaline cartilage and not likely to resorb, restrictions from sports and training are advised, as is a referral to a spine surgeon for evaluation. Surgical excision of the offending portion of the ring apophysis is likely required. After the surgery and healing, return to sports can be considered with selective rehabilitation.[35]

CONGENITAL ABNORMALITIES OF THE CERVICAL SPINE

Certain odontoid abnormalities and congenital fusion of the C1 to C2 area can be associated with catastrophic injuries or progressive deformities, and resultant sudden-onset neurologic loss or instant death are common. Therefore these lesions, in isolation or in combination with other congenital lesions, are contraindications to participation in sports.

Klipple-Feil anomalies are congenital fusions of the cervical spine. If there are limited fusions in the C3 to C4 area with full range of motion, sports can be allowed without worry of increased injury risk. However, if there are multiple levels of fusion in the cervical spine, the forces can lead to increased risk of injury. In these cases the participation in sports should be restricted. Fusions limited to 1 or 2 levels with associated limited range of motion are also at an increased risk, indicating an absolute contraindication to participation in sports.[43]

STINGERS AND BURNERS

Burners or stingers in the high-school population are caused by brachial plexus stretch in about 50% of the high-school-age football players who sustain them; the other 50% of this age group, as well as most college and professional players with burners or stingers, exhibit compression within the foramina of the cervical spine. If the first-time burner completely resolves, return to sports without restriction can be allowed. However, persistent numbness, neck pain, or motion restriction, especially with a repeat injury, should restrict the player from sports until a further evaluation is performed.[44]

REFERENCES

1. Klepper S. Making the case for exercise in children with juvenile idiopathic arthritis: what we know and where to go from here. Arthritis Rheum 2007;57(6): 887–90.
2. Klepper S. Exercise in pediatric rheumatic diseases. Curr Opin Rheumatol 2008; 20:619–24.
3. Arthritis Foundation. Juvenile Arthritis Alliance school success. Available at: http://www.arthritis.org/ja-school-success.php. Accessed January 27, 2010.
4. Lelieveld O, Armbrust W, van Leeuwen M, et al. Physical activity in adolescents with juvenile idiopathic arthritis. Arthritis Rheum 2008;59(10):1379–84.
5. Long AR, Rouster-Stevens KA. The role of exercise therapy in the management of juvenile idiopathic arthritis. Curr Opin Rheumatol 2010;22:1–5.
6. Takken T, van der Net J, Helders P. Do juvenile idiopathic arthritis patients benefit from an exercise program? A pilot study. Arthritis Care Res 2001;41:81–5.
7. Takken T, van der Net J, Helders PJ. Aquatic fitness training for children with juvenile idiopathic arthritis. Rheumatology 2003;42(11):1408–14.
8. Singh-Grewal D, Schneiderman-Walker J, Wright V, et al. The effects of vigorous exercise training on physical function in children with arthritis: a randomized, controlled, single-blinded trial. Arthritis Rheum 2007;57(7):1202–10.
9. Takken T, Van Brussel M, Engelbert RH, et al. Exercise therapy in juvenile idiopathic arthritis: a Cochrane Review. Eur J Phys Rehabil Med 2008;44(3):287–97.
10. Minden K, Niewerth M, Listing J, et al. Long-term outcome in patients with juvenile idiopathic arthritis. Arthritis Rheum 2002;46(9):2392–401.
11. Huffman EA, Yard EE, Fields SK, et al. Epidemiology or rare injuries and conditions among United States high school athletes during the 2005–2006 and 2006–2007 school years. J Athl Train 2008;43(6):624–30.
12. Youn J, Sallis RE, Smith G, et al. Ocular injury rates in college sports. Med Sci Sports Exerc 2008;40(3):428–32.
13. Filipe JAC, Rocha-Sousa A, Falcao-Reis F, et al. Modern sport eye injuries. Br J Ophthalmol 2003;87:1336–9.
14. Jeffers JB. Eye injuries. In: Harris SS, Anderson SJ, editors. Care of the young athlete. 2nd edition. Elk Grove Village (IL): American Academy of Pediatrics; 2010. p. 193–200.
15. Baker RJ. Conditions and injuries of the eyes, nose, and ears. In: Patel DR, Greydanus DE, Baker RJ, editors. Pediatric practice: sports medicine. New York: McGraw-Hill; 2009. p. 446–55.
16. American Academy of Pediatrics and American Academy of Ophthalmology. Policy statement: protective eyewear for young athletes. Pediatrics 2004; 113(3):619–22.
17. Anderson CR. Solitary kidney and sports participation. Arch Fam Med 1995;4: 885–8.
18. Grinsell MM, Showalter S, Gordon K, et al. Single kidney and sports participation: perception versus reality. Pediatrics 2006;118(3):1019–27.
19. Sharp DS, Ross JH, Kay R. Attitudes of pediatric urologists regarding sports participation by children with a solitary kidney. J Urol 2002;168:1811–5.

20. Gerstenbluth RE, Spirnak JP, Elder JS. Sports participation and high grade renal injuries in children. J Urol 2002;168:2575–8.

21. Wan J, Corvino TF, Greenfeld SP, et al. The incidence of recreational genitourinary and abdominal injuries in the western New York pediatric population. J Urol 2003; 170:1525–7.

22. Wan J, Corvino TF, Greenfeld SP, et al. Kidney and testicle injuries in team and individual sports: data from the National Pediatric Trauma Registry. J Urol 2003;170:1528–32.

23. Johnson B, Christensen C, DiRusso S, et al. A need for reevaluation of sports participation recommendations for children with a solitary kidney. J Urol 2005;174:686–9.

24. American Academy of Pediatrics. Council on sports medicine and fitness. Medical conditions affecting sports participation. Pediatrics 2008;121(4):841–8.

25. Basler RSW. Skin problems in athletes. In: Mellion MB, Walsh WM, Madden C, et al, editors. Team physician's handbook. 3rd edition. Philadelphia: Hanley & Belfus; 2002. p. 311–25.

26. Basler RSW. Skin conditions. In: Anderson SS, Harris SJ, editors. Care of the young athlete. 2nd edition. Elk Grove Village (IL): American Academy of Pediatrics; 2010. p. 249–60.

27. Pecci M, Comeau D, Chawla V. Skin conditions in athletes. Am J Sports Med 2009;37(2):406–18.

28. Agel J, Ransone J, Dick R, et al. Descriptive epidemiology of collegiate men's wrestling injuries: National Collegiate Athletic Association injury surveillance system, 1988–1989 through 2003–2004. J Athl Train 2007;42(2):303–10.

29. National Collegiate Athletic Association. NCAA guideline 2j Skin infections in athletes. Available at: www.NCAA.org. Revised June 2008. Available at: http://ncaa.org/wps/portal/ncaahome?WCM_GLOBAL_CONTEXT=/ncaa/ncaa/academics+and+athletes/personal+welfare/. Accessed January 11, 2010.

30. National Federation of State High School Associations Sports Medicine Advisory Committee. Sports related skin infections position statement and guidelines. Available at: www.nfhs.org. Revised October 2006. Available at: http://www.nfhs.org/content.aspx?id+3325. Accessed January 11, 2010.

31. Centers for Disease Control and Prevention. FAQ about methicillin-resistant Staphylococcus aureus (MRSA) among athletes. Available at: www.cdc.gov. Updated Nov 2008. Available at: http://www.cdc.gov/ncidod/dhqp/ar_MRSA_AthletesFAQ.html. Accesses January 11, 2010.

32. Sedgwick PE, Dexter WW, Smith CT. Bacterial dermatoses in sports. Clin Sports Med 2007;26:383–96.

33. Baker R, Patel D. Lower back pain in the athlete: common conditions and treatment. Prim Care 2005;32:201–29.

34. Omey M, Micheli L, Gerbino P. Idiopathic scoliosis and spondylolysis in the female athlete. Clin Orthop Relat Res 2000;372:74–87.

35. Patel D, Rowe D. Thoracolumbar spine injuries. In: Patel DR, Greydanus DE, Baker RJ, editors. Pediatric practice: sports medicine. New York: McGraw-Hill; 2009. p. 377–95.

36. Green B, Johnson C, Moreau W. Is physical activity contraindicated for individuals with scoliosis? A systematic literature review. J Chiropr Med 2008;8:25–37.

37. Wood K. Spinal deformity in the adolescent athlete. Clin Sports Med 2002;21(1):77–92.

38. Sys J, Michielsen J, Bracke P, et al. Nonoperative treatment of active spondylolysis in elite athletes with normal X-ray findings: literature review and results of conservative treatment. Eur Spine J 2001;10(6):498–504.

39. Bono C. Low-back pain in athletes. J Bone Joint Surg Am 2004;86:382–96.
40. Lemire JJ, Mierau DR, et al. Scheuermann's juvenile kyphosis. J Manipulative Physiol Ther 1996;19(3):195–201.
41. Torg J, Guille J, Jaffe S. Injuries to the cervical spine in American football players. J Bone Joint Surg Am 2002;84:112–22.
42. McTimoney CA, Micheli LJ. Current evaluation and management of spondylolysis and spondylolisthesis. Curr Sports Med Rep 2003;2(1):41–6.
43. Torg J, Ramsey-Emrhein J. Suggested management guidelines for participation in collision activities with congenital, developmental, or postinjury lesions involving the cervical spine. Med Sci Sports Exerc 1997;27(7):256–72.
44. Cantu R, Bailes J, Wilberger J. Guidelines for return to contact or collision sport after a cervical spine injury. Clin Sports Med 1998;17(1):137–46.

Vitamin D, Muscle Function, and Exercise Performance

Magdalena Bartoszewska, BA[a,b], Manmohan Kamboj, MD[c,d,*],
Dilip R. Patel, MD, FAAP, FACSM, FAACPDM, FSAM[b,c]

KEYWORDS

- Vitamin D • Vitamin D deficiency • Physical performance
- Muscle strength • Exercise

Vitamin D is currently a topic of great interest among researchers. Increasing evidence suggests that exposure to a few minutes of sun daily may strengthen the immune system, maintain cardiovascular health, protect against certain cancers, and possibly even enhance athletic performance. Researchers propose that these are among the nonskeletal benefits of vitamin D.[1–6] Recent data also indicate that vitamin D deficiency is pandemic; the healthy and the young are not excluded.[1]

Muscle tissue was among the first nontraditional vitamin D target organs to be identified.[6–8] Much attention has since been paid to the effects of vitamin D on muscle strength, exercise capacity, and physical performance. Numerous studies have reported a correlation between vitamin D and muscle function.[3,6–10] These findings raise many important clinical questions, especially in the area of sports medicine.

If vitamin D does improve muscle function, what implications does this have on the performance of athletes who have vitamin D deficiency? Is routine screening necessary? What is the role of vitamin D supplementation to enhance performance in these athletes? Although the issue of vitamin D deficit may have been recognized, controversy exists regarding what constitutes normal serum levels, the amount of supplementation required to restore normal levels, and the relative effect of such supplementation on our overall health. This review summarizes the current

[a] Michigan State University College of Human Medicine, East Lansing, MI, USA
[b] Michigan State University Kalamazoo Center for Medical Studies, 1000 Oakland Drive, Kalamazoo, MI 49008, USA
[c] Department of Pediatrics and Human Development, Michigan State University College of Human Medicine, East Lansing, MI, USA
[d] Pediatrics Residency Program, Division of Pediatric Endocrinology, Michigan State University Kalamazoo Center for Medical Studies, 1000 Oakland Drive, Kalamazoo, MI 49008, USA
* Corresponding author. Pediatrics Residency Program, Division of Pediatric Endocrinology, Michigan State University Kalamazoo Center for Medical Studies, 1000 Oakland Drive, Kalamazoo, MI 49008.
E-mail address: kamboj@kcms.msu.edu

Pediatr Clin N Am 57 (2010) 849–861
doi:10.1016/j.pcl.2010.03.008
0031-3955/10/$ – see front matter
pediatric.theclinics.com

understanding of the functions of vitamin D, describes its role in muscle function, and explores the possible implications of its deficiency and supplementation on exercise performance in individuals who are vitamin D deficient and nondeficient.

SEARCH STRATEGY

The authors performed a literature search using PubMed/Medline, Ovid, EMBASE, and ScienceDirect databases indexed under the Medical Subject Heading (MeSH) terms; "Vitamin D OR Vitamin D supplementation OR Vitamin D deficiency" combined with the terms; "athletic performance" OR "performance enhancement" OR "strength" OR "exercise" OR "muscle strength" OR "muscle function" OR "physical performance" OR "in normal individuals" OR "chronic fatigue" OR "myalgia." The literature search was limited to articles dating back to January 2000 and written in the English language. All types of articles were reviewed, based on their direct relevance to the aims of this review. In addition, we searched the reference lists of all identified articles, and latest editions of standard texts. Additional sources written before the year 2000 were included for completeness as part of background information on the topic.

THE BASICS ABOUT VITAMIN D
Sources

Vitamin D is a steroid hormone that regulates various tissue processes by way of specific cell receptors.[10,11] 25-Hydroxy vitamin D (25-OHD) is the main storage form of vitamin D, whereas 1,25-dihydroxy vitamin D (1,25-DiOHD or 1,25(OH)$_2$D) is the main biologically active metabolite responsible for calcium homeostasis. The main forms of vitamin D are listed in **Table 1**. The main source of vitamin D in the human body is cutaneous synthesis via the effects of ultraviolet radiation on the vitamin D precursor, 7-dehydrocholesterol. This mechanism is well regulated and accounts for most of vitamin D synthesis in the body. Anything that reduces the number of solar UVB photons penetrating the skin or alters the amount of 7-dehydrocholesterol in the skin affects production of vitamin D$_3$.[3] Examples of factors that interfere with 1 or both of these processes, thus causing vitamin D deficiency, are listed in **Table 2**. On the contrary, protective mechanisms such as pigment in skin and formation of inactive isomers (luminosterol, tachysterol) prevent its overproduction.

The alternative source of vitamin D is from dietary intake (**Table 3**). However, most modern diets contain inadequate vitamin D; even those rich in fortified dairy or cereal products. Vegetarian and vegan diets are lacking in this regard.[12–14] Thus, whenever sufficient cutaneous production is poor, vitamin D deficiency likely ensues.[15]

Vitamin D Requirements and Normal Levels

The present recommendation for adequate daily vitamin D for all age groups is 400 IU.[16] Despite clear recommendations, there is still controversy about the normal serum level of serum vitamin D. From studies looking at the physiology of the vitamin

Table 1 Main forms of vitamin D	
Type of Vitamin D	**Source**
Vitamin D$_2$ (ergocalciferol)	Plant
Vitamin D$_3$ (cholecalciferol)	Animal
Dihydrotachysterol	Synthetic

Table 2
Factors that predispose to vitamin D deficiency
Dark skin
Inadequate sun exposure
Sun exposure at dawn and dusk
Insufficient surface area of skin exposed to sun
Cloudy (typically winter) outdoors
Northern latitudes
Consistent use of sunscreens or sun block lotions
Low dietary intake

D cycle (**Fig. 1**), it is surmised that serum levels of less than 30 ng/mL are consistent with relative vitamin D deficit, whereas levels of 30 ng/mL or more may be considered to be sufficient.[17] Using these guidelines, it is estimated that 50% of children and adolescents have vitamin D deficiency. The importance of adequate vitamin D levels for the maintenance of good bone health and prevention of osteoporosis is clearly

Table 3	
Major dietary sources of vitamin D	
For Every 100 g (3.5 ounces) of:	**IU of Vitamin D:**
Cod liver oil (~2 teaspoons)	10,000
Lard (pork fat)	2800
Atlantic herring (pickled)	680
Eastern oysters (steamed)	642
Catfish (steamed/poached)	500
Skinless sardines (water packed)	480
Mackerel (canned/drained)	450
Smoked chinook salmon	320
Sturgeon roe	232
Shrimp (canned/drained)	172
Egg yolk (fresh)	148 (one yolk contains about 24)
Butter	56
Lamb liver (braised)	20
Beef tallow	19
Pork liver (braised)	12
Beef liver (fried)	12
Beef tripe (raw)	12
Beef kidney (simmered)	12
Chicken livers (simmered)	12
Small clams (steamed/cooked moist)	8
Blue crab (steamed)	4
Crayfish/crawdads (steamed)	4
Northern lobster (steamed)	4

Source: United States Department of Agriculture Database.

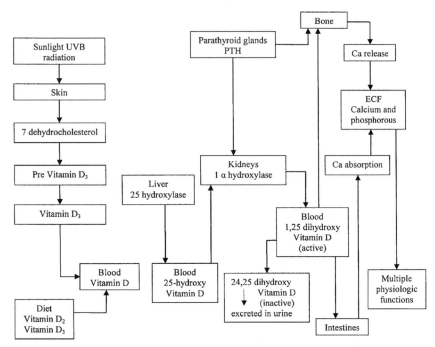

Fig. 1. The vitamin D cycle.

documented.[1,3,4,9,12,18,19] The presence of insufficient vitamin D levels in such a large proportion of the population therefore has significant implications for prevalence of disorders of calcium, phosphorus, bone metabolism, and the resultant pathology.

Mechanism of Vitamin D Action

Vitamin D exerts its effects by binding to the vitamin D receptor (VDR), which is a nuclear hormone receptor.[11,20] VDRs belong to the family of nuclear hormone receptors and are structurally homologous to the other members of the group, including retinoic acid, retinoid X, and thyroid hormone receptors. The VDR acts by forming a heterodimer with retinoid-X receptor, binding to the DNA elements, and recruiting coactivators in a ligand-dependent fashion.[11,21] Vitamin D acts mainly to amplify transcription by way of upregulatory response elements, although some of its effects may also include transcription repression. In addition, the hormone promotes DNA protein interactions of various other transcription factors.[14]

VDRs are found in many tissues and organs, including the small intestine, colon, osteoblasts, activated T and B lymphocytes, pancreatic β islet cells, brain, heart, skin, gonads, prostate, breast, mononuclear cells, as well as skeletal and smooth muscle.[3]

Functions of Vitamin D

Vitamin D has been long-recognized for its calciotropic properties, acting at the level of the kidney, intestine, and bone.[8,11] Vitamin D is a pleiotropic hormone, influencing other body processes in addition to calcium metabolism.[7,9,11] In the last few years, new data have revealed a correlation between vitamin D levels and several significant diseases, including hypertension, diabetes, depression, and cancer.[1,3–5,9,18,22] Studies suggesting a likely protective role of vitamin D in these conditions have placed it at the frontline of current scientific endeavors, earning it a potential claim to being the new miracle drug.[23]

The concept of vitamin D pleiotropism originated in 1985 with the identification of VDRs outside bone from cultured rat myoblast cells, proving that, in addition to bone, muscle is also a direct target organ for 1,25(OH)2D.[6] The VDR has subsequently been described in tissues such as smooth muscle, heart muscle, liver, lung, colon, gonads, and skin, and was also recently isolated from human skeletal muscle.[3,6,24]

The expanded role of vitamin D was further supported by the discovery of an independent photoendocrine system in epidermal keratinocytes.[22] In addition to synthesizing the prehormone vitamin D destined for kidney activation, epidermal keratinocytes were also found to produce their own, local vitamin D 24-hydroxylase enzyme capable of activating it, as well as epidermal VDRs.[22,25] These findings suggest local paracrine and autocrine effects of vitamin D in addition to its role as an endocrine hormone.[22,25] This intracellular autocrine function has also been identified in various organs including bone, brain, muscle, pituitary gland, and liver. The main functions of vitamin D are summarized in **Table 4**.[11,26–29]

Vitamin D is believed to affect the body's immune system, endocrine system, cardiocirculatory system, neuromuscular performance, and neuropsychological functioning.[1,3,4,9] It is also believed to act as a potent antioxidant protecting against free radical damage, as well as being an inducer of cellular differentiation, protecting against carcinogenesis.[1,3,4,9]

ROLE OF VITAMIN D IN MUSCLE
Vitamin D–deficiency Myopathy

The first associations between vitamin D and muscle function were made from observations of muscle weakness in children with rickets as well as adults with osteomalacia.[8] Vitamin D deficiency has been known to cause muscle weakness, hypotonia, and prolonged time to peak muscle contraction, as well as prolonged time to muscle relaxation.[24,30,31] Varying patterns of muscle weakness, proximal myopathy, generalized musculoskeletal pain, and hypotonia occur in children who have vitamin D deficiency. Muscle weakness and hypotonia, in turn, cause a waddling gait and difficulty in walking, sitting, standing, and climbing stairs.[32]

Ahmed and colleagues[33] studied patients who were treated with statins, vitamin D deficient, and had myalgias, and found that vitamin D supplementation, while continuing statin therapy, reversed the myalgia in 92% of these patients. Sixty-four

Table 4 Main functions of vitamin D	
Site	**Function**
Intestine	Production of calbindin (the calcium-binding protein in the intestine) Promotes calcium and phosphorus absorption in the intestine Regulates gene transcription and cell proliferation in the parathyroid gland
Bone	Role in synthesis of type 1 collagen: evidence is equivocal Stimulates synthesis of osteocalcin Promotes differentiation of osteoclasts
Muscles	Increases amino acid uptake in muscles Alters phospholipid metabolism in muscles Vitamin D deficiency causes myopathy Nongenomic effects on muscles Increases troponin C in muscles

percent of the 128 patients with myalgia had low vitamin D, versus 43% of the patients who were asymptomatic. Of the 82 patients who were vitamin D deficient and myalgic, while continuing statins, 38 received vitamin D (50,000 IU/wk for 12 weeks), with a resultant increase in serum vitamin D and resolution of myalgia in 35 (92%) of them. The study concluded that hypovitaminosis D was associated with myalgia in patients treated with statins, and that this myalgia can be reversed by vitamin D supplementation. These results indicate that vitamin D probably has an advantageous effect on muscle function.

Vitamin D deficiency is also associated with musculoskeletal pain.[34] One study found that 89% of subjects with chronic musculoskeletal pain were deficient in vitamin D.[34] Another study revealed that 93% of patients presenting to a community clinic with nonspecific musculoskeletal pain were found to have vitamin D deficiency.[35] Of these patients, all less than 30 years of age were vitamin D deficient, with 55% being severely deficient.[35] Patients with vitamin D deficiency and musculoskeletal pain may often be misdiagnosed with fibromyalgia, chronic fatigue syndrome, myositis, or other nonspecific collagen vascular diseases.[5] It is estimated that 40% to 60% of patients with fibromyalgia may have vitamin D deficiency.[5]

These observations suggest not only the likely association of vitamin D in muscle functioning but also the importance of vitamin D–deficiency screening and treatment in patients with myalgias. Many of the patients presenting with myalgias are also athletes who may potentially benefit from an intervention as simple as vitamin D replacement.

Molecular Mechanisms of Vitamin D Actions in Muscles

Adequate muscle function and contraction uses genomic and nongenomic actions. Genomic actions are mediated by the nuclear VDRs. Normocalcemia, which is facilitated by vitamin D sufficiency, is essential for normal muscle contraction. Nongenomic actions are performed via VDRs present on cell membranes. The actions of vitamin D on muscle are also believed to be effected by vitamin D–binding protein.[36] Studies have shown that vitamin D facilitates the adenosine triphosphate (ATP)–dependent calcium uptake in sarcoplasmic reticulum, increases the concentrations of phosphorus Y and ATP in the cell, and leads to increased protein synthesis.[37,38] These findings support the manifestation of myopathy and generalized weakness seen in hypovitaminosis D and rickets. In muscle tissue, the genomic pathway is believed to influence muscle calcium transport and phospholipid metabolism.[7]

Nongenomic functions of vitamin D are also being increasingly recognized.[39] These are characterized by rapid effects that do not result from gene transcription. A proposed mechanism of initiation of these rapid effects is the binding of $1,25(OH)_2D$ to another vitamin D–specific receptor; a cell surface receptor.[7] Receptor binding activates a network of second-messenger pathways that transmit the signal to the cytoplasm.[7] This is also believed to direct intracellular calcium regulation in muscle cells.[7] Another speculated effect of vitamin D in muscle cells includes activation of the mitogen-activated protein kinase (MAPK) signaling pathways.[8] In humans, MAPK pathways regulate cell processes such as myogenesis, cell proliferation, differentiation, and apoptosis. In this way, vitamin D is believed to stimulate muscle cell proliferation and growth.[7]

VDR Knockout Mice Model

VDR null mutant mice are characterized by growth retardation, osteomalacia, muscle impairment, and systemic metabolic changes such as secondary hyperparathyroidism and hypocalcemia.[7] VDR null mutant mice have muscle fiber diameters that are 20% smaller and more variable in size than those of wild-type mice at 3 weeks of age (before weaning).[7] These VDR mutant mice also had abnormally high expression of myogenic differentiation factors compared with wild-type mice, suggesting alterations in muscle cell differentiation pathways resulting in abnormal muscle fiber development and maturation.[7]

VDR Polymorphisms in Muscle

Subtle variations in the DNA sequence of the VDR gene, also known as VDR polymorphisms, are associated with a series of biologic characteristics including muscle strength.[7] *BsmI*, a restriction fragment length polymorphism of the VDR gene, has been associated with muscle performance.[7] In a cross-sectional study of nonobese women, the VDR *BsmI* polymorphism was associated with differences in quadriceps muscle strength, but not in grip strength.[40]

Another recent, population-based cross-sectional study has found an association of the poly A repeat and the *BsmI* polymorphisms with hamstring cross-sectional area, but not with quadriceps or grip strength.[40] Young women with the bb allele, which may be associated with higher VDR activity, were found to have lower fat-free mass and hamstring (but not quadriceps) strength compared with those with the BB allele.[7] Why the allele associated with higher VDR activity would have reduced muscle strength remains unknown.[7]

Vitamin D and Histologic Changes in Muscle

Muscle biopsies obtained in patients with osteomalacia reveal an atrophy of type II muscle fibers with enlarged interfibrillar spaces and infiltration of fat, fibrosis, and glycogen granules.[24,30] In sudden movements, the fast and strong type II fibers are the first to be recruited to avoid falling. Primarily type II fibers are affected by vitamin D deficiency, which probably explains the falling tendency of elderly individuals who are vitamin D deficient.[24,30] Oh and colleagues[41] assessed the role of vitamin D as a factor accounting for fatty degeneration and muscle function in the rotator cuff. Lower serum vitamin D levels were related to higher fatty degeneration in the muscles of the rotator cuff ($P = .001$, $P = .026$, $P = .001$ for supraspinatus, infraspinatus, and subscapularis muscles, respectively).[41] Serum levels of vitamin D were also found to have a significant positive correlation with isokinetic muscle torque.[41]

Vitamin D and Cardiovascular Smooth Muscle Effects

In addition to its effect on skeletal muscles, vitamin D also plays an important role in the functioning of the cardiovascular system smooth muscle. Studies show that 1,25-DiOHD increases active stress generation in arteries, therefore affecting blood pressure.[13,42] In a study of elderly patients, parathyroid hormone (PTH) and 1,25-DiOHD were reported to be independent determinants of blood pressure, and a decrease in blood pressure and heart rate was observed after short term vitamin D and calcium supplementation.[43,44] The specific role of PTH versus 1,25-DiOHD on blood pressure and heart rate has not been clearly elucidated.

Recent data from the long-term National Health and Nutrition Examination Survey (NHANES) findings, which included 3577 adolescents aged 12 to 19 years, show low serum vitamin D to be associated with an increased risk of high blood pressure, high blood sugar, and metabolic syndrome. The average serum level of 25(OH)D was 28.0 ng/mL in whites, 15.5 ng/mL in blacks, and 21.5 ng/mL in Mexican Americans.[22] After adjusting for age, sex, race, body mass index, socioeconomic status, and physical activity, adolescents with 25(OH)D levels in the lowest quartile (<15 ng/mL) were 2.36 times more likely to have high blood pressure, 2.54 times more likely to have high blood sugar, and 3.99 times more likely to have metabolic syndrome than those with vitamin D levels in the highest quartile (>26 ng/mL).[22] These findings may have important bearings on a young athlete's ability to perform.

VITAMIN D DEFICIENCY (INSUFFICIENCY) IN ATHLETES

Vitamin D deficiency is pandemic, including a high prevalence among the young and the healthy.[1,3,4,15,45–48] Concurrently, vitamin D deficiency is also reported in otherwise healthy athletes.[15,45–48] Because cutaneous synthesis of vitamin D is the main source of adequate vitamin D supply, factors that limit sunlight exposure pose the greatest risk for developing vitamin deficiency, especially in athletes. Therefore, among those at greatest risk are athletes competing in northern latitudes (especially during the winter months), athletes practicing indoors, those who consciously avoid sun exposure or use sunscreen, and those of darker skin pigmentation.[15]

Several studies have documented the high rate of vitamin D deficiency or insufficiency in athletes. A cross-sectional survey of elite gymnasts at the Australian Institute of Sports[49] highlighted the high prevalence of vitamin D deficiency or insufficiency even in elite athletes who otherwise would be assumed to be healthy. Of 18 female, adolescent gymnasts, 13 had low dietary calcium intakes, and 6 had vitamin D levels less than 50 nmol/L (20 ng/mL). This finding underlines the importance of surveillance for vitamin D insufficiency in athletes, especially those who train indoors and have inadequate sun exposure. The study also revealed the high prevalence of stress injuries of bone in these girls in the year before the study. Recommendations for vitamin D supplementation were implemented in this group following the study.[49]

In a group of German gymnasts training predominantly indoors, 77% were found to have vitamin D levels less than 35 mg/mL, with 37% having levels less than 10 mg/mL.[50] Contrary to expectations, a French study also revealed low levels of 25-hydroxyvitamin D in cyclists.[30] A Finnish study reported unequivocal results, with no difference in vitamin D status between a group of cyclists and controls.[51]

Ward and colleagues[45] assessed serum 25(OH)D in girls aged 12 to 14 years, and measured muscle power with jumping monography; a novel outcome sensitive for assessing the muscles most often affected by vitamin D deficiency. Vitamin D levels were significantly associated with muscle power and force in adolescent girls. Vitamin D myopathy is associated with fatigue induction and nonparticipation in physical education or organized sports.[45] A reduced motivation to exercise resulting from vitamin D myopathy may, in turn, alter psychosocial development and health during the adolescence, contributing to low mechanical bone stimulus for bone-mass gain.[22]

Studies in the elderly population provide insights that are important in establishing the role of vitamin D in neuromuscular and skeletal muscle function. A meta-analytical study of the elderly population concluded that vitamin D supplementation appeared to reduce the risk of falls by 20%.[52] Improvement in the musculoskeletal function indicated by a reduction in the number of falls was also documented in a double-blind, randomized, control trial by a 3-month treatment trial with calcium and vitamin D supplementation, in the elderly age group.[53] The role of vitamin D supplementation in improving muscular performance, balance, and reaction time, but not muscular strength, was shown in one study, suggesting a neuromuscular or neuroprotective role of vitamin D.[54] Several studies also show an increase in type 2 muscle fibers and improvement in muscle atrophy with vitamin D treatment.[55–57]

VITAMIN D AND ATHLETIC PERFORMANCE

If vitamin D affects neuromuscular functioning, the logical question is whether it will affect skeletal, muscular, and neuromuscular functioning in athletes, and how much that would affect their performance levels? The effect of vitamin D levels on athletic performance has rarely been studied. Once vitamin D insufficiency is identified, potential interventions for improvement include dietary supplementation with vitamin D and calcium or increased sun exposure. Exposure to sun is increased by increasing the amount of time spent in the sun, modifying the sun exposure for maximally appropriate ultraviolet radiation exposure, or increasing the surface area of skin exposed to the sun.

UV Radiation and Increased Physical Performance

The athletic benefits of UV radiation were described as early as the 1930s, linking UV exposure to improvements in motor performance, strength, and speed.[15,16,58] In 1938, Russian investigators reported that a course of UV irradiation improved speed in the 100-m dash in 4 students undergoing daily physical training. Mean times improved by 1.7% in the nonirradiated controls versus 7.4% in the irradiated students undergoing identical training.[15] In the late 1960s, American researchers found that even a single dose of ultraviolet irradiation improved the strength, speed, and endurance of college women.[15]

Seasonality of Physical Performance

The seasonality of athletic ability has also been observed.[15] European studies dating back to the 1950s were among the first to analyze changes in fitness associated with the time of the year.[15] Significant seasonal variation in $25(OH)D_3$ levels has also been shown.[22] In the northern hemisphere, vitamin D stores peak in the summer, begin to decline by the autumn, and reach their nadir during the winter months.[15,22] Based on our current assumption that vitamin D may increase athletic capacity, the authors expect the results of the early European observational studies to correlate with the pattern of seasonal variability of vitamin D stores. Several such studies revealed a peak in physical performance during the summer months.[5,15,59]

A 1956 study, cited by Cannell and colleagues[15] in their review, attempted to quantify a seasonal variation in the trainability of musculature. The major criticism of the observed seasonality of physical fitness is that people tend to be more active when it is warm outside. For this reason, the study also controlled for the time spent exercising. The researchers found that there was a significant peak in trainability in the summer, followed by a sharp autumn decline, and lowest trainability in the winter.[15] The distinct pattern of increased performance in the summer followed by a sharp decline in the early autumn closely resembles the pattern of seasonal variability of vitamin D, suggesting a possible association between them.

In 1979, a large cross-sectional survey of 1835 healthy Norwegian men (age 40–59 years) also found a small, but significant, overall seasonal variability in physical performance ($P = .04$) with a peak in fitness occurring during the summer ($P<.001$).[59] However, in contrast with the previous study, no difference in physical performance was established between winter and autumn.[59]

Vitamin D Deficiency and Obesity

Factors that perpetuate low vitamin D levels may also significantly hinder athletic performance. Limited mobility and increased storage of vitamin D in fat tissue have been postulated as potential causes, but obesity is a consequence of low vitamin D levels.[22] Moreover, obese individuals only produce half the amount of vitamin D produced by nonobese individuals in response to sun exposure.[22] Vitamin D absorption following oral supplement administration is not impaired in obese individuals. These results suggest a decreased passage of vitamin D formed in the skin into the general circulation due to its subcutaneous accumulation in obese people.[22] As such, hypovitaminosis D not only impedes muscle function but also contributes to obesity.

SUMMARY

Although there is some evidence that an adequate level of vitamin D is positively correlated with improvement in exercise performance, key questions still remain: How does vitamin D enhance skeletal muscle function? What is the optimal vitamin D level, if any, that will maximize exercise performance? It is generally agreed that persons who have vitamin D deficiency should receive vitamin D supplementation. It is unclear whether vitamin D supplementation by otherwise healthy athletes would be of benefit. The fundamental debate about the optimal daily dietary intake and adequate levels of vitamin D continues. Studies suggest a daily intake ranging between 400 IU and 2000 IU.[60] More research and clinical trials addressing these issues will be important, especially in the pediatric and adolescent population and in athletes.[7]

If vitamin D does improve muscle function, the implications of this on the performance of athletes who may be vitamin D deficient need to be established. Other important questions include whether there is a role for vitamin D supplementation in enhancing performance in such individuals; whether oversupplementation could potentially be used to boost performance in nondeficient athletes; and whether such supplementation would be effective, safe, or fair.

ACKNOWLEDGMENTS

The authors thank Kim Douglas, Kalamazoo Center for Medical Studies, for assistance in preparing this manuscript.

REFERENCES

1. Hutchinson MS, Grimnes G, Joakimsen RM, et al. Low serum 25-hydroxyvitamin D levels are associated with increased all-cause mortality risk in a general population. The Tromso study. Eur J Endocrinol 2010;162(5):935–42.
2. Holick MF. Vitamin D: the other steroid hormone for muscle function and strength. Menopause 2009;16(6):1077–8.
3. Holick MF. The vitamin D deficiency pandemic and consequences for nonskeletal health: mechanisms of action. Mol Aspects Med 2008;29(6):361–8.
4. Melamed ML, Michos ED, Post W, et al. 25-Hydroxyvitamin D levels and the risk of mortality in the general population. Arch Intern Med 2008;168(15):1629–37.
5. Holick MF. Sunlight and vitamin D for bone health and prevention of autoimmune diseases, cancers, and cardiovascular disease. Am J Clin Nutr 2004;80(Suppl 6): 1678S–88S.
6. Hamilton B. Vitamin D and human skeletal muscle. Scand J Med Sci Sports 2010; 20(2):182–90.
7. Ceglia L. Vitamin D and its role in skeletal muscle. Curr Opin Clin Nutr Metab Care 2009;12(6):628–33.
8. Ceglia L. Vitamin D and skeletal muscle tissue and function. Mol Aspects Med 2008;29(6):407–14.
9. Verstuyf A, Carmeliet G, Bouillon R, et al. Vitamin D: a pleiotropic hormone. Kidney Int 2010. [Epub ahead of print]. DOI:10.1038/Ki.2010.17.
10. Stewart JW, Alekel DL, Ritland LM, et al. Serum 25-hydroxyvitamin D is related to indicators of overall physical fitness in healthy postmenopausal women. Menopause 2009;16(6):1093–101.

11. Bringhurst FR, Demay MB, Kronenberg HM. Hormones and disorders of mineral metabolism. In: Larsen PR, Kronenberg HM, Melmed S, et al, editors. Williams textbook of endocrinology. 10th edition. Philadelphia: Saunders; 2003. p. 1317–20.

12. Chapuy MC, Arlot ME, Duboeuf F, et al. Vitamin D_3 and calcium to prevent hip fractures in elderly women. N Engl J Med 1992;327(23):1637–42.

13. Bian K, Ishibashi K, Bukoski RD. 1,25(OH)$_2$D$_3$ modulates intracellular Ca^{2+} and force generation in resistance arteries. Am J Physiol 1996;270(1 Pt 2):H230–7.

14. Inoue T, Kamiyama J, Sakai T. Sp1 and NF-Y synergistically mediate the effect of vitamin D_3 in the p27^{kip1} gene promoter that lacks vitamin D response elements. J Biol Chem 1999;274(45):32309–17.

15. Cannell JJ, Hollis BW, Sorenson MB, et al. Athletic performance and vitamin D. Med Sci Sports Exerc 2009;41(5):1102–10.

16. Wagner CL, Greer FR, American Academy of Pediatrics Section on Breastfeeding, American Academy of Pediatrics Committee on Nutrition. Prevention of rickets and vitamin D deficiency in infants, children, and adolescents. Pediatrics 2008;122(5):1142–52.

17. Dawson-Hughes B, Heaney RP, Holick MF, et al. Estimates of optimal vitamin D status. Osteoporos Int 2005;16(7):713–6.

18. Bischoff-Ferrari HA, Giovannucci E, Willett WC, et al. Estimation of optimal serum concentrations of 25-hydroxyvitamin D for multiple health outcomes. Am J Clin Nutr 2006;84(1):18–28.

19. Dawson-Hughes B, Harris SS, Krall EA, et al. Effect of calcium and vitamin D supplementation on bone density in men and women 65 years of age or older. N Engl J Med 1997;337(1):670–6.

20. Baker AR, McDonnell DP, Hughes M, et al. Cloning and expression of full-length cDNA encoding human vitamin D receptor. Proc Natl Acad Sci U S A 1988; 85(10):3294–8.

21. Rachez C, Freedman LP. Mechanisms of gene regulation by vitamin D_3 receptor: a network of coactivator interactions. Gene 2000;246(1–2):9–21.

22. Pérez-López FR. Vitamin D and its implications for musculoskeletal health in women: an update. Maturitas 2007;58(2):117–37.

23. Parker-Pope T. The miracle of vitamin D: sound science, or hype? NY Times 2010 Feb 1. [Online Edition].

24. Pfeifer M, Begerow B, Minne HW. Vitamin D and muscle function. Osteoporos Int 2002;13(3):187–94.

25. Luder HF, Demas MB. The vitamin D receptor, the skin and stem cells. J Steroid Biochem Mol Biol 2010. [Epub ahead of print].

26. Kaplan FS, Hayes WC, Keaveny TM, et al. Form and function of bone. In: Simon DR, editor. Orthopaedic basic science. Rosemont (IL): American Academy of Orthopaedic Surgeons; 1994. p. 127–94.

27. Kumar R. Vitamin D and calcium transport. Kidney Int 1991;40(6):1177–89.

28. Massheimer V, Fernandez LM, Boland R, et al. Regulation of Ca^{2+} uptake in skeletal muscle by 1,25-dihydroxyvitamin D_3: role of phosphorylation and calmodulin. Mol Cell Endocrinol 1992;84(1–2):15–22.

29. Pointon JJ, Francis MJ, Smith R. Effect of vitamin D deficiency on sarcoplasmic reticulum function and troponin C concentration of rabbit skeletal muscle. Clin Sci (Lond) 1979;57(3):257–63.

30. Maïmoun L, Manetta J, Couret I, et al. The intensity level of physical exercise and the bone metabolism response. Int J Sports Med 2006;27(2):105–11.

31. Rodman JS, Baker T. Changes in the kinetics of muscle contraction in vitamin D depleted rats. Kidney Int 1978;13(3):189–93.

32. Gloth FM 3rd, Lindsay JM, Zelesnick LB, et al. Can vitamin D deficiency produce an unusual pain syndrome? Arch Intern Med 1991;151(8):1662–4.

33. Ahmed W, Khan N, Glueck CJ, et al. Low serum 25 (OH) vitamin D levels (<32 ng/mL) are associated with reversible myositis-myalgia in statin-treated patients. Transl Res 2009;153(1):116.

34. Gerwin RD. A review of myofascial pain and fibromyalgia–factors that promote their persistence. Acupunct Med 2005;23(3):121–34.

35. Heath KM, Elovic EP. Vitamin D deficiency: implications in the rehabilitation setting. Am J Phys Med Rehabil 2006;85(11):916–23.

36. Boland R. Role of vitamin D in skeletal muscle function. Endocr Rev 1986;7(4):434–48.

37. Curry OB, Basten JF, Francis MJ, et al. Calcium uptake by sarcoplasmic reticulum of muscle from vitamin D deficient rabbits. Nature 1974;249(452):83–4.

38. Birge SJ, Haddad JG. 25-Hydroxycholecalciferol stimulation of muscle metabolism. J Clin Invest 1975;56(5):1100–7.

39. Caffrey JM, Farach-Carson MC. Vitamin D_3 metabolites modulate dihydropyridine-sensitive calcium currents in clonal rat osteosarcoma cells. J Biol Chem 1989;264(34):20265–74.

40. Stewart CE, Rittweger J. Adaptive processes in skeletal muscle: molecular regulators and genetic influences. J Musculoskelet Neuronal Interact 2006;6(1):73–86.

41. Oh JH, Kim SH, Kim JH, et al. The level of vitamin D in the serum correlates with fatty degeneration of the muscles of the rotator cuff. J Bone Joint Surg Br 2009;91(12):1587–93.

42. Merke J, Hofmann W, Goldschmidt D, et al. Demonstration of 1,25(OH)$_2$vitamin D_3 receptors and actions in vascular smooth muscle cells in vitro. Calcif Tissue Int 1987;41(2):112–4.

43. St. John A, Dick I, Hoad K, et al. Relationship between calcitrophic hormones and blood pressure in elderly subjects. Eur J Endocrinol 1994;130(5):446–50.

44. Pfeifer M, Begerow B, Minne HW, et al. Effects of a short-term vitamin D_3 and calcium supplementation on blood pressure and parathyroid hormone levels in elderly women. J Clin Endocrinol Metab 2001;86(4):1633–7.

45. Ward KA, Das G, Berry JL, et al. Vitamin D status and muscle function in post-menarchal adolescent girls. J Clin Endocrinol Metab 2009;94(2):559–63.

46. Foo LH, Zhang Q, Zhu K, et al. Low vitamin D status has an adverse influence on bone mass, bone turnover, and muscle strength in Chinese adolescent girls. J Nutr 2009;139(5):1002–7.

47. Foo LH, Zhang Q, Zhu K, et al. Relationship between vitamin D status, body composition and physical exercise of adolescent girls in Beijing. Osteoporos Int 2009;20(3):417–25.

48. Hamilton B, Grantham J, Racinais S, et al. Vitamin D deficiency is endemic in Middle Eastern sportsmen. Public Health Nutr 2010;15:1–7.

49. Lovell G. Vitamin D status of females in an elite gymnastics program. Clin J Sport Med 2008;18(2):159–61.

50. Heaney RP, Armas LA, Shary JR, et al. 25-Hydroxylation of vitamin D3: relation to circulating vitamin D_3 under various input conditions. Am J Clin Nutr 2008;87(6):1738–42.

51. Lehtonen-Veromaa M, Möttönen T, Irjala K, et al. Vitamin D intake is low and hypovitaminosis D common in healthy 9- to 15-year-old Finnish girls. Eur J Clin Nutr 1999;53(9):746–51.

52. Bischoff-Ferrari HA, Dawson-Hughes B, Willett WC, et al. Effect of vitamin D on falls: a meta-analysis. JAMA 2004;291(16):1999–2006.

53. Bischoff HA, Stähelin HB, Dick W, et al. Effects of vitamin D and calcium supplementation on falls: a randomized controlled trial. J Bone Miner Res 2003;18(2): 343–51.
54. Dhesi JK, Jackson SH, Bearne LM, et al. Vitamin D supplementation improves neuromuscular function in older people who fall. Age Ageing 2004;33(6):589–95.
55. Young A, Edwards R, Jones D, et al. Quadriceps muscle strength and fibre size during treatment of osteomalacia. In: Stokes IAF, editor, Mechanical factors and the skeleton, vol. 12. London: John Libbey; 1981. p. 137–45.
56. Sato Y, Iwamoto J, Kanoko T, et al. Low-dose vitamin D prevents muscular atrophy and reduces falls and hip fractures in women after stroke: a randomized controlled trial. Cerebrovasc Dis 2005;20(3):187–92.
57. Sørensen OH, Lund B, Saltin B, et al. Myopathy in bone loss of ageing: improvement by treatment with 1 alpha-hydroxycholecalciferol and calcium. Clin Sci (Lond) 1979;56(2):157–61.
58. Rosentsweig J. The effect of a single suberythemic biodose of ultraviolet radiation upon the strength of college women. J Assoc Phys Ment Rehabil 1967;21(4): 131–3.
59. Erikssen J, Rodahl K. Seasonal variation in work performance and heart rate response to exercise: a study of 1,835 middle-aged men. Eur J Appl Physiol 1979;42:133–40.
60. Hollis BW. Circulating 25-hydroxyvitamin D levels indicative of vitamin D sufficiency: implications for establishing a new effective dietary intake recommendation for vitamin D. J Nutr 2005;135(2):317–22.

Index

Note: Page numbers of article titles are in **boldface** type.

Pediatr Clin N Am 57 (2010) 863–877
doi:10.1016/S0031-3955(10)00084-2
0031-3955/10/$ – see front matter © 2010 Elsevier Inc. All rights reserved.

pediatric.theclinics.com

Moving?

Make sure your subscription moves with you!

To notify us of your new address, find your **Clinics Account Number** (located on your mailing label above your name), and contact customer service at:

Email: journalscustomerservice-usa@elsevier.com

800-654-2452 (subscribers in the U.S. & Canada)
314-447-8871 (subscribers outside of the U.S. & Canada)

Fax number: 314-447-8029

Elsevier Health Sciences Division
Subscription Customer Service
3251 Riverport Lane
Maryland Heights, MO 63043

*To ensure uninterrupted delivery of your subscription, please notify us at least 4 weeks in advance of move.

ELSEVIER